Comparative Pathobiology

Volume 1
BIOLOGY OF
THE MICROSPORIDIA

Comparative
Pathobiology

Comparative Pathobiology

Volume 1
BIOLOGY OF
THE MICROSPORIDIA

Edited by **Lee A. Bulla, Jr.**
United States Department of Agriculture
Manhattan, Kansas

and

Thomas C. Cheng
Lehigh University
Bethlehem, Pennsylvania

Contributing editors

Jiří Vávra
Czechoslovak Academy of Science
Prague, Czechoslovakia

and

Victor Sprague
University of Maryland
Solomons, Maryland

Plenum Press · New York and London

Library of Congress Cataloging in Publication Data

Main entry under title:

Biology of the microsporidia.

    (Comparative pathobiology, v. 1)
    Includes index.
    1. Microsporidia. 1. Bulla, Lee A. II. Cheng, Thomas Clement. III. Series
[DNLM: 1. Invertebrates. 2. Pathology. QL362.C737]
QL368.M5B56   593'.19   76-46633
ISBN 0-306-38121-4

©1976 Plenum Press, New York
A Division of Plenum Publishing Corporation
227 West 17th Street, New York, N.Y. 10011

Printed in the United States of America

Acknowledgments

Technical and clerical help in preparing Volume 1 was provided by National Science Foundation Grant GB-26519 to Victor Sprague.

We thank Aileen Berroth, whose skillful attention to the typing and assembly of the material in this volume helped make the publication possible.

FOREWORD

This is the introductory volume of a new series to be issued under our general editorship. With the development of an unprecedented increase in interest in comparative pathobiology, we are of the opinion and intent that *Comparative Pathobiology* should become the focal point for the publication of definitive reviews and the proceedings of significant symposia in this area of modern biomedical science.

Although the term is now in common use, the question is still sometimes raised as to what "pathobiology" includes. This broad area of modern biology includes but extends beyond traditional pathology. It also encompasses studies directed at understanding the biology, chemistry, and physics of infectious agents, including how they contact and invade the effected organism; the reactions of hosts to such agents, as well as to abiotic invaders; the ecologic parameters which facilitate infection; and the development of tools essential for the understanding of host-pathogen interactions. In other words, pathobiology is interdisciplinary and incorporates all of those aspects of biology, chemistry, and physics which directly or indirectly permit greater understanding of the nature of infectious and noninfectious diseases and the possible implications of such in biomedicine, agriculture, and environmental science.

By "comparative" is meant an analytical and critical evaluation of comparable processes as they apply to all categories of animals, invertebrates as well as poikilothermic and homeothermic vertebrates. Furthermore, we would like to accentuate the idea that the study of diseases, infectious and noninfectious, among other pathologic phenomena, should be viewed from a broader spectrum than is customarily the case.

Some comments relative to this volume appear appropriate. The Microsporida has become recognized as an important group of microorganisms which are not only interesting parasites but are also being promoted by some as biological control agents against certain invertebrate vectors of disease. Also, there is some evidence that certain species are pathogenic to vertebrates. Consequently, it appears timely to present in two volumes, this and the subsequent volume of *Comparative Pathobiology*, authoritative reviews of various aspects of the biology of micro-sporidans. Persons familiar with the literature will readily appreciate the contributing authors to this volume are the most active investigators and the recognized authorities on the micro-sporidans.

In editing this volume, we have made it a point to retain the styles of the individual contributors. This may have resulted in some minor inconsistencies, but, in our opinion, this has been compensated for by permitting the individualism of the authors to become visible.

As the general editors, we wish to acknowledge the expert cooperation of Dr. Victor Sprague of the University of Maryland and Dr. Jiří Vàvra of the Czechoslovak Academy of Sciences who were responsible for selecting and inviting their colleagues to contribute to this volume.

We wish to take this opportunity to announce that individuals who are planning symposia to deal with some aspect of comparative pathobiology and who wish the publication of the proceedings to be considered in this series should contact either one of us. In addition to symposia, we are also interested in considering lengthy review papers by recognized authorities.

It is our hope that the launching of *Comparative Pathobiology* will represent a major step in the maturation of this important area of modern biology.

Lee A. Bulla, Jr.

Thomas C. Cheng

Editors

PREFACE

Microsporidiology is a field of science with a rather long
history. Although it evolved as a part of the general field of
zoology, and especially of protozoology and parasitology, it is
now rapidly growing into a scientific discipline sufficiently
distinct as to justify the application of the distinctive name.
During the past few years it has captured the interests of many
hundreds of biologists and is now growing at a rapidly accelerating
rate. This growth trend is clearly evident when we examine, for
example, the last four quarter-century periods of its history as
reflected in the increase in the number of named species.
A few of the microsporidia were observed over a century and a
half ago but members of this group first became objects of
concentrated scientific interest just over a century ago when
Pasteur and others made historic studies on pebrine disease of
silkworm. At that time the etiological agent of silkworm disease,
Nosema bombycis Naegeli, 1857*, was the only microsporidian species
that had been named. Soon thereafter an order, Microsporidia
Balbiani, 1882, was created for this and a few related (then unnamed) species. By 1899, Labbé, who gave the first complete
review of the literature on this group, was able to list in the
order only one family, three genera, 33 named species, and 20
unnamed ones.
Exactly a quarter of a century after Labbé's work, Kudo (1924a)
published tis famous monograph, in which one objective was "to
collect in one paper for easy reference all the published information on Microsporidia, now very widely scattered." Meantime,
judging from the numbers of new taxa that had become established,
the first 25 years of 20th century was a period of remarkably
rapid increase in knowledge of the microsporidia. Kudo listed
four families, 14 genera, about 170 recognized species, and a
number of "ambiguous forms." Thus, the increase in the number of
recognized species was about 137. Possibly, the stimulating influence that Pasteur and other noted students of pebrine disease
had on their colleagues, especially on their own countrymen, was
a very significant factor in the great increase of knowledge
during that period. This influence is suggested by the fact that

a majority of the publications in that period were written by
French workers and that the overwhelming majority of the new taxa
were proposed by these workers.

Judging from the number of new species described, the next
quarter of a century was a period of relatively little activity in
the study of microsporidia. In 1947, Weiser published a key to
the recognized species that included 215 names. This was an increase of only 45 species as compared with about three times that
many in the previous period. Undoubtedly, many factors (including
the paralysis of European science during World War II) interacted
to account for the apparent decline in activity. In any case,
this apparently was a period that, for a number of reasons,
offered relatively little reward to students of microsporidia.
During that period these parasites appeared to have little or
no medical or veterinary significance. Aside from their destruc-
tive effects on silkworms and honey bees, they were not known to
have much economic emportance. Their theoretical value as biological control agents (which had been advanced as early as 1905
by Pérez) was not very appealing during these years when chemical
agents offered very great promise. The microsporidia then
appeared to have little more than an academic importance and Kudo
(1924a) had already done the definitive work on them. At the same
time, the knowledge had already advanced to such a state that the
limitations of the tools of research then available (especially,
the light microscope) had become serious impediments to further
research activities in some important areas relating to these
extremely small protozoans.

Now, there are about 525 named species. Besides, about 200 unnamed ones have been reported. Thus, the number of known species
has increased by about 300 during the past quarter of a century.
This has been really phenomenal growth as compared with any
similar period of time. The growth was doubtless due to a number
of interacting factors with cause and effect relationships. One
factor was the general upsurge of interest in invertebrate
pathology that led to the founding of the Society for Invertebrate
Pathology in 1967, with its Division on Microsporidia organized
in 1969. Another was the use of new or improved tools that added
new dimensions to the study of these minute organisms; especially
important among these were the electron microscope, tissue culture
techniques, new methods in cytochemistry, and immunological
techniques. Still another was renewed interest in microsporidia
as possible biological control agents while chemical pesticides
were becoming increasingly unsatisfactory. It was in this same
period that Nelson (1962), Weiser (1964), and Lainson *et al.*,
(1964) independently rediscovered *Encephalitozoon cuniculi*
Levaditi, Nicolau, and Shoen, 1923, in laboratory rodents and
substantiated the generally rejected claim of the original authors
that this parasite is a microsporidium. Petri and Schiødt (1966)
and Arison *et al.* (1966) demonstrated that infection with this

same parasite inhibits various kinds of cancer in mice. More
recent research (summarized by Shadduck and Pakes, 1971) shows that
Encephalitozoon is a very frequent parasite, not only seriously
interfering in experimental work with laboratory rodents but also
affecting other animals (*e.g.*, carnivores from zoological gardens)
as well. There were also a few reports of microsporidia in man,
although the first fully substantiated report was published only
recently by Margileth *et al.* (1973). Thus, the microsporidia
became important in human and veterinary medicine. Finally,
microsporidia have proved to be especially interesting to parasi-
tologists who are concerned with different aspects of host-
parasite interaction as exhibited at the cellular level (Weidner,
1972; Trager, 1974; Weissenberg, 1976).

Indications are that the recent great upsurge of activity only
marks the beginning of a period that offers unprecedented promise
of reward to students of microsporidia. We can now dare to
conjecture that the microsporidia constitute the largest group
of parasitic animals, and one of the largest groups of animals,
with respect to number of species. This conjecture rests on the
fact that microsporidia occur as parasites in nearly all major
animal groups, and furthermore, are extremely common in such
large groups as Insecta and Crustacea. The existence of an almost
endless number and variety of species offers essentially unlimited
opportnuity for studies in systematic zoology. We can now also
dare to suggest that the microsporidia are the most important
group of parasitic animals with respect to their total effect on
other animals. This idea is supported by their common occurrence,
their wide zoological distribution (from protozoa to man), and the
notoriously lethal effects of many species on their hosts. Thus,
the largest part of the general field of animal parasitology may
still be very largely unexplored. For these and many other reasons,
it seems highly probable that the foreseeable future will be a
period of great activity and discovery in microsporidiology.

The increasing activity in this relatively new branch of biology
is accompanied by a number of difficulties that become increasingly
serious. Many of the type species are so poorly defined that they
do not serve their intended purpose as standards of reference.
The classification that has been in general use for a half-century
was so poorly conceived that it cannot adequately accommodate the
known taxa and has become almost useless. Many terms applying to
the microsporidia are used with such a variety of meanings that
they are more likely to hinder clarity of communication than to
enhance it. Methodology is so poorly standardized that reliability
of such important data as spore measurements is usually questionable
and their reproducibility seldom possible. The literature is so
voluminous and so scattered that access to it is excessively
difficult. These and other problems plague the student of microsporidia. A single source of information that will alleviate such
difficulties is badly needed.

Volumes 1 and 2 of "Comparative Pathobiology" represent an attempt to provide a convenient, general reference work that will facilitate the efforts of both students and researchers who are pursuing an interest in the microsporidia. Fifty years after Kudo (1924a) published his famous monograph, it is no longer feasible to collect all published information. Furthermore, we now know that much of the published information is misinformation. Therefore, the present aim is to make a critical review, stressing not only the areas in which information is questionable or lacking. At the same time, special attention is given to such major problem areas as classification, terminology, and methods.

Originally, we solicited contributions by specialists on microsporidia of all the different host groups, and the following authors actually submitted manuscripts: E. U. Canning (Platyhelminthes. Ambhibia and Reptilia. Mammalia), F. Coste-Mathiez and O. Tuzet (Chironomidae), C. Kalavati (Isoperta), J. Maurand (Simuliidae), and E. Vivier (Protozoa). Because we were unable to obtain, within a reasonable time, contributions on most of the host groups, plans to include these papers were reluctantly abandoned. Since then, three of those that were submitted have been published elsewhere. These are papers by Canning (1975), Maurand (1975), and Vivier (1975). Other specialists could make valuable contributions by publishing critical reviews of microsporidia in the remaining host groups.

The treatise was conceived as a single unit, covering in a comprehensive way our present knowledge of the microsporidia. Because of its length it had to be divided into two volumes. The subject matter was apportioned roughly according to two broad areas, biology and systematics. One chapter, Erickson's contribution on type slides, quite logically belongs with the volume on systematics but was, for several practical reasons, placed in the volume on biology. The chapter on methods and the Glossary are needed in both volumes and could just as logically appear in one as the other. We think that some lack of logic in apportionment of the subject matter will have little practical significance, however, because we anticipate that the two parts will become equally available to individuals who need access to a general reference work on the microsporidia.

We are fully aware that this is not in any sense a definitive work. We anticipate that many omissions and errors will be noted by users. Omissions are inevitable, not due so much to oversight as to the impossibility of keeping abreast of the flood of current literature. Newly published papers on microsporidia appear literally every few days and tend to render this treatise obsolete faster than revisions can be made in the final stages

of its preparation. Nevertheless, the treatise will have served
a useful purpose if it provides a large nucleus of organized
information and ideas that will facilitate the work of our
colleagues in further pursuit of their studies on microsporidia.
We urge the readers to be critical of the shortcomings and to
offer suggestions for improvement of possible future editions.

Victor Sprague

Jiří Vávra

*Literature cited here will be found among the References at the
end of Volume 2.

Contents

Structure of the Microsporidia

Jiří Vávra

INSTITUTE OF PARASITOLOGY
CZECHOSLOVAK ACADEMY OF SCIENCES
PRAGUE, CZECHOSLOVAKIA

I. INTRODUCTION

Considerable knowledge of microsporidian structure has been accumulated during 150 years of research. Critical evaluation of this knowledge reveals, however, that most progress has been achieved during the past fifteen years after electron microscopic application. Although some light microscope observations have contributed amazingly accurate data on microsporidian structure, the extreme smallness of microsporidia (the spores of which are probably the smallest eukaryotic cells) as well as the compactness and complexity of their structural organization requires better resolution than that obtained with the light microscope.

Electron microscopy combined with ultrathin sectioning was introduced into microsporidiology around 1960 and has proved to be a milestone in the understanding of microsporidian structure. Since then nearly a hundred papers on the fine morphology of microsporidia have been published. The general structure of the spore and of various developmental stages, as well as the fine structural aspects of microsporidian life cycle, are known. The material contained within this chapter is based mainly on the contributions of electron microscopy. My goal is to summarize the present state of knowledge and to show some perspectives for further research of microsporidian morphology.

Hopefully, the reader will recognize the fact that although we have progressed quite far in our comprehension of microsporidian morphology, there are still gaps in our understanding of some structures and in the explanation of their functional significance. Unfortunately, in some respects, we are already approaching the technical limits of electron microscopy and it becomes more and more obvious that if any further significant progress is to be made, new techniques, particularly cytochemical and biochemical, should be applied to these organisms.

It is fully appropriate to ask whether any future research of microsporidian structure is still worth the effort. The answer to this question is positive. The theoretical value of microsporidia is enormous due to the fact that these organisms are so well adapted to intracellular parasitism and yet they represent structurally a relatively simple system of one cell living inside another cell. During their long history of parasitism, microsporidia have also evolved some structures unique in the realm of eukaryotic

organisms. However, at some stages of development they look like
simple, nonspecialized cells. Due, in part, to both these features
microsporidia represent an extremely valuable material for the
study of various aspects of host-parasite relations at the cellular
level as well as for the study of cellular differentiation.

II. STRUCTURE OF MICROSPORIDIAN DEVELOPMENTAL STAGES (EXCLUDING SPORES)

All microsporidian cells other than spores are structurally
simple, nonspecialized cells. The sporoblasts are the inter-
mediary stage between these simple cells and the structurally
complicated spores. As mentioned in the chapter on microsporidian
development, each microsporidian has a nucleus – or a diplokaryon –
(several of these being present in plasmodial stages). The
microsporidian cytoplasm has the usual organelles such as the endoplasmic reticulum, ribosomes, Golgi zone of a special type, and
cytoplasmic microtubules. There are no mitochondria, no reserve
substances in the microsporidia as well as no structures comparable
to kinetosomes, peroxisomes, or typical lysozomes. The cell
membrane is a simple unit membrane in early developmental stages.
Later in the life cycle a more complicated cell wall is formed
(Fig. 1).

A. NUCLEUS

The microsporidian nucleus is typically round or oval and its
fine structure corresponds to that of a typical eukaryotic
nucleus.

1. Nuclear membrane

The nuclear membrane is a double unit membrane perforated with
pores (Vávra, 1965) which are sometimes closed by a diaphragm
(Vivier & Schrevel, 1973; Hildebrand, 1974). The outer membrane is
studded with ribosomes, has continuities with the endoplasmic
reticulum (Maurand, 1966), and occasionally forms vesicular blebs.
Infrequently, pores have not been recognized in the microsporidian
nucleus (Szollosi, 1971; Vávra, 1968a). This condition is very
unusual for a eukaryotic nucleus (Stevens and André, 1969) and it
needs further examination.
The nuclear membrane is a persistent structure in microsporidia.
The observations suggesting that the nuclear membrane is absent
in some stages of the life cycle (Schubert, 1969b) seem to result
from a poor preservation of the material. Detailed anatomy of the
nuclear membrane in *Thelohania bracteata* was revealed by freeze-
etching (Liu, 1972). The membrane exhibits the same characteristics
as observed in other cytomembranes. Particles are mostly found in

Fig. 1.   Schematic representation of the fine structural organi-
          zation of microsporidian developmental stages other than
          spores. Various configurations of the cell limiting
          membrane (1-11): 1, Simple unit membrane typical of
          meronts; 2, unit membrane with vesicular protrusions
          (meronts of *Caudospora* and *Telomyxa*); 3, unit membrane
          with filiform projections (meronts of *Pleistophora
          debaisieuxi*); 4, cell wall of two unit membranes of
          Inodosporus (ESM, exosporont membrane); 5, the cell wall
          of early sporogonial stages of *Pleistophora debaisieuxi*
          showing the secretion of dense material on the surface
          of the sporont cell wall and the formation of the pan-
          sporoblast membrane, PM; 6, fully differentiated cell
          wall of *P. debaisieuxi*. The complex of two unit membranes
          is covered with a dense cell coat differentiated into
          tubular appendages confined to the pansporoblast cavity
          or chamber (PCH) which itself is limited by the pansporo-
          blast membrane, PM; 7, cell wall of sporogonial stages of
          Nosema algerae. Sporont unit membrane is covered by a
          thick dense coat and a thin membranous layer; 8, cell
          wall of *Nosema apis* sporonts from winter bees where the
          exosporont membrane forms tubular out-pocketings; 9,
          cell wall of sporogonial stages of typical *Nosema* or
          Caudospora. The membranous complex is covered by a thin
          cell coat; 10, cell wall of *Pleistophora* sp. from
          Daphnia showing the relation of the cell wall to the
          scindosome (s). 11, *Thelohania bracteata*, sporogonial
          plasmodium. The cell wall is covered by granular
          secretion (SE) which fills a large part of the pan-
          sporoblast chamber, PCH.
             The cytoplasmic organization of the developmental
          stages are: CT, cytoplasmic microtubules; EV, endocytic
          vesicle; G, Golgi apparatus; N, nucleus, NB, blebs on
          the nuclear membrane, NC, nucleolus; PV, polar vesicles;
          RER, rough endoplasmic reticulum; S, scindosome; SER,
          smooth endoplasmic reticulum; S, spindle plaque; ST,
          spindle tubules; SV, secretory vesicle.

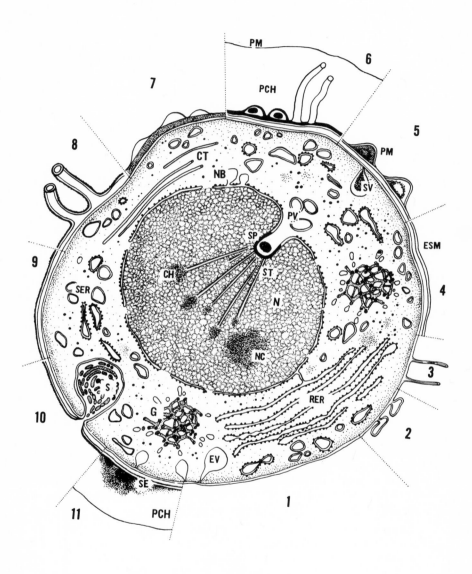

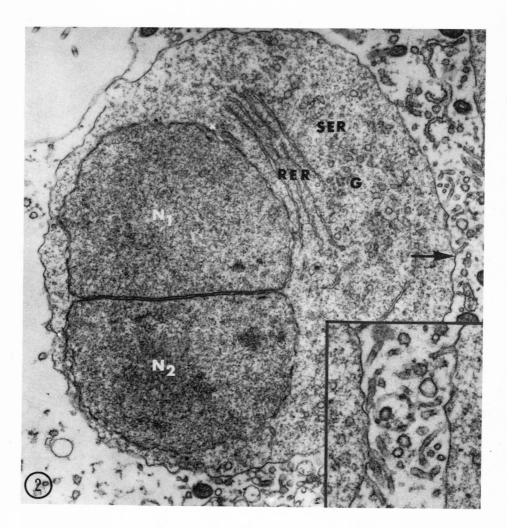

Fig. 2.   Meront of *Pleistophora debaisieuxi* containing a diplo-
          karyon (N_1-N_2), rough endoplasmic reticulum (RER), smooth
          endoplasmic reticulum (SER).   The cell membrane is a unit
          membrane forming microvillosities (arrow). x 19,600. Inset:
          detail of the cell membrane with microvillosities. X
          28,000.

the fractured face of the inner nuclear membrane viewed from the cytoplasmic side and on the fractured face of the outer nuclear membrane viewed from the nucleoplasmic side. The nuclear pore complex generally has a central granule and is ringed by eight substructures arranged in eight-fold symmetry. The diameter of the nuclear pore complex and the occurrence of the central granule in the pore is different in various developmental stages which suggests a different nuclear-cytoplasmic exchange. The pores are also present in nuclei of freshly discharged sporoplasms (Ishihara, 1968).

2. Nucleoplasm

The nucleoplasm is usually homogenous in the early developmental stages (sporoplasm, early meronts), whereas later, especially during sporulation, a more dense nucleolus is observed (Lom and Corliss, 1967; Richards and Sheffield, 1970). Chromatin is usually finely dispersed in microsporidian nuclei (euchromatin). Aggregates of heterochromatin were reported in older meronts (Youssef and Hammond, 1971) and sporonts (Weidner, 1970) and were sometimes clearly identifiable as chromosomes (Sprague and Vernick, 1968b; Canning and Sinden, 1973). Rod-like, dense structures, probably chromatids, were observed in nuclei of meronts in *Pleistophora debaisieuxi* (Fig. 4) (Joyon and Vávra, unpublished).

3. The diplokaryon

Sometimes the microsporidian nuclear component is represented by two closely adjacent nuclei in an intimate relationship--the diplokaryon. Both nuclei of the diplokaryon are structurally identical and behave synchronously during the cell cycle. Both nuclei have their own membranes (Vávra, 1965; 1968, Fig. 2). In the area of contact the nuclei are flattened, there are no pores in this region (Liu, 1972; Walker and Hinsch, 1972). The nuclear membranes are thicker and more electron dense along the plane of apposition (Sprague *et al.*, 1968; Ormieres and Sprague, 1973). Sometimes in the region of contact, the double membranes of each diplokaryon nucleus seem to be fused (Youssef and Hammond, 1971; Canning and Sinden, 1973). In *Ameson* (syn. *Nosema*) *michaelis* the nuclei of the diplokaryon are separated by a narrow bridge of cytoplasm and an internuclear sac with a number of vesicles (Weidner, 1970).

An unconventional explanation of the diplokaryon structure was proposed by Cossins and Bowler (1974) who interpret the diplokaryon of *Thelohania contejeani* as a single, U-shaped nucleus with a deep cleft. The authors claim that they have confirmed this configuration in serial sections of sporoblasts. Cossin and Bowler's data need critical reexamination. Maurand and Vey (1973) found that there is only a single nucleus in the sporoblasts of the same microsporidian and that the U-shaped nucleus occurs in the spores only.

Fig. 3.   The spindle apparatus of *Thelohania bracteata*. The
           chromosomes (CH) are attached by the spindle microtubules
           (ST) to the spindle plaque with associated dense material
           (arrow) situated in a depression of the nuclear membrane
           double arrow). X 36,000.

Fig. 4.   Dense structures (chromosome chromatids?) in the nucleus
           of *Pleistophora debaisieuxi* are shown at arrows. Some of
           the structures seem to be paired (a). The pairs may be a
           actually synaptonematic complexes. (Joyon and Vavra,
           unpublished). X 30,000.

Fig. 5.   Detailed view of the spindle plaque in *Stempellia sp.*
           Note that the plaque is a multilayered structure. Polar
           vesicles (PV) are separated from the plaque by a layer
           (d) of dense cytoplasm. Mm, nuclear membrane. X
           106,000.

Fig. 6.   Two closely situated spindle plaques (arrows) in the
           nucleus of *Stempellia sp.* X 32,000.

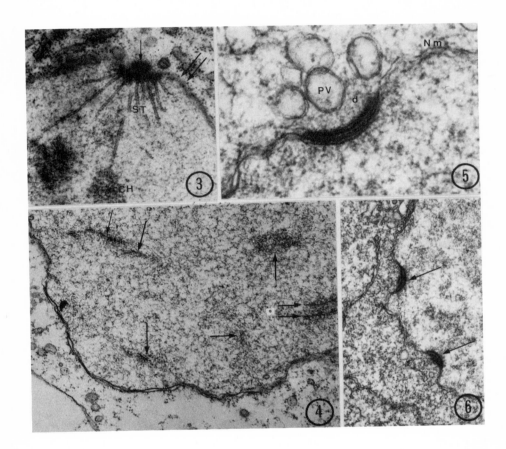

As discussed in the chapter on microsporidian development, in some microsporidia, stages with diplokaryon and with single nucleus alternate in the life cycle. Electron microscopy so far has not produced any suggestive evidence of nuclear fusion in stages where the monokaryotic condition is reached.

4. *Nuclear division*

Division of the microsporidian nucleus proceeds as acentriolar pleuromitosis (Hollande, 1972) during which the nuclear membrane is preserved (Vávra, 1965; Vinckier *et al.*, 1971; Sprague and Vernick, 1968b; Hildebrand, 1974; Vivier and Schrevel, 1973, Fig. 7).

5. *Spindle plaque and spindle tubules*

There is no centriole in the microsporidian cell. Instead, a specialized area on the nuclear membrane serves as an attachment point for the intranuclear spindle apparatus (Figs. 3, 5, and 6). This structure, first observed by Vávra (1965), was originally given the unappropriate name "centrosome" but later Vávra and Undeen (1970) and Sprague and Vernick (1971) recognized its structural similarity with the kinetic center of yeasts. The latter authors adopted the name "centriolar plaque" for the spindle terminus. However, a better and less confusing name would be "spindle plaque" which was recently used for spindle terminus in yeast (Moens and Rapport, 1971).
The microsporidian spindle plaque is a dense circular area of about 180 nm (Canning and Sinden, 1973) closely associated with the nuclear membrane. In well fixed specimens, two dark layers are resolved in the plaque (Vávra, unpublished, Fig. 5). At the site of the plaque the nuclear membrane is modified, being more electron dense and its layers indistinct (Vivier, 1965; Vinckier *et al.*, 1971b) and the perinucle – or space being narrower (Youssef & Hammond, 1971). During the division, the spindle plaque, together with the adjacent nuclear membrane, is invaginated into the nucleus for some distance (Vávra, 1965). The spindle plaque persists in early sporoblasts, although spindle microtubules are no longer apparent (Walker and Hinsch, 1972). It is not known whether the plaque persists also in the spore. The plaque so far has not been reported in the sporoplasm. The division of the plaque has not been observed although the occurrence of two closely adjacent plaques (Vávra, unpublished) suggests that it takes place (Fig. 6).
In dividing diplokaryon nuclei the spindle microtubules are parallel with the line of apposition of the two nuclei (Sprague and Vernick, 1969a; Canning and Sinden, 1973). However, sometimes stages can be found possessing a diplokaryon in which the spindle plaques are at the side of the nucleus opposite to the line of diplokaryon apposition. According to the latter authors, this situation suggests that such stages begin their development as

uninucleate cells. Such an explanation, however, does not take
into account that new spindle plaques are probably derived from
the preexisting ones and that after each division of the nucleus,
at least one of the plaques has to migrate along the nuclear
surface. There are indications, however, that the behaviour of
spindle plaques might be more complicated. Light microscope
observations of *Pleistophora debaisieuxi* (Vávra, unpublished) seem
to indicate that there are more than just two plaques in the dividing
nucleus. It seems that at least two other plaques are ready in the
place where the spindle of the future nuclear division will terminate (Fig. 3 in Chapter 2, this monograph. Serial sections will be
necessary to prove this hypothesis.

The spindle tubules which converge from the chromosomes toward
the plaques are 15-30 nm in diameter (Vivier, 1965; Vinckier
et al., 1971; Walker and Hinsch, 1972; Sprague and Vernick, 1968b,
Fig. 3). The spindle microtubules extend across the perinuclear
space (Youssef and Hammond, 1971) and converge on the dark material
of the plaque on the outside of the nuclear membrane. There is
either a dark granule (Vávra, 1965; Vávra and Undeen, 1970) or
sometimes several (usually three) opaque vesicles with double walls
("polar vesicles" of Youssef and Hammond, 1971) in the vicinity of
the spindle plaque (Figs. 3, 5). Their significance is unknown.
As will be mentioned later, the Golgi zone also is often associated
with the spindle plaque.

B. *CYTOPLASM*

The microsporidian cytoplasm contains endoplasmic reticulum, free
and bound ribosomes, Golgi zone, vesicles of endocytosis, and some
inclusions not properly classified (Fig. 1). The sporoblasts also
contain some organelles of the future spore. These structures will
be discussed in the section dealing with the structure of the spore.

1. *Endoplasmic reticulum*

Both conventional types (rough and smooth) of endoplasmic
reticulum occur in microsporidian cells. Only with exception was
the endoplasmic reticulum not identified (Burke, 1970).

Rough endoplasmic reticulum (RER) is present in the developmental
stages in the form of cisternae and vesicles. Usually there are
four to six cisternae in a meront (Milner, 1972). The cisternae are
arranged in a stack and are parallel to the surface of the nucleus.
Vesicles of the RER are irregularly distributed in the cytoplasm
(Figs. 2 and 7). Under certain conditions, the RER vesicles are
the predominant type of reticulum, whereas in other cases the
cisternal type is more developed. As a rule there are more RER
cisternae in sporulation stages than in meronts and their
arrangement is also more orderly in late developmental stages
(Youssef and Hammond, 1971; Cali, 1970; Lom and Corliss, 1967).

Fig. 7.   Nuclear division and cytoplasmic cleavage in the sporont
           of *Pleistophora debaisieuxi*. The nuclear membrane is
           preserved, the dividing nuclei are connected by an isthmus
           (NI) through which are stretching the spindle micro-
           tubules attached at the spindle plaque (SP). RER, rough
           endoplasmic reticulum; G, Golgi apparatus. There are
           no specialized structures associated with the cleavage
           zone (arrow). X 16,000.

Fig. 8.   Structures resembling mitochondria (arrows) in a young
           spore of *Nosema locustae*. SPW, spore wall. X 44,500.
           Courtesy Dr. A Huger, unpublished.

Fig. 9.   Two Golgi apparatuses (G_1, G_2) in the cytoplasm of a
           meront of *Thelohania bracteata*. The Golgi is situated in
           the close vicinity of the nucleus (N) and is associated
           with (arrows) the lamellae of endoplasmic reticulum
           (RER). Close apposition of both Golgi is suggestive of
           dictyokinesis. X 29,000.

Fig. 10.   Same material as in Fig. 9. The outer zone of the Golgi
           apparatus consists of larger vesicles (cisternae)
           frequently associated with the endoplasmic reticulum
           (arrow). X 58,000.

Fig. 11.   Dividing meront of *Thelohania bracteata* with a conspic-
           uous structure in the isthmus between the daughter cells.
           It is believed that the structure represents Golgi zone
           associated with the endoplasmic reticulum and in a
           special configuration when distributed into two cells
           (dictyokinesis) X 19,000.

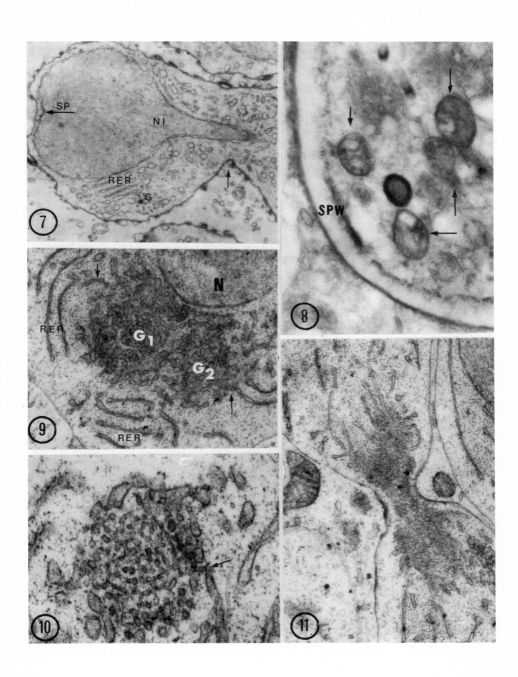

In some microsporidia, the presence of RER was not ascertained.
Whereas the RER is abundant in *Metchnikovella wohlfarthi*
(Hildebrand and Vivier, 1971), there is no RER in *Metchnikovella
hovassei* (Vivier, 1965; 1966). Similarly Szollosi (1971) was not
able to find any association between endoplasmic reticulum and
ribosomes in *Pleistophora* sp., although other species of the same
genus have the RER well developed (Vávra, 1965; Lom and Corliss,
1967).

There are numerous vesicles with smooth membranes in the
microsporidian cell. Those vesicles which are freely distributed
and have a transparent content are thought to belong to the
smooth endoplasmic reticulum (SER). In those cells in which the
nucleus is undergoing karyokinesis, the vesicles of the SER are
more abundant and are larger in size (Vivier and Schrevel, 1973).
In *Pleistophora* sp. only SER was reported although parallel
cisternae, which belong in other microsporidia to the RER are quite
abundant in this particular microsporidian (Szollosi, 1971).

2. *Ribosomes*

Developmental stages exhibit ribosomes attached to the endoplasmic reticulum or freely dispersed in the cytoplasm (Vávra,
1965; Sprague and Vernick, 1969a; Sprague and Vernick, 1968b;
Lom and Corliss, 1967; Ishihara, 1968; Szollosi, 1971; Youssef
and Hammond, 1971; Walker and Hinsch, 1972). In some species and
in some stages most of the ribosomes are in the dispersed state
and this phenomenon was considered a sign of active cell differentiation (Weidner, 1970). There is general agreement that the quantity
of ribosomes increases during the development, especially at the
sporoblast stage and during spore morphogenesis (Lom and Corliss,
1967; Liu and Davies, 1972b). Polyribosomes arranged in tight
spirals often occur in sporoblasts and in young spores (for more
details see the section on spore structure) (Fig. 26). Exceptionally
meronts are reported as having more ribosomes than the sporulation
stages (Weidner, 1970).

As far as the physical characters of the microsporidian ribosomes
are concerned, the only existing data are those of Ishihara and
Hayashi (1968) who found that in extruded sporoplasm of *Nosema bombyc*
there are only 70 S monoribosomes with two subunits of 50 and 30 S
respectively. The occurrence of 70 S ribosomes in an eukaryotic
organism is an exception. If the sedimentation coefficient values
represent a real feature specific to microsporidians, it may have
taxonomic implications (Weidner, 1970). Ishihara and Hayashi also
found that the RNA content of microsporidian ribosomes resembles the
RNA values of prokaryotic organisms more than those of protozoa.
The ribosomes of *Metchnikovella* are structurally similar to those
of their gregarine hosts (Vivier and Schrevel, 1973).

3. Microtubules and filaments

Rarely observed structures of microsporidian cytoplasm are microtubules (Fig. 1). To date, they have been reported only in the cytoplasm of meronts of *Nosema bombycis* (Ishihara, 1970) and in the cytoplasm of dividing meronts of *Metchnikovella* (Vivier and Schrevel, 1973) where they are represented by classical microtubules (20-25 nm in diameter) arranged laterally to the dividing nucleus. There has been no record of cytoplasmic filaments in microsporidia and the mechanism of the cytoplasmic constriction during cytokinesis is unknown (Szollosi, 1971).

4. Mitochondria

Mitochondria are not present in microsporidian cells at my stage of development (Vávra, 1965) and this fact has been confirmed by all investigators of the microsporidian fine structure. However, there are reports of the presence of "mitochondria-like structures" in several microsporidia. Maurand (1973) observed such structures in sporogonial plasmodium and young spores of *Thelohania moenadis*. It seems, however, that these structures are identical with the dense inclusion ("posterosome") containing tubuli that occurs regularly in the posterior vacuole and which is discussed in the section dealing with this organelle. Structures "somewhat resembling mitochondria" were depicted by Richards and Sheffield (1970) in sporoblasts of *Steinhausia (Syn. Coccospora) brachynema*. It is impossible to say whether these structures are actually mitochondria. Huger (personal communication) found a structure closely resembling a mitochondrion in a body which might be a young but atypical *Nosema locustae* spore (Fig. 8).

Sometimes there occur vesicular structures with internal tubuli ("scindosomes") contained in sporogonial plasmodia that constrict into individual sporoblasts (Figs. 19, 20, 21, 22). These entities superfically resemble mitochondria, although, as will be discussed later, they probably are produced by invagination of the cell limiting membrane.

5. Other inclusions

There are no reserve substances in microsporidian cells (Maurand and Loubes, 1973) and spores. Their absence is evidently due to the fact that microsporidia as obligatory intracellular parasites have no metabolically active stages outside the host cell. Electron dense inclusions ("posterosome") occurring in the posterior part of the sporoblasts will be discussed in the section dealing with the fine structure of the posterior vacuole. Inclusions occurring during sporulation around and on the surface of sporonts and sporoblasts will be dealt with in the section on the cell limiting membrane.

6. *Golgi apparatus*

In the cytoplasm of microsporidian developmental stages there is one or several areas that contain small opaque vesicles limited by a single membrane (Vávra, 1965, 1968) (Fig. 1). The vesicles form a meshwork in a homogenous matrix having a density greater than that of the surrounding cytoplasm (Youssef and Hammond, 1971). There are no ribosomes present in the matrix (Vávra, unpublished) (Figs. 9, 10). In some microsporidian species the area of vesicles has a double appearance: the center of the area is occupied by small vesicles, while its marginal portion is formed by larger and less dense vesicles. Cisternae and vesicles of rough endoplasmic reticulum are closely associated with the marginal portion (Vávra, unpublished) (Figs. 9, 10).

The afore mentioned area of vesicles has been called "primitive Golgi zone" (Vávra, 1965), the word primitive being used because the structure has little resemblance to stacks of flattened saccules of typical Golgi. The concept of microsporidan Golgi is gradually being accepted although with some reluctance (Sprague and Vernick, 1968b). In accordance with the present knowledge of Golgi apparatus (Morré, *et al.* 1971), there is no reason to doubt that this area of vesicles is a true Golgi zone. The dense matrix in which the vesicles are embedded obviously corresponds to the "zone of exclusion" so typical for Golgi apparatus. In many generative or resting cells, Golgi zone consists of small vesicles, e.g. prestages of Golgi apparatus in frog oocytes (Ward and Ward, 1968) are extremely similar to microsporidian Golgi. As will be shown later, the microsporidian Golgi is the site of endomembrane differentiation and has thus the same function as a typical Golgi.

In developmental stages other than sporoblasts, one to several Golgi apparati may be scattered in the cytoplasm. Only exceptionally has the Golgi not been observed (Lom and Corliss, 1967; Sprague *et al.*,1968; Maurand *et al.*, 1971). In *Metchnikovella* sp., the Golgi vesicles are closely associated with the spindle plague (Vivier, 1965; Hildebrand, 1974) and they increase in number during plasmotomy (Vivier and Schrevel, 1973). In *Nosema apis*, the Golgi apparati are located at opposite poles of the nucleus or are adjacent to each nucleus of the diplokaryon. In multinucleate meronts, the Golgi is more developed than in earlier stages; its vesicles are joined to form a tubular network closely associated with endoplasmic reticulum channels (Youssef and Hammond, 1971). During the life cycle, the Golgi apparatus becomes more prominent and more numerous as the development progresses (Vivier and Schrevel, 1973). The individual vesicles also form a more interconnected meshwork (Fig. 12). There are no firm data on the number of Golgi apparati in microsporidian cells at various stages of development.

There is some evidence that the Golgi apparatus is involved in the synthesis of the surface coat of sporonts. Usually, the surface coat is formed first in areas overlying Golgi (Canning and Nicholas, 1974). Also, there is evidence that the dark material packaged within Golgi vesicles is secreted on the surface of sporogonial stages of *Pleistophora debaisieuxi* and later assembled into tubular expansions characteristic of this species (Vávra, unpublished). During spore morphogenesis the Golgi assumes a central role in the elaboration of various spore organelles (see section on spore structure). Positive reaction to silver methenamine by microsporidian Golgi (Walker and Hinsch, 1972) may be an indication of Golgi involvement in cellular carbohydrate metabolism (Favard, 1969).

Continuity of microsporidian Golgi during a complete life cycle is not established. Undifferentiated Golgi has not been observed in microsporidian spores except for that reported by Gassouma and Ellis (1973). It has been suggested that the polaroplast -polar cap complex- could be interpreted as Golgi (Sprague and Vernick, 1968a, 1969a). As will be shown in the section dealing with the fine structure of the spore we presently consider the polaroplast as a derivative of the Golgi. There is no Golgi in freshly discharged sporoplasm (Ishihara, 1968; Weidner, 1972; Weidner and Trager, 1973). Due to the perinuclear position of the microsporidian Golgi its origin has been sought in the nuclear envelope (Vinckier, 1973).

Light microscope observations indicate that dictyokinesis exists in microsporidia (Sprague and Vernick, 1969a); electron micrographs with two closely adjacent Golgi zones (Vávra, unpublished) seem to confirm such observations (Fig. 9). An unusual formation of lamellar stacks stemming from a dense trunk-like region has been observed occasionally in the isthmus connecting two dividing merunts in *Thelohania bracteata* (Vávra, unpublished; Fig. 11). Presumably, this structure represents microsporidian Golgi in a special configuration when distributed into two daughter cells.

7. *Cell limiting membrane*

The cell limiting membrane has special importance in microsporidia because it is the only membrane separating the parasite from the host cell cytoplasm. Only rarely does the host cell form additional membranes enclosing the parasite in the so-called parasitophorous vacuole (Canning and Nicholas, 1974: Barker, 1975). The microsporidian cell membrane reflect varying degrees of interaction between the parasite and the host; its configuration changes during the life cycle with such regularity that different stages can be identified according to its structure.

While inside the spore the sporoplasm does not exist as a preformed cell and therefore is not limited by a membrane (Weidner, 1972; Petri, 1974). However, after passage through the

Fig. 12.   Vesicular meshwork representing the Golgi apparatus
            in sporoblast of *Stempellia sp.* This configuration of
            Golgi is found in cells where the polar filament is
            being formed. X 66,000.

Fig. 13.   Freshly extruded sporoplasm of *Ameson* (syn. *Nosema)*
            michaelis still attached to the polar tube (arrow).
            The sporoplasm is a simple cell with nucleus (N) and
            cytoplasm in which arrays of membranes (CM) can be
            recognized. The cell is limited by single membrane
            which is coated with a dense material. X 35,000.
            From Weidner (1972).

Fig. 14.   Early sporulation stages of *Pleistophora debaissieuxi.*
            The stage at A is a very young sporont the membrane of
            which is only slightly thicker than that of the meront
            in Fig. 2. The cell at B is a more advanced sporont
            in which the exosporont membrane, the secretion and the
            pansporoblast membrane start to differentiate. X 17,000.

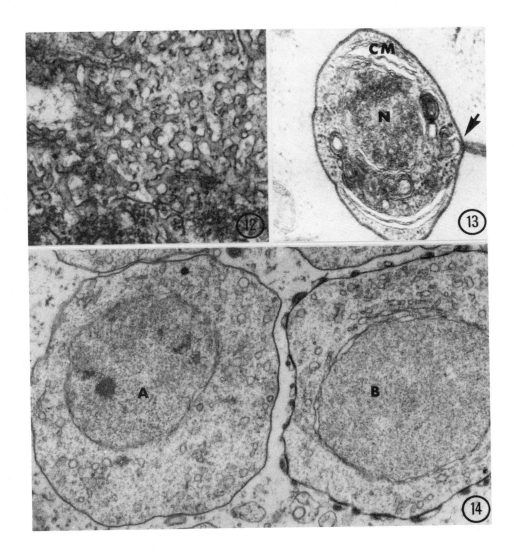

polar tube the sporoplasm is limited by a membrane (Fig. 13).
There are two envelopes around a freshly discharged sporoplasm,
the outer one being continuous with the outer sheath of the
discharged polar tube (see also the chapter on microsporidian
physiology by E. Weidner, this monograph). When inoculated into
a host cell, one of the envelopes disappears and the sporoplasm
remains surrounded by single membrane (Weidner, 1972).

Most microsporidologists agree that meronts are limited by a
single unit membrane (Vávra, 1968a; Sprague, Vernick and Lloyd
1968; Weidner, 1970; Youssef and Hammond, 1971; Canning and
Nicholas, 1974; see Fig. 2). Only exceptionally has the meront
membrane been reported as having a more complicated structure.
Canning and Sinden (1973) found that in *Nosema algerae* the cell
membrane is covered with a thin layer of dense material interspersed
with microtubuli. Milner (1972) observed a multilayered outer
coat in *Nosema whitei*. However, it remains to be confirmed that
the stages with such unusual membrane configuration are truly
meronts.

The limiting membrane of many microsporidian meronts exhibits
structural evidence of an active interaction with host cell
cytoplasm. The surface area of the meront membrane can be
substantially increased by vesicular or tubular projections
interdigitated with host cell cytoplasm (Vávra, 1968a; Codreanu
and Vávra, 1970; Vivier and Schrevel, 1973; Fig. 2). These projections are more numerous in parasites situated within host
nuclei (Takizawa *et al.*, 1973). Meront membrane often forms
vesicles that may be encytotic (Vávra, 1968a). Continuity between
microsporidian cell membrane and the membranous system inside the
host cell has been suggested by Sprague and Vernick (1968b).

The cell limiting membrane of sporont and of sporogonial
plasmodia is markedly different from the unit membrane of meronts
(Figs. 14-19). In fact, the difference in membrane configuration
is used as a criterion for distinguishing the early stages of the
sporulation phase from meronts (Cali, 1970). The beginning of the
sporulation phase in the life cycle is marked by thickenning of the
cell membrane (Vávra, 1965). Apparently, there are two mechanisms
of thickenning. According to Canning and Nicholas (1974), an
electron dense coat is initially deposited in irregular thin patches
on the outside of the meront plasmalemma. During later development,
the extramembranous material is disseminated more uniformly until
it forms a continuous coat of about 20-30 nm over the surface
of the cell. In some species the thickenning of the sporont
membrane apparently is due to the appearance of an additional unit
membrane (Vávra, 1965) which could be the "exosporont membrane"
described by Overstreet and Weidner (1974). Alternatively, it may
thicken because of the laying down of an additional complex of
two or three unit membranes (Maurand, 1973). The membrane complex
on the surface of the sporont is later covered or impregnated by
dense material that renders a thick, dense cell wall characteristic
of sporulation stages (Figs. 15, 16, 17, 18).

In many species the sporont transforms into a multinucleate plasmodium from which individual finger-like sporoblasts are cleaved. Large vesicles filled with a whirl of tubuli are found in several species at the base of the cleavage furrow (Fig. 19). The structure of these vesicles is comparable to a large mesosome (Maurand, 1973). Detailed observations of Vávra (unpublished) show that the vesicles are formed by invagination of the inner membrane (plasmalemma) of the plasmodium. The name scindosome (*scindo* is Latin for cleave) is proposed for this structure. The neck of the invaginated vesicle is open to the exterior and the dense cell coat seems to be synthesized at this site (Fig. 20). There are indications that the tubuli inside the vesicle furnish material from which the extramembranous coat is formed (Figs. 21, 22). Several scindosomes may be found near the surface of each sporoblast cleaved from the plasmodium. They persist in the sporoblast for a long time and may structurally imitate a mitochondrion.

In microsporidian suborders Diplokaryonina and Monokaryonina (Sprague, this monograph), sporont membrane morphogenesis ends with the formation of a dark extramembranous coat already described. However, in microsporidians of the suborder Pansporoblastina, an additional membrane is formed in early sporulation external to the sporont cytoplasmic membrane (Vávra, 1965). This so-called pansporoblast membrane has two characteristics: 1. it is a thin membrane probably of the unit type, and 2. the membrane surrounds the sporont cell or the sporogonial plasmodium in a loose fashion (Figs. 15-19). The pansporoblast membrane appears as a sachet enshrouding sporoblasts or spores originating from a single sporont. Electron microscopy of freeze-etched preparations reveals that the pansporoblast membrane is 17-19 nm thick with a rough outer surface densely covered with particles of 15-17 nm (Liu *et al.*, 1971).

Two modes of pansporoblast membrane formation are observable with electron microscopy. In *Pleistophora debaisieuxi,* the appearance of the pansporoblast membrane occurs simultaneously with the formation of the exosporont membrane. The original plasmalemma of the early sporont becomes thicker and diffuse and later separates into two distinct unit membranes (membrane complex of the sporont). At the same time small blisters of a very fine membrane appear on the exterior of the sporont membrane complex (Fig. 15). These blisters grow and merge to form a complete envelope (Vávra, 1965 and other unpublished observations). According to Szollosi (1971), the pansporoblast membrane in *Pleistophora* sp. is a transformed membrane of the meront and an additional neoformed membrane appears at the surface of the sporogonial plasmodium.

The pansporoblast membrane occurs in two forms during sporogony. It appears as a loose sachet around the sporogony stages of some microsporidia. In other species the pansporoblast membrane more closely outlines the sporogonial plasmodium and cleaves synchronously

Fig. 15.   Detail of the cell limiting wall in a young sporont of
           Pleistophora debaisieuxi. The cell membrane is thicker
           at the site of exosporont membrane synthesis (double
           arrow). Pansporoblast membrane (PM) is formed as
           blisters on the surface of the sporont. Dense secretion
           material (S) is deposited in the future pansporoblast
           cavity (PC). N, nucleus of the parasite. X 132,000.

Fig. 16.   Cell wall of the advanced sporogonial plasmodium of
           Pleistophora debaisieuxi. The cell membrane (arrow) is
           covered by a membranous layer (exosporont membrane)
           impregnated by electron dense coat (double arrow) which
           also forms the external tubuli (ET) reaching into the
           pansporoblast cavity which is delimited by pansporoblast
           membrane (PM). X 116,000.

Fig. 17.   Detail of the cell wall in young sporoblast of *Stempellia
           sp*. The cell wall (SCW) is a dark layer in which no
           substructure is shown. Pansporoblast membrane (PM)
           delimits the pansporoblast cavity (PC) in which dark
           secretion material in form of short tubuli with crenu-
           lated outline is dpposited. X 48,000.

Fig. 18.   Cell wall of a late sporogonial stage in *Tuzetia sp.* is
           formed by three layers of membranes to which the pan-
           sporoblast membrane (PM) is closely applied. X 54,000
           (Courtesy of Drs. J. Maurand and A. Fize).

Fig. 19.   Cleaving sporogonial plasmodium of *Pleistophora sp.* from
           Daphnia. Two scindosomes (S) are present in the cleavage
           furrow; (SCW, plasmodium cell wall; PM, pansporoblast
           membrane; PC, pansporoblast cavity). X 6,000.

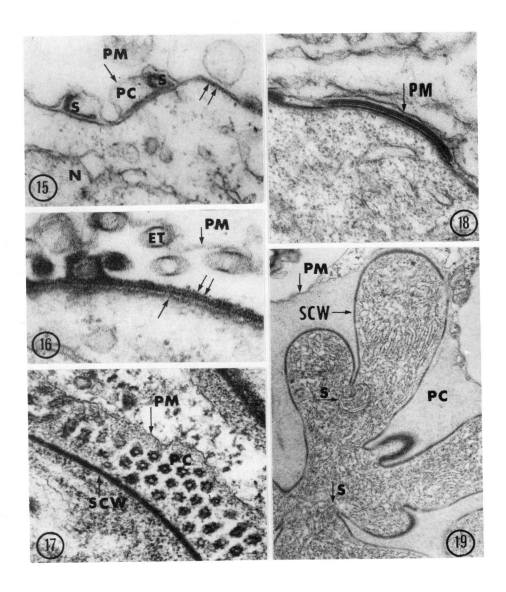

Fig. 20.   Detail of the scindosome from Fig. 19. The continuity
            of the scindosome membrane with the inner membrane
            (plasmalemma) of the plasmodium is clearly shown. The
            cavity of the scindosome is open into the pansporoblast
            cavity. X 100,000.

Figs. 21
 and 22.   Scindosomes of *Stempellia sp.* apparently emptying their
            contents into the pansporoblast cavity. Note that at
            the neck of the scindosome the dense sporogonial cell
            wall is discontinuous. X 114,000.

Fig. 23.   Part of the pansporoblast of *Glugea daphniae*. The
            secretion material is deposited in the pansporoblast
            cavity (PC) in the form of short microtubuli which
            sometimes aggregate into clumps. S_1-S_2, spores; PM,
            pansporoblast membrane. X 33,000.

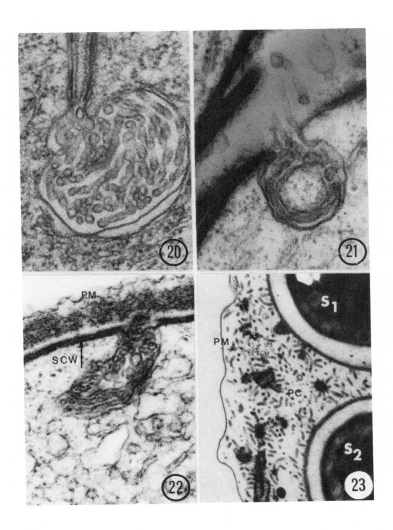

with it (family Tuzetiidae). In the latter case each sporoblast
and spore is enclosed by an individual pansporoblastic envelope
derived from the fission of the common pansporoblast. During late
sporulation, the pansporoblast may or may not persist until spores
are mature. If the membrane does persist, spores issued from a
single sporont are held togethe rin a characteristic configuration.
In the absence of membrane, the spores lie freely in the cytoplasm as is exemplified by the apansporoblastic species.

Only rarely is the pansporoblast membrane modified to bear
projections or form a thick cystic envelope. In *Trichoduboscquia,*
the membrane is drawn into four spines (Leger, 1926), the formation
of which is controlled by the nuclei inside the pansporoblast.
When the number of spores formed inside the pansporoblast is less
than 16, there is a correspondingly fewer number of spines. For
example, in pansporoblasts with 12 spores there are only three
spines and in pansporoblasts with eight spores there are 2 spines
(Weiser, 1961). Triangular pansporoblasts with two to three
flagelliform filaments occur in the genus *Mitoplistophora*
(Codreanu, 1964).

In some species the pansporoblast membrane is transformed into
a cystic envelope. The membrane of *Pleistophora hyphessobryconis*
is thick and contains a vesicular layer beneath it. This
arrangement occurs in young pansporoblasts whereas with mature
spores only a thin pansporoblastic membrane persists (Lom &
Corliss, 1967). In *Hessea squamosa,* the pansporoblast membrane
is changed into a thick-walled cyst that displays a mosaic of
polygonal plates from which lamellar projections extend. The wall
of the cyst consists of two distinct zones: an outer, dense zone
and a subjacent, moderately dense, laminated one (Ormieres and
Sprague, 1973). Apparently, the outer zone is the original
pansporoblast membrane (appears during early sporulation) whereas
the inner zone is formed later during sporoblast formation. The
inner zone may be homologous to the "secretion" material of other
pansporoblast-forming microsporida. Two kinds of cysts appear
in *Chytridiopsis* sp. One is a thin-walled ("fragile") cyst; its
wall probably corresponds to the limiting membrane of the original
sporogonial plasmodium. The other type is a thick-walled
("durable") cyst with walls of high electron density (Sprague,
Ormieres and Manier, 1972). The formation of thick-walled cysts
is also known to occur in the family Metchnikovellidae for which
the shape of the cyst characterizes the three genera of this
family. In addition to a normal cycle that involves schizonts
growing into large plasmodia which, in turn, dissolve to form
uninucleate sporoblasts and spores, the genus *Metchnikovella*
commonly has plasmodia enveloped by a thick-walled cyst. The cyst
originates as a dark material secreted at the outside of the
limiting membrane of the plasmodium. The cyst envelope later
differentiates into two layers: an inner envelope formed from
tightly packed fibres (approximately 0.25 µm thick) and an outer
loosely reticulated zone about 1 µm thick.

Between the pansporoplast membrane and the underlying membrane
of the sporont or of the sporogonial plasmodium or sporoblast)
is a space called either the pansporoblast cavity or, "pansporoblast determinate area", or "pansporoblastic chamber" (see
Overstreet and Weidner, 1974). The pansporoblast cavity is an
"empty" space in which some electron dense material is deposited
during development. Vávra (1965) observed that this dense material
is secreted into the pansporoblast cavity from the surface of the
cell(s) contained within. The name "secretion" applied to this
substance seems to be substantiated by the observations of
Maurand (1973) and Vávra (unpublished) of dense material crossing
the membrane of the sporogonial plasmodium. The secretion
apparently does not represent material of the host organism
taken up by the pansporoblast as suggested by Liu and Davies
(1972d). The secreted material varies (even within the same
species) from granules of different size and density to tubules,
filaments, or aggregates of particles. Freeze-etched preparations
reveal the secretion material of *Thelohania bracteata* sporoblasts
as vesicles with finger print like profiles (Liu *et al.*, 1971).
Undoubtedly, the secreted material is identical with what
Debaisieux in 1919 described as "granules de differentiation"
or "granules intercalaires chromatiques" (see Glossary).

A highly conspicuous feature of the secreted material is its
tendency to assemble itself into tubules. These formations may
be species specific and may be similar to classical microtubules
(Dwyer and Weidner, 1973, Fig. 23); Fig. 16 depicts some large
tubules in *Pleistophora debaisieuxi*. Results of cytochemical
investigations indicate that the secreted material is protein
rich in sulfhydryl groups. Secretion of proteinaceous material
into the pansporoblast cavity should not be confused with another
secretion of acid mucoploysaccharides that is formed only during
sporoblast formation (Maurand and Loubes, 1973). In most instances the material secreted during early sporogony disappears
while the spores are being formed. Occasionally, however, the
secreted material remains in the form of tubular appendages
ornamenting the surface of the spores (Vávra, 1965). The mucous
layer covering the surface of some spores (Lom and Vavra, 1962b)
also may originate as material secreted into the pansporoblast
cavity during sporulation.

The material secreted into the pansporoblast cavity of *Telomyxa
glugeiformis* probably serves as a cement. Two sporoblasts and two
spores originate from one sporont and these two cells remain permanently glued together inside the pansporoblast membrane by a
dark material homologous to the secretion already described for
other microsporidia. In such a manner a permanent couple of spores
("diplospore') is formed (Codreanu and Vávra, 1970, Fig. 72c and
also Fig. 1 of Vávra's section on Development of Microsporidia,
this monograph).

The significance of the pansporoblast is not readily apparent.
Numerous species lack a pansporoblast and compete well with those

that do. In some species, depending on environmental conditions, there is alteration of life cycles that involves the presence and absence of a pansporoblast (see chapter on microsporidian development, this monograph). Overstreet and Weidner (1974) hypothesize that the pansporoblast functions to regulate the flow of material from host to parasite. These authors assume that the pansporoblast is a kind of "growth chamber" for the cells contained within. It may have a protective function when developed as a thick envelope.

What function the secretion material has remains unknown. Based on its tubular nature, we may presume that it operates to transport material within the pansporoblast cavity, i.e. between the pansporoblast membrane and the membrane of the microsporidian. Sporoblast appendages function in a similar manner for some microsporidia (Overstreet and Weidner, 1974). The secretion probably plays a role in spore morphogenesis (Liu et al., 1971) and aids lysis of the surrounding host tissue. That it contains substances that influence the physiology of the host organism is another possibility (Maurand and Bouix, 1969).

Typically, the cell wall of the sporoblast has the same structure as in the sporogonial plasmodium. However, the dense coat is more developed and its opacity is greater. In some species, future spore appendages start to appear as expansions of the exosporont membrane covered with the cell coat (Vávra, 1968a). Whether the sporoblast wall may have special premeability characteristics is not known. At a certain point in sporoblast development there appears a highly crenulated periphery. This feature could be an artifact associated with some peculiar physical property of the sporoblast membrane and may be due, in part, to fixation and preparation for electron microscopy (Sprague and Vernick, 1968b). When the sporoblast membrane transforms to a thick wall, the inner plasma membrane of the sporoblast remains as the cytoplasmic membrane of the spore. The thin lucent layer separating the plasmalemma from the exosporont membrane and from the extramembranous coat thickens gradually during endospore development. The outer dense coat (sometimes with an additional layer of bristles and tubules or other structures) changes into the exospore.

III. SPORE STRUCTURE

The spore is the terminal stage of development and its structure is peculiarly adapted to its function of transmitting infectious material to a new host. The microsporidian spore is a unicellular entity in which all specialized organelles originate by cytoplasmic differentiation from the sporoblast. At one time the spore was thought to be similar to myxosporidian and actinomyxidian spores which are truly multicellular structures. Jírovec (1932) was the first to demonstrate convincingly that the entire microsporidian spore is a single cell containing a single nucleus (or a diplokaryon in some species). More recently, ultrastructural investigations on myxosporidian and actinomyxidian spores have demonstrated that their structural and functional principles are completely different from those of microsporidia. Also, the spores of Haplosporidia, although unicellular in nature, are structurally dissimilar to microsporidia (see Vávra, 1974a).

Microsporidian spores observed in the light microscope exhibit a variety of shapes and sizes (Kudo, 1924; Weiser, 1961). However, all the different types of spores are rather similar in having three basic components: the sporoplasm, the extrusion apparatus, and the spore envelope (Fig. 28).

A. SPOROPLASM

Information on the fine structure of the intrasporal sporoplasm is incomplete. All that is known for sure is that the spore has a nucleus (Figs. 28, 29) and that the nucleus (or diplokaryon) is the only one present in the spore; it is identical with the nucleus of the future germ. Some investigators have been unable to distinguish the nucleus within the spore (Sprague and Vernick, 1968b; Stanier, et al., 1968; Scholtyseck and Daneel, 1962; Schubert, 1969a) probably due to technical difficulties specific to their material. In some species, especially after permanganate fixation, the sporoplasm nucleus can be recognized easily (Gassouma and Ellis, 1973). It has a typical fine structure being covered by a double membrane with pores (Weidner, 1972; Liu, 1972). The convex face of the inner nuclear membrane bears numerous particles that can be observed in freeze-etched preparations (Liu and Davies, 1972c).

Apparently, there is no specialized area of the cytoplasm surrounding the spore nucleus that might represent the germ cytoplasm and there is no plasmatic membrane other than the plasmatic membrane associated with the spore wall surrounding such cytoplasm. It has been suggested but not proven that the microsporidian germ represents a minute cell within the spore (Lom and Vávra, 1963a,c). Recently, however, Weidner (1972) and Petri (1974) challenged this view claiming that there is no preformed germ and that the intrasporal sporoplasm is freely dispersed. The extrasporal sporoplasm limiting membrane is acquired during the hatching of the spore and during the passage of the sporoplasm through the filament. This means that most, if not all, of the cytoplasm within the spore belongs to the germ.

The spore content is usually so dense that with the exception of several rough endoplasmic reticulum lamellae, practically no details can be observed in the cytoplasmic part of the spore. In young spores that are more transparent, spirally arranged rows of polyribosomes are sometimes observed (Schubert, 1969a; Canning and Sinden, 1973; Ormieres and Sprague, 1973; Canning and Nicholas, 1974). In some cases, the ribosomal nature of these formations have not been recognized and various names such as "spiral structures" (Schubert, 1969a) or "organized structures of

Figs. 24
 and 25.   Sporoblasts of *Pleistophora debaisieuxi* being cleaved
            from the sporogonial plasmodium. While the sporoblasts
            are still connected by an isthmus, they start to form
            organelles of the future spore. (N, nucleus; BER, rough
            endoplasmic reticulum; SER, smooth endoplasmic reticulum;
            AD, primordium of the future anchoring disc; PF, polar
            filament; PM, pansporoblast membrane enclosing the
            pansporoblast cavity with tubular material inside).
            X 16,000.

Fig. 26.   Sporoblast of *Ameson* (syn. *Nosema) michaelis* being
            cleaved from a moniliform sporogonial plasmodium. In
            this species the formation of spore organelles is very
            advanced. (N, nucleus; PF, polar tube; PL, polaroplast;
            arrow points to the membrane complex of two overlying
            membranes impregnated with dense material and covered by
            microtubules). Courtesy of Dr. E. Weidner. X 40,000.

Fig. 27.   Endoplasmic reticulum-associated ribosomes arranged into
            tightly packed helices in a sporogonial stage of
            Octosporea muscae-domesticae. X 53,000.

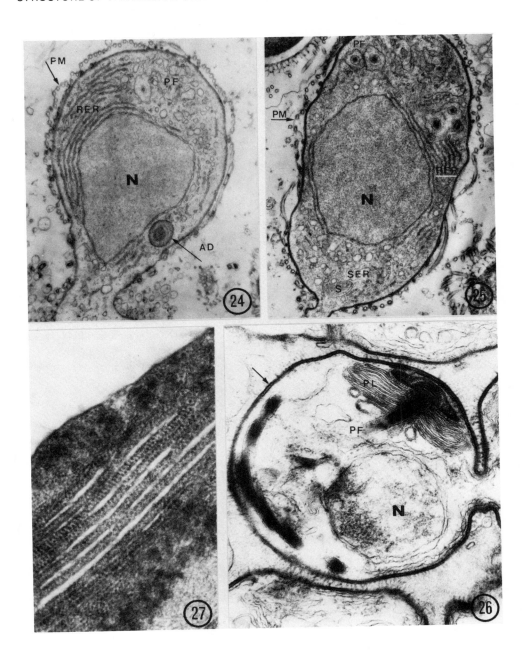

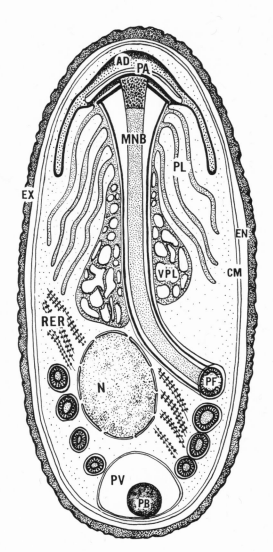

Fig. 28.   Schematic representation of the fine structure of the
           microsporidian spore. AD, anchoring disc of the polar
           tube; CM, cytoplasmic membrane of the spore content; EN,
           endospore; EX, exospore; MNB, manubroid part of the
           filament; N, nucleus; PA, polar aperture; PB, posterior
           body; PF, polar tube; PL, lamellae of the lamellar
           polaroplast; PV, posterior vacuole; RER, endosplasmic
           reticulum densely populated with ribosomes; VPL,
           vesicular part of the polaroplast.

undetermined nature" (Ormieres and Sprague, 1973) were given to them. The report of Vinckier (1973) clearly shows that an aggregation of ribosomes on endoplasmic reticulum lamellae is at the origin of such a polyribosome arrangement (Fig. 30). The arrangement of ribosomes in young spores of *Octosporea muscae-domesticae* closely resembles the arrangement of RNA particles in the chromatoid body of *Entamoeba* (Vávra, unpublished). How long the polyribosome spirals persist during spore maturation and its subsequent dormancy is not known. Freshly discharged sporoplasms have only free monoribosomes as shown by ultrastructural observations (Weidner, 1972) and ultracentrifugation analysis (Ishihara and Hayashi, 1968).

A conspicuous quality of the cytoplasmic content of the dormant spore is its extreme electron density that suddenly diminishes when the spore is activated for extrusion (Lom, 1972). This loss of density, which is also confirmed by the loss of refractivity of the spore in phase-contrast optics, has not been satisfactorily explained (see also Weidner, this monograph). Due to the limited permeability of the spore to electrons, no firm information is available on the Golgi apparatus in the mature spore. It is known that most of the organelles in the sporoblast are elaborated by the Golgi but there is only one report of a structure similar to Golgi in a mature microsporidian spore (Gassouma and Ellis, 1973). Freshly extruded sporoplasms contain no trace of this organelle.

B. EXTRUSION APPARATUS

Most of the microsporidian spore is occupied by its extrusion apparatus that comprises three distinct parts: the polaroplast, the polar tube with associated organelles (anchoring disc, polar aperture), and the posterior vacuole (Fig. 28).

The anterior part of the spore is occupied by the polaroplast which in mature and dormant spore occupies about 25 to 35 percent of the total spore volume (Figs. 28, 29, 37). In the light microscope, the area of the polaroplast resembles a vacuole and has incorrectly been called "anterior vacuole." Because this "anterior vacuole" has the same position in the spore as the sporont cytoplasmic polar capsule in myxosporidian spores, both structures were thought to be identical before they were compared in the electron microscope. The polaroplast has a conspicuous structure of tightly packed electron dense lamellae between which less dense layers are interposed (Huger, 1960; Figs. 37, 38). In perspective, the lamellae are extremely flattened vesicles (or hollow discs) stacked one upon the other and lie perpendicular to the anterior-posterior axis of the spore. The basal part of the polar tube penetrates through the center of the lamellar stack (Fig. 38). The structure of the polaroplast is easily influenced by handling of spores during specimen preparation. In well

Fig. 29.   Total view of the spore of *Pleistophora debaisieuxi*
            still enclosed in the pansporoblast membrane (PM). The
            spore content is generally dense but some organelles can
            be recognized: N, nucleus; CT, cytoplasm; PL, polaro-
            plast with a more dense lamellar and less dense,
            vesicular part; AD, anchoring disc; PF, polar filament.
            Numerous tubuli radiate from the spore exospore into the
            pansporoblast cavity (PC). X 10,000.

Fig. 30.   Part of a macrospore of *Nosemoides* (syn. *Nosema*) *vivieri*
            showing ribosomes arranged in tight rows on the endo-
            plasmic reticulum. PF, polar filament; PV, posterior
            vacuole. X 58,000. Courtesy of Dr. D. Vinckier.

Fig. 31.   Filaments in negatively stained mucus of *Gurleya elegans*
            (S, spore from which the mucus filaments stretch out).
            X 25,000.

Fig. 32.   Endospore layers obtained by alkaline hydrolysis of
            spores of *Nosema plodiae*. Note that the spore case is
            a completely closed structure although thinner at the
            anterior end (arrow). X 13,000.

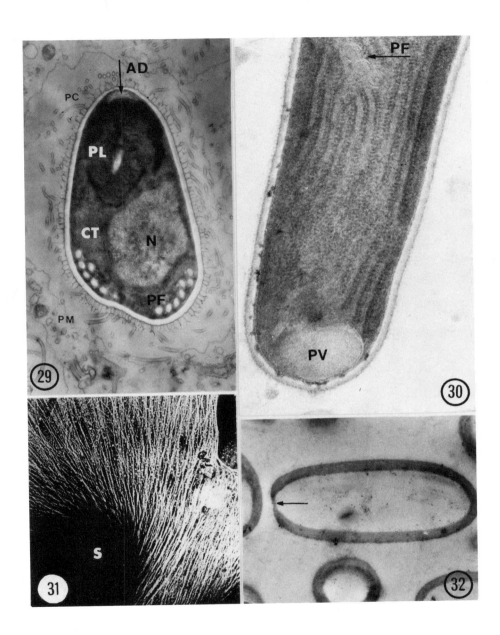

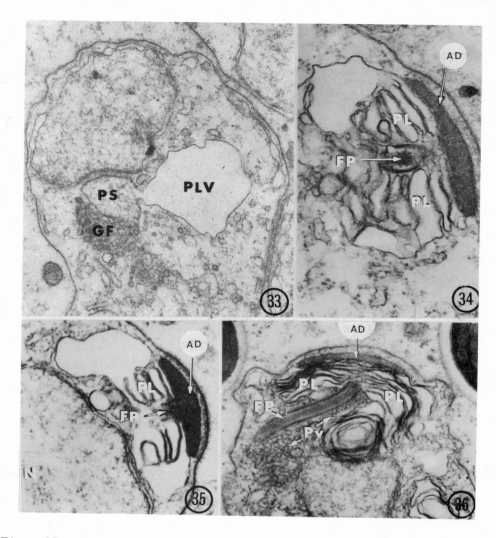

Figs. 33
– 36.   Progressive development of the polaroplast in *Nosemoides*
           (syn. *Nosema) vivieri*. The large vacuole (PLV) is
           situated close to the nucleus (N) and is connected with
           the vesicle of the polar sac (PS).   The Golgi apparatus
           which will form the polar tube (GF) is closely
           associated with the polar sac. By progressive folding
           of the walls of the vacuole the lamellar polaroplast
           (PL) is formed. FP, polar tube; AD, anchoring disc
           of the filament (=transformed polar sac). X 35,000
           (Fig. 33); X 62,000 (Fig. 34); X 60,000 (Fig. 35); X
           42,000 (Fig. 36). From Vinckier (1973).

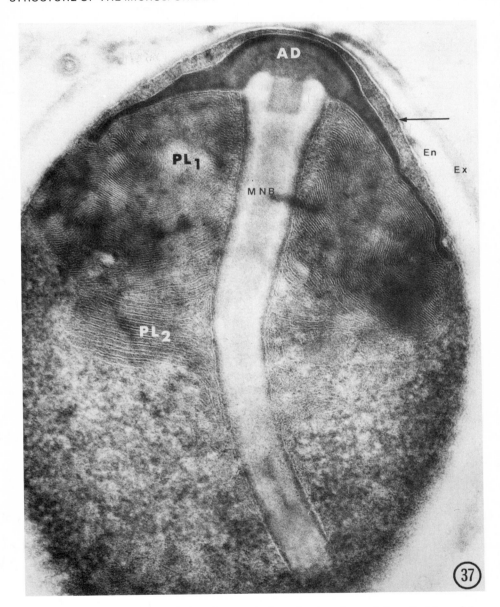

Fig. 37. Spore of *Thelohania contejeani* showing the relationship
between the manubroid part of the polar filament (MNB),
the anchoring disc of the polar filament (AD) and the
polaroplast. The latter organelle has two parts
(PL_1, PL_2) which differ in the arrangement of the
lamellae. X 85,000. Courtesy of Drs. J. Maurand and
A. Vey.

Fig. 38.   Sporoblast of *Ameson* (syn. *Nosema) michaelis* showing
the manubroid part of the polar tube (MNB), the
anchoring disc (AD), polar aperture with septa (PA) and
the polaroplast (PL). Note that the lamellae of the
polaroplast are arranged in bundles of three membranes.
X 189,000. (Enlarged in the inset; X 400,000). From
Weidner (1970).

Figs. 39
  - 41.   *Steinhausia* (syn. *Coccospora) brachynema.* The polar
filament (PF) is ensheated by a honeycomb layer
(arrows) apparently representing a special kind of
polaroplast. X 25,000 (Fig. 39); X 17,000 (Fig. 40;
X 15,000 (Fig. 41). From Richards and Sheffield
(1970).

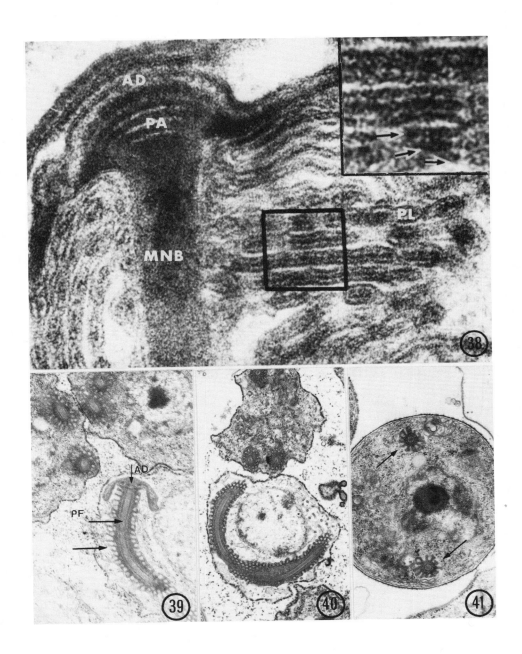

preserved specimens the lamellae are tightly packed and regularly spaced; hypotonic fixatives cause the transparent intralamellar matrix to swell and consequently the regular arrangement of the polaroplast is disturbed. The lamellae also are loosely arranged in sporoblasts and young spores. As will be discussed later, the polaroplast originates by flattening of expanded sacs (probably of Golgi origin) surrounding the anterior part of the polar tube (Liu and Davies, 1972a). These sacs have smooth surfaces and are limited by a double membrane. Alteration of dark and light lamellae occurs because of compression of the sacs and their membranes. Weidner (1970) considers the polaroplast as an accordion-like folding of a single membranous continuum in which each polaroplast lamella is formed by a loop of double membranes.

Although the polaroplast is essentially lamellar, there is some variation in the detailed arrangement of the lamellae at various levels of the polaroplast. The apical part of the organelle typically consists of tightly packed lamellae ("lamellar polaroplast") whereas the posterior region of the organelle is more vesicular ("vesicular polaroplast"). In *Thelohania contejani*, the dark and light layers are of the same thickness in the anterior region whereas every second dark zone in the posterior part is twice as thick as the light zone (Maurand and Vey, 1973; Fig. 37). In *Nosemoides* (syn. *Nosema*) *vivieri*, the lamellar part of the polaroplast follows the inner contour of the spore shell and protrudes in a large arc as far as the middle of the spore. The vesicular part of the polaroplast is situated in the cavity formed by the lamellar part (Vinckier, 1973; Fig. 36). The vesicular part of the polaroplast in several other microsporidian species is represented by long tubules (Stanier *et al.*, 1968; Schubert, 1969a; Lom, 1972). In *Pleistophora simulii*, there is a granulo-vesicular anterior part of the polaroplast and a lamellar posterior part that is continuous with small vesicles of the endoplasmic reticulum ("polaroplaste ergastoplasmique"; see Maurand, 1966). The polaroplast in *Ameson* (syn. *Nosema*) *michaelis* differentiates from two types of saccules into an extremely dense lamellar portion in which the lamellae are very tightly packed (originally it was suspected that this region was a fluid filled cavity; see Sprague *et al.*, 1968) and a posterior region also laminated but much less electron dense (Weidner, 1970). The anterior two-thirds of the polaroplast in *Nosema lophii* is occupied by regularly spaced, alternating dark and light layers whereas the remaining portion consists of less regularly spaced thick, electron dense plates delimited by membrane (Weidner, 1972).

In some microsporidia, the polaroplast is vesicular rather than lamellar. Maurand (1973) found this type of polaroplast in several species of the genus *Gurleya* and *Pyrotheca*. A similar type of polaroplast was observed in some representatives of the genus *Stempellia* (Hazard and Fukuda, 1974; Vávra, unpublished observations).

The polaroplast is closely associated with the manubroid portion of the polar tube during its formation and continued development. Some investigators believe that both organelles are parts of the same membrane system, hence the term "polar filament-polaroplast complex" (Lom and Corliss, 1967). In *Nosemoides* (syn. *Nosema*) *vivieri* the primitive polar sac is connected by a narrow channel with a large transparent vacuole (Vinckier, 1973). Apparently, this vacuole is the primordium of the polaroplast, or at least of its lamellar part. According to Vinckier's photomicrographs (Figs. 33-36) this vacuole positions itself just below the central part of the polar sac thus encircling the basal part of the polar tube. The wall of the vacuole differentiates into lamellar folds protruding deeply into the interior cavity of the vacuole. These folds subsequently increase in number and length. The whole vacuole, which has transformed into lamellar leaflets, elongates and extends deeply into the spore. The vesicular part of the polaroplast in *Nosemoides* seems to originate from Golgi vesicles that were left behind during the formation of the polar filament (Vinckier, 1973). The membranes of the polaroplast are smooth and both the Golgi apparatus and the smooth endoplasmic reticulum may contribute to their origin. Possibly, the polaroplast is a specialized derivative of the endoplasmic reticulum (Lom and Corliss, 1967; Sprague and Vernick, 1967; 1968b Sprague *et al.*, 1968; Weidner, 1970) or it is simply a reoriented package of remnants of the Golgi membrane complex (Szollosi, 1971, Canning and Sinden, 1973). Sprague and Vernick (1969a) hypothesize that the outer portion of the polaroplast is derived from the cisternae of the Golgi and that the inner zone is derived from vesicles of the Golgi. The intimate relationship of the large primoridial vacuole with the polar sac, which itself is a Golgi product, and the close association of the vesicular part of the polaroplast with Golgi vesicles left over after the polar filament formation, seem to support the concept of the polaroplast being entirely derived from the Golgi apparatus.

Each polaroplast lamella consists of a pair of unit-like membranes (Weidner, 1970). Whether the polaroplast membranes are really identical with unit membranes is, however, questionable. Polaroplast membranes are consistently well preserved by embedding with glycolmethacrylate, a poor preservative of unit membranes (Barker, 1975) and, during freeze etching, the polaroplast membranes do not split in the manner typical of unit membranes (Liu and Davies, 1972a). As already mentioned, each lamella consists of a loop of two closely apposed double membranes. When compressed during later stages of spore differentiation, a pattern of regularly alternating dark and light zones occur. The periodicity of dark and light lines is different in various species (Lom and Corliss, 1967; Huger, 1960; Schubert, 1969a; Stanier *et al.*, 1968). A conspicuous, but not yet fully understood feature of the polaroplast membranes is that under some conditions (partial activation of the spore?) the

lamellae are arranged in bundles of three dense membranes (Fig. 38).
This arrangement is also evident in freeze-etched spores (Fig. 8
in Liu and Davies, 1972a), indicating that the relatively simple
arrangement of polaroplast lamellae in young spores is transformed
during spore maturation.

The polaroplast is capable of changing its volume, most
probably by swelling (Lom and Vávra, 1963b). The change in the
polaroplast volume is evidenced by the increase in the distance
between individual lamellae. Swelled polaroplasts possess lamellae
arranged as irregular, transparent vacuoles encircled by electron
dense borders (Vávra, 1968a). Microcinematographic recordings of
the spore extrusion process reveal that the swelling of the
polaroplast is the first event in spore extrusion. The swelling
polaroplast increases intrasporal pressure. This phenomenon can
be visualized in spores of *Pleistophora hyphessobryconis* wherein
the swelled polaroplast often bulges the spore envelope. The
increased pressure forces the basal part of the filament out of
the spore (Lom and Vávra, 1963b). The fate of the polaroplast
lamellae during the extrusion is not clear. Either they are
pushed with the spore content into the lumen of the everting
polar tube or, as suggested by Weidner (1972), they are incorporated
into the polar tube and contribute to its elongation. When extruding spores are observed under the light microscope, the swelling
of the polaroplast appears to proceed from the anterior tip of
the spore back to the posterior vacuole. The structural relationship of the polaroplast to the posterior vacuole is however not
well understood. According to Sprague and Vernick (1969a), the
polaroplast and the posterior vacuole are parts of the same membrane system.

There are some microsporidia in which a polaroplast has not been
observed. Curiously, all species lacking polaroplast have spores
of subspherical shape. In *Steinhausia* (syn. *Coccospora)*, a honeycomb layer of Golgi origin surrounds the entire length of the
polar filament (Richards and Sheffield, 1970; Figs. 39-41). The
alveolar character of this layer and its close association with
the filament seems to indicate that the honeycomb layer is a
special kind of polaroplast and perhaps its primitive type.
Similar structure ensheaths the polar filament in *Chytridiopsis*
(Sprague, Ormieres and Manier, 1972). *Steinhausia* is able to
extrude its filament (Fig. 42) but it is not known whether other
species lacking a typical polaroplast are capable of the same. As
discussed in the section on polar tube structure, the outermost
layer of the polar tube may be a giant polaroplast lamella
ensheathing the length of the filament.

C. *POLAR TUBE (POLAR FILAMENT)*

The most conspicuous but also the most enigmatic organelle of the
microsporidian spore is the polar tube. Typically, the filament is

a thread-like structure attached to the inner side of the apical portion of the spore shell by an umbrella-shaped bulge called the anchoring disc (See Glossary; Figs. 37, 38). The filament descends from the attachment site along the longitudinal axis of the spore. The straight basal part of the filament (manubroid) is thicker than its other parts (Fig. 37). In some microsporidia (family Mrazekidae), the basal part is thickened into a rod-like structure, the manubrium. The filament descends in a straight line for some distance and makes a sharp turn to form coils arranged in one or several layers at the posterior end of the spore. The number of coils is variable in different species; less variation occurs within the same species. As few as three to four coils are present in the spores of *Encephalitozoon cuniculi* (Petri and Schiodt, 1966) whereas up to 44 coils may occur in spores of *Nosema apis* (Scholtyseck and Danneel, 1962). Generally, most microsporidians have about 11 coils. Nine out of 15 species examined by Milner (1972) possessed 11-15 coils. The number of coils and their angle of tilt to the long axis of the spore can be used as taxonomic criteria (Burges *et al.*, 1974). Filament thickness measured under the light microscope is about 0.1 µm. The electron microscope, however, shows that the basal part of the filament is thicker and that the filament is tapered slightly toward the distal end. Some variation in the thickness of the filament occurs among different species.

The structure of the polar tube and the mode of its eversion from the spore has been of prime concern since Stempell's (1909) recognition that the exit of the germ from the spore is closely associated with filament eversion. Stempell believed that the polar filament is an evaginable hollow tube through which the germ flows out. Several subsequent studies corroborated this idea; others did not, indicating that the filament is not a tube but a solid structure (for details see Lom and Vávra, 1963b).

Krieg (1955) observed whole extruded filaments and concluded that they are solid structures. Huger (1960) was the first to use ultrathin sections of well preserved spores to reveal filament structure "*in situ*" and to demonstrate that the filament is an organelle of rather complicated structure. This fact is now well recognized.

All studies performed with the aid of the electron microscope have shown that (1) the polar tube consists of several concentric layers, (2) the proportion of individual layers varies somewhat along the longitudinal axis, and (3) the layering is very similar in all microsporidian polar filaments (Vávra *et al.*, 1966). High resolution electron micrographs reveal the presence of 11 different layers in cross-sectioned filament (Schubert, 1969a; Figs. 55, 56). The filament is limited from the outside by a thin (3-4nm) membranous layer (A) lying next to a transparent space (B) of 2-2.5 nm. Another very electron dense layer (C)

Fig. 42.   Spore of *Steinhausia* (syn. *Coccospora*) *brachynema* with
           its filament extruded. X 21,700.   From Richards and
           Sheffield (1970).

Fig. 43.   Young spore of *Duboscquia sp.* from *Diacyclops*.   The
           polar filament (PF) has different structure in different
           coils.   GF, rest of the Golgi apparatus after the polar
           tube formation; N, nucleus; RER, endoplasmic reticulum
           with ribosomes; PV, membranes at the site of the future
           posterior vacuole. X 41,000.

Fig. 44.   Spore of *Nosema algerae* after embedding into glycol-
           methacrylate.   The outer filament membrane of the polar
           filament (PF) is well preserved which speaks against its
           unit membrane nature.   Spirals of polyribosomes are
           shown at arrow.   EN, endospore layer of the spore wall;
           EX, exospore layer. X 30,000.   Courtesy of Drs. E. U.
           Canning and R. E. Sinden.

Fig. 45.   Polar tube of *Stempellia sp.* which has been expelled
           from the spore without eversion.   The three principal
           strata of the filament are clearly shown in longitudinal
           and in cross section(inset).   OFT, outer filament tube;
           IFT, inner filament tube; PFL, polar filament lumen.
           X 130,000.

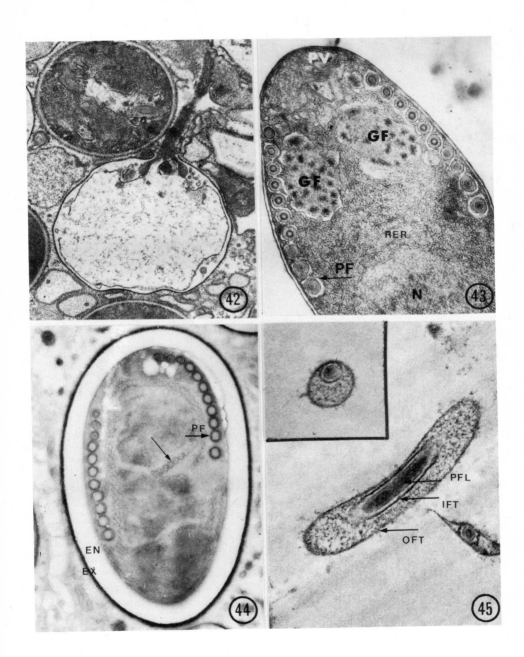

then follows and is 4-5 nm thick. The next transparent interspace (D) has a thickness of 2-2.5 nm. Another ring (E) of medium electron density occurs and is about 2.5-3.5 nm thick. This one is adjacent to a large electron transparent layer (F) of 6-10 nm. Next to the center are two closely adjacent dense rings (G and I), each 3-4 nm thick. They are separated by a more transparent layer H of 1-2 nm. The inner ring I makes the outer limit of a central, less dense field (K) of 45-55 nm, the center of which sometimes contains a more dense spot (L) not defined by Schubert. Similar layers, although of slightly different proportions, can be distinguished in filaments of *Pleistophora debaisieuxi* and the manubrium of *Bacillidium cyclopis* (Vávra, unpublished). In low resolution electron micrographs only a few of the above mentioned layers can be resolved and in cross section the filament usually appears as a double dense ring (layers one and two of the internal dense zone of Vávra *et al.*, (1966) which are probably identical to the ensemble of rings C.D.E and G.H.I, respectively) surrounded by a lighter area ("couche externe", presumably identical to rings A and B described by Schubert). Occasionally, a high density spot appears in the center of the filament ("organite axiale" of Vávra *et al.*, 1966, that probably corresponds to layer L). The proportion of individual layers is not the same along the length of the filament. The relatively transparent layers between layer C and the double dense ring G and I are much thicker in the manubroid part of the filament; they reach extreme thickness in the manubrium. In other respects, the manubrium has essentially the same ultrastructure as a typical polar filament (Vávra *et al.*, 1966; Goetz, 1974).

The polar filament in a few microsporidia is atypical. The outer filament envelope in the genus *Steinhausia* (syn. *Coccospora)* is represented by a honeycomb layer (Richards and Sheffield, 1970; Figs. 39-41 and 72 I). A similar layer is present around the filament of *Chytridiopsis* (Sprague *et al.*, 1972). These unusual polar filaments may be quite similar to normal filaments if their outermost layer is homologous to the polaroplast membrane. In spores of the genus *Metchnikovella*, there is no polar filament but rather a short cylindrical structure (also called manubrium; Fig 72 K) presumably homologous to the polar filament. Electron microscope studies show that the manubrium of Metchnikovellidae also has a composite structure of several concentric rings (Hildebrand and Vivier, 1971; Vivier and Schrevel, 1973).

Interpretation of the polar filament fine structure is extremely difficult because of the smallness of its internal structures. The polar filament becomes extensively reorganized during spore maturation; also it is somewhat different before and after eversion (Lom, 1972, Weidner, 1972). It is generally believed that the polar filament is a composite structure of two tubes

one within the other (Lom, 1972; Weidner, 1970; Walker and
Hinsch, 1972; Sprague and Vernick, 1974) that appear membranous
in cross-section. The outer filament tube in mature spores is
probably identical with the layers C,D,E of Schubert (1969a)
whereas the inner filament tube seems to be identical to the
layers G,H,I. The outer filament tube is not to be confused with
a membrane that is later added to the polar tube from the cytoplasmic side ("filament cytoplasmic sheath"). This sheath is
probably identical to layer A described by Schubert (Figs. 45-49)
and its significance will be discussed later.

In osmium fixed specimens, the outer filament tube appears as
a single membrane (Vávra, 1965) whereas glutaraldehyde fixation
of newly formed filament reveals it to be composed of two unit-
like membranes (Weidner, 1970; Vinckier, 1973; Canning and
Nicholas, 1974; see Figs. 45-49). The outer filament tube does
remain preserved after embedding with glycolmethacrylate (Fig.
44), a fact that speaks against its unit membrane nature (Canning
and Sinden, 1973). The bimembranous feature of the outer
filament tube is lost during filament maturation and the mature
filament seems to be limited by a single unit-like membrane
(Vinckier, 1973; probably layers C,D,E of Schubert, 1969a).

The inner filament tube is usually eccentrically located within
the outer tube (Walker and Hinsch, 1972); this arrangement is
thought to be occasioned by the resiliency of the microtubules
presumably present within the inner filament tube (Sprague and
Vernick, 1974). Interpretation of the inner tube is an extremely
controversial issue of the polar tube fine structure. Most of
the controversy is due to the fact that the inner filament tube
often appears discontinuous in cross sections. This phenomenon is
particularly apparent in young filaments or in filaments of activated spores. Consequently, some authors have interpreted the
inner filament tube as a fibrillous (or microtubullar) cylinder
composed of nine subunits (Scholtyseck and Daneel, 1962) each consisting of a fibrillar doublet (Huger, 1960). These investigators compared the fine structure of the filament to that of a
ciliary axoneme and concluded that the filament could not evert.
Liu and Davies (1972b, 1973b) observed 12 microcylinders in a
freeze-etched filament of *Thelohania bracteata*. Similar configuration of the polar filament interior was seen in ultrathin
sections by Vivares and Tuzet (1974). Sprague and Vernick
(1968b) as well as Canning and Nicholas (1974) have observed a
ring with 18 subunits at the site of the inner filament tube.

The possibility that the inner tube is fibrillar was first
mentioned by Vávra (1965) who noticed that spirally twisted
fibres are arranged in a sheath-like manner within the polar
filament. This observation has since been confirmed in a number
of species (Vávra, unpublished; Sprague and Vernick, 1971; Akao,
1969). Fibrillar structures were also seen by Vavra
(1972b) in negatively stained extruded filaments. Lom

Figs. 46
- 48.   Initial stage of the polar filament formation in
          Pleistophora debaisieuxi. After osmium fixation, the
          canal of the young filament is widely distended   (com-
          pare with Fig. 49). The principal strata of the filament
          (OFT, outer filament tube; IFT, inner filament tube;
          PFL, polar filament lumen) are clearly shown. In longi-
          tudinal or tangential sections the IFT reveals a
          fibrillar substructure (arrow). X 55,000 (Fig. 46);
          X 40,000 (Fig. 47); X 90,000 (Fig. 48).

Fig. 49. The initial stage of polar tube formation in *Nosemoides*
          (syn. *Nosema*) *vivieri* showing coalexcence of Golgi
          vesicles with opaque content into the double tube of the
          polar filament. The lumen of the tube is occupied by
          the dark material. This is a typical aspect of the young
          polar tube when glutaraldehyde is used as primary fixa-
          tive. X 50,000. Courtesy of Dr. D. Vinckier.

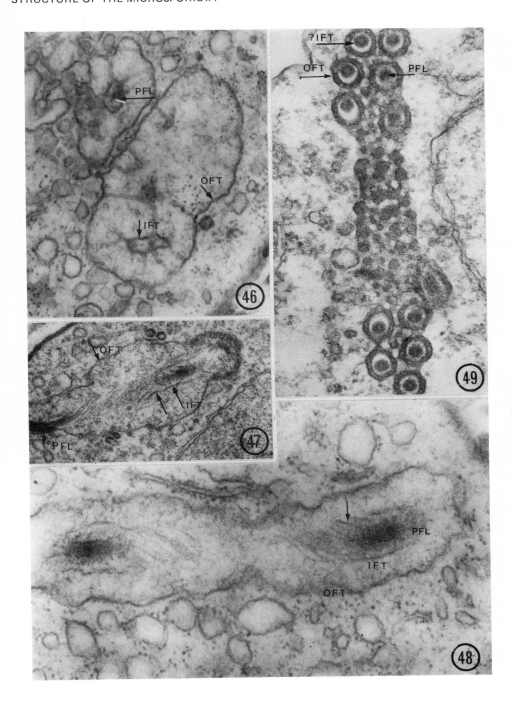

Figs. 50
and 51.   Cross section of the polar filament in *Nosema sp.* from
           Hippocampus erectus. Resting spore (Fig. 50), spore
           activated for extrusion (Fig. 51). Both figures are
           reproduced in the same magnification in order to demon-
           strate the changes in the polar tube during activation.
           There is an increase of the volume of the layer between
           the polar filament cytoplasmic sheath (FCS) and the polar
           outer filament tube (OFT). The volume of the polar
           filament itself (=from the layer OFT inwards) is also
           reduced. X 182,000. From Lom (1972).

Fig. 52.   Cross sections of the polar tube of *Glugea daphniae*
           stained with Thiery's periodic acid-thiosemicarbazide-
           silver proteinate method. Two layers of the tube are
           positive: the outer one (1) very weakly, the inner one
           (2) staining heavily. X 200,000.

Fig. 53.   Cross section of the polar tube in a young spore of
           Caudospora stained with Thiery's reaction for 1, 2 glycol
           groups. The glycoprotein substance is loosely scattered
           in some coils whereas in others it is concentrated into
           a tube. This clearly demonstrates that adjacent coils
           have different structure during development. X 80,000.

Fig. 54.   Cross section of the polar tube of *Glugea daphniae* at
           the level of the entrance of the filament into the anchor-
           ing disc (Thiery's reaction). The two positive layers of
           the filament (1, 2) are surrounded by positively stained
           material of the disc. X 74,000.

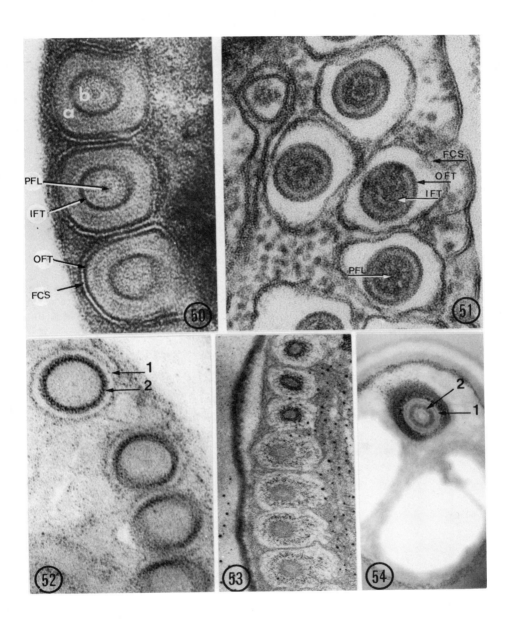

Fig. 55. Cross section of the polar tube in *Heterosporis finki*
          (probably synonym of *Pleistophora hyphessobryconis*).
          Eleven different layers in the filament can be recog-
          nized. From Schubert (1969 a). X 228,000.

Fig. 56. Schematic drawing of the polar tube layers shown in
          Fig. 55.

Fig. 57. Half-everted polar tube of *Nosema whitei*, negatively
          stained. The tube has six layers and the end of the tube
          where the layers are turning upon themselves is indicated
          by arrows. X 146,000.

Fig. 58. Fully everted polar tube of *Nosema whitei* stained
          negatively after a short digestion by trypsin. The
          meshwork of very fine fibres is clearly revealed. X
          292,000.

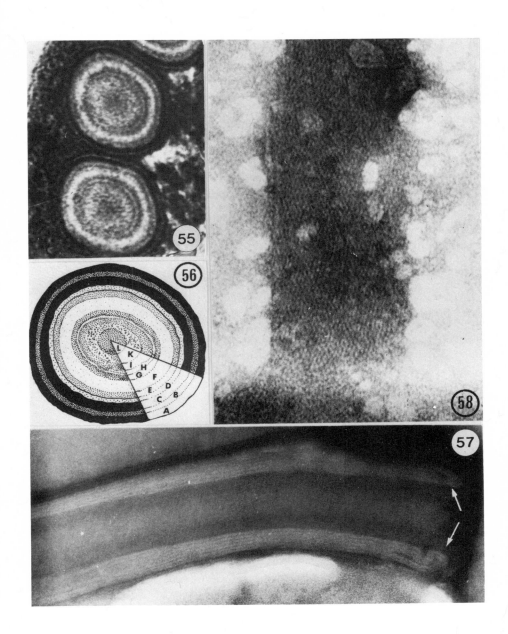

and Corliss (1967) on the other hand, believe that spirally wound
fibres in the filament interior are an artifact caused by fixation-
induced shrinkage of membranous structures. The absence of any
fibrillar structures inside the discharged and negatively stained
polar tube (Lom; 1972) seems to corroborate the membranous nature
of the filament. Membranous laminae (up to five pairs) have
been viewed in filaments extruded from spores with hydrogen
peroxide (Lom and Vávra, 1963a,c).

The internal filament tube delimits the internal lumen of the
filament. This lumen is not clearly defined as a cavity because
it contains electron dense material (Figs. 45-49); the filament
has been interpreted as a solid structure (Huger, 1960;
Scholtyseck, and Daneel, 1962). However, the presence of
material within the lumen of the filament does not necessarily
preclude a hollow tube. Functional characteristics of the
filament as well as electron microscopic observations of passage
of the spore content through the filament clearly indicates the
tubular nature of the filament. This fragmentary consideration
of the polar filament reveals that an understanding of its
structure is certainly incomplete. Though it has been demonstrated that the filament is essentially a double tube, what is
not known is the structure of the inner tube and of the material
lying between both the outer and inner filament tubes.

The structure of the inner filament membrane sometimes is
fibrillar or tubular or membranous. Observations of extruded,
negatively stained filaments of *Nosema whitei* (Vávra, 1972b and
unpublished results) provide some understanding of its architecture. Negatively stained extruded polar filament appears
membranous (Fig. 57); however, mild proteolytic digestion before
staining, renders a meshwork of very fine fibres (ca. 1.5 nm thick)
as the main component of the filament (Fig. 58). The fibres make
a tight coil with a pitch of about 25 degrees and optical
diffraction analysis (Vávra, unpublished) suggests that their
course is slightly undulatory. Apparently, at least one of the
filament layers is made from tightly wound fibres that probably
are cemented together into a membranous structure. The resistance
of fibres to proteolytic digestion suggests that they may contain
substances other than protein.

The polar filament contains material that reacts positively
with periodic acid - Schiff reagent (Sprague and Vernick, 1968b)
which can be observed in the electron microscope (Vávra, 1971;
1972; Figs. 52-54). There are two layers that presumably contain
carbohydrate. One of these is either identical to or lies
very closely to the double ring G-I of Schubert (1969a), the
other being identical to Schubert's layer E (see Fig. 52).

Very little is known about the core substance of the filament.
Weidner (1972) believes that the filament matrix is glycoprotein
and that this substance, after extrusion, envelopes the polar
filament as a sheath. This sheath does not stain with silver

methenamine although it is sensitive to trypsin and binds ferritin-conjugated concavalin A. It is continuous with the outer envelope of the vesicle in which the sporoplasm occurs after extrusion. Weidner speculates that the core material in the lumen of the filament contributes to its structural rigidity during extrusion. He also believes that the core component is the vehicle by which the surrounding membrane of the filament passes in convey or belt fashion out of the spore (see also Weidner, this monograph). Another hypothetical function of the filament matrix may be to lubricate the filament interior during the eversion process. One unresolved question is which filament layers belong to the eversible portion of the organelle and which ones represent the non-evaginable envelope. Schubert (1969a) does not think that his described layer A is evaginable; Lom (1972) has demonstrated that the transparent layer B denoted by Schubert becomes much larger in spores ready for extrusion (Figs. 50, 51). I have compared the dimensions of some of the polar filament layers in Lom's (1972) Figs. 8 and 9 (see Figs. 50 and 51, this chapter) showing dormant and activated spores, respectively. Analysis of these pictures clearly reveals the total volume of the polar filament, including the filament cytoplasmic sheath that remains practically unchanged in activated spores and the entire polar filament that lies below the cytoplasmic membrane and is greatly compressed during spore activation. This situation is especially apparent in the inner filament membrane which appears wrinkled in activated spores. The transparent layer between the cytoplasmic membrane and the polar filament seems to be greatly enlarged in activated spores and the dark center of the filament also is slightly increased in size.

It is apparent from the above described changes that the cytoplasmic membrane probably represents the nonevaginable sheath mentioned by Schubert (1969a). The light zone immediately below this membrane is capable of considerable swelling during spore activation. Possibly, the cytoplasmic membrane around the filament is homologous to the polaroplast membrane and transparent layer B beneath belongs to the polaroplast swelling material. If this hypothesis is true, the swelling of the polaroplast is not limited to the polaroplast itself but progresses further along the whole length of the filament. The presence of a swelled area around the polar filament in activated spores might reduce filament friction during its uncoiling from the spore. The alveolar layer surrounding the polar filaments in *Steinhausia* (syn. *Coccospora*) (Richards and Sheffield, 1970) and in *Chytridiopsis* (Sprague *et al.*, 1972) is positioned exactly as is the filament cytoplasmic sheath in other microsporidia. Apparently the alveolar layer, at least in *Steinhausia*, has the same function as the polaroplast, which in its typical form is absent in both species. This fact may support the idea that the polaroplast and the filament cytoplasmic sheath are homologous.

Just how the polar filament is terminated is not known
Whether it is open or closed at the distal end is in question and
no firm data are available to resolve the problem. An intriguing
observation has recently been made by Vinckier (1973) who observed that the posterior vacuole in *Nosema vivieri* has some fine
structure traits very similar to that of the polar tube. Both
structures originate as derivatives of the Golgi apparatus.

Various authors have traced the origin of the polar filament
to one or two of the following cell structures: (1) the Golgi
zone, (2) the endoplasmic reticulum, (3) the nucleus, and (4)
the ribosomes. Vávra (1965) first noticed that the filament is
formed inside a large and irregular vesicular canal that originates
by coalescence of vesicles derived from the Golgi apparatus (Figs.
46-48). Several authors have endorsed this view (Jensen and Wellings,
1970; Liu and Davies, 1972b; Szollosi, 1971; Walker and Hinsch,
1972; Devauchelle, Vinckier and Prensier, 1970; Vinckier, 1973).
Other investigators, however, are of the opinion that the polar
filament originates from the endoplasmic reticulum (Lom and
Corliss, 1967). Weidner (1970) and Youssef and Hammond (1971) seek
the origin of the polar filament in both the Golgi (which
supposedly gives rise to the core of the filament) and in the
endoplasmic reticulum (which supposedly forms the outer envelope).
Jensen and Wellings (1972) believe that the posterior part of the
polar filament develops from the Golgi complex whereas the
anterior part is formed from the electron dense material located
in the perinuclear cisterna and in the agranular endoplasmic
reticulum. Some authors suppose that ribosomes are involved in
the formation of the polar tube. Canning and Sinden (1973) concluded
that the filament forming material in *Nosema algerae* may have
arisen by secretion from Golgi vesicles or that it may have been
produced by closely packed layers of polyribosomes. Milner (1972)
also believes that the filament forming material in *Nosema whitei*
is of ribosomal origin. According to Sprague and Vernick (1968b),
the filament is of nuclear origin and develops by the transformation of the isthmus connecting two daughter nuclei after division.
From other work, the same authors modified their hypothesis by
assuming that both the nuclear isthmus and Golgi are involved in
polar filament formation (Sprague and Vernick, 1969; 1974).

Although there is no unanimous agreement concerning the origin
of the polar filament, more recent data support the idea that it
originates from the Golgi zone. The observations of Vinckier
(1973) furnish clear evidence for such a beginning. Apparently,
vesicles of the Golgi apparatus coalesce to form a tube limited
by two unit membranes separated by opaque material (Fig. 49).
The center of the tube is filled with dense material probably
derived from dense Golgi vesicles. This mode of polar filament
formation is in agreement with the observations of Jensen and
Wellings (1972) and of Walker and Hinsch (1972). The latter
authors concluded that the similar positive reaction for polysaccharides exhibited by the Golgi and the membranes of the polar

filament provides good evidence for the polar tube originating from the Golgi.

The filament is built from the basal end. First, the bulbous part representing the future polar sac appears in the vicinity of the nuculeus. Later the coils are synthesized and their formation progresses down from the basal part toward the terminal portion. The core of the filament and its envelope appear first; later additional layers are formed inside of the filament. The internal differentiation of the filament again progresses down from the basal portion. Thus, several adjacent coils may have slightly different structure (Figs. 43, 53). Finally, the filament cytoplasmic sheath is added.

The filament is considerably elastic. During extrusion. it can be as much as three times longer than when coiled inside the spore. This extreme increase in length was thought to be due to the contribution of the polaroplast membranes to the filament during extrusion (Weidner, 1972). This idea, however, does not explain why in the Mrazekidae, which have a well developed polaroplast, there is no significant increase in the length of the manubrium and of the filament during extrusion. For this reason, it appears that the increase in filament length is due simply to its elasticity. Microcinematographic recordings of extruding filaments show them to retract within a few seconds after extrusion is completed (Lom and Vávra, 1963b). The filament is also elastic transversally. When the germ traverses the filament, its diameter increases two-fold at the site of germ passage (Lom and Vavra, 1963b; Weidner, 1972). A layer(s) of twisted fibres may be requisite to this two dimensional elasticity.

The basal end of the filament is terminated by a specialized structure that attaches the filament to the inner side of the apical part of the spore shell. This structure appears in the light microscope as a granule ("polar cap") stainable with basic dyes and reactive with periodic acid-Schiff reagent (Vávra, 1959; Huger, 1960; Fig. 67). Electron microscopic observations demonstrate that this structure originates prior to polar filament formation and appears as a large vesicle ("polar sac") limited by a unit membrane. The vesicle is filled by finely granulated matter of medium density. The polar sac is originally situated in close proximity to the sporoblast nucleus between the nuclear membrane and the Golgi zone. Vinckier (1973) demonstrated that the polar sac is partially embedded in a depression of the nuclear membrane and is separated from the membrane by a thin layer of material of medium density (Fig. 33). The position of the polar sac during its formation have led some authors to believe that it represents transformed nuclear material (Jensen and Wellings, 1972; Vinckier, 1973). However, Vávra (1968a) interpreted the polar sac as an integral part of the filament and not as a special organelle to which the polar filament is ooupled (Jensen and Wellings, 1972). The close perinuclear position of the polar sac is changed during

Figs. 59
  - 61.   Formation of the polar sac (Future anchoring disc) in
             Nosemoides (syn. *Nosema) vivieri.* The polar sac is
             closely associated with the nucleus (N) and is situated
             in the invagination of the latter. The Golgi apparatus
             which forms the polar tube (GF) is situated in the im-
             mediate vicinity of the polar sac (PS). Fig. 61 dem-
             onstrates the insertion of the polar tube into the polar
             sac. The outer filament tube (OFT) is continuous with
             the membrane around the sac whereas the inner filament
             tube IFT) delimiting the polar filament lumen (PFL)
             penetrates deeply into the sac. X 36,000 (Fig. 59);
             X 50,000 (Fig. 60); X 76,000 (Fig. 61). From Vinckier
             (1973).

Fig. 62.   Polar sac of *Pleistophora debaisieuxi* in the phase of
             transformation into the anchoring disc. The dark,
             collarlike structure HI is the point around which the
             polar filament tursn during filament eversion. The
             three principal strata of the filament are also shown.
             X 56,000.

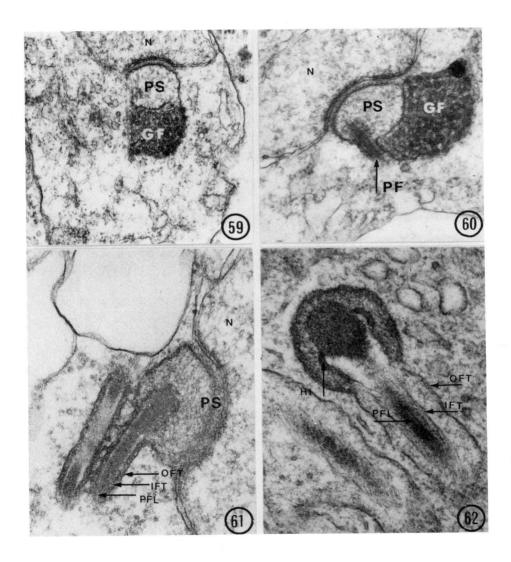

Fig. 63. Partially differentiated anchoring disc in *Stempellia sp.*
from *Megacyclops*. The same structures as in Fig. 62
are present although in different proportions. SCW,
sporoblast cell wall. X 72,000.

Fig. 64. Fully differentiated anchoring disc in *Caudospora*
simulii stained by Thiery's method. The material of the
disc itself (including the "hinges" HI) is PAS positive.
The polar aperture and septa (PA), the manubroid part of
the filament (MNB) stain very weekly. X 140,000.

Fig. 65. Total view of the anchoring disc in *Glugea daphniae*
stained by Thiery's method. Note the heavy silver deposit
in the anchoring disc in which a less dense polar aperture layer is present. The polar filament (PF) is
weakly positive. Other spore components such as the
polaroplast (PL), spore cytoplasm, exospore (Ex) and
endospore (En) are negative. X 10,000.

Fig. 66. Extruding spore of *Stempellia sp.* stained by Thiery's
method. The apical portion of the anchoring disc is
ruptured by the filament and forms a sheath on the
surface of the proximal portion of the polar tube (arrow).
The distal portion of the anchoring disc holds the polar
tube attached in the spore case. Uneverted part of the
filament can be seen (PF). X 50,000. From Vávra (1972a).

Fig. 67. Light micrograph of *Nosema lepiduri* spores stained with
the PAS method. The polar cap is revealed in each spore.
X 3,500.

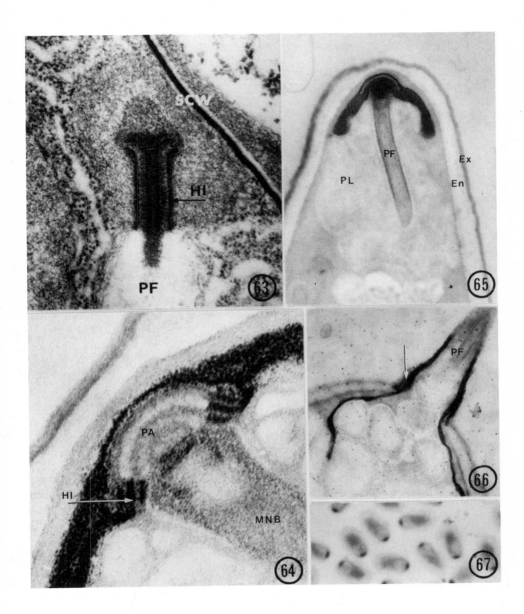

the time when the coils of the polar tube are formed. At that time, the polar sac migrates toward the anterior pole of the spore where it flattens into a mushroom shaped anchoring disc that fits into the inner contour of the spore apex.

The polar sac is, in the beginning, a circular structure. The outer filament membrane is continuous with the polar sac whereas the inner structures of the filament penetrate into the polar sac for a short distance. Later, a dark structure shaped like a collar develops between the polar sac and the polar filament. This structure functions as a hinge during filament eversion (Lom, 1972). A dense granular material caps the top of the polar filament inserted into the polar sac (Fig. 62). When the polar sac is flattened into its final shape, the point of insertion of the polar filament ("polar aperture") becomes covered by a series of alternate dark and light lamellae ("septa of the polar aperture"). This arrangement characterizes the fully formed anchoring disc (Fig. 64). The anchoring disc reacts positively with periodic acid-Schiff and Thiery's periodic acid-thiosemi-carbazide reagents (Vávra, 1972a). However, the electron micro-scope shows that there are several layers in the anchoring disc that vary in their degree of reactivity. There is a thin layer covering the top of the anchoring disc that reacts very strongly. Beneath this layer is a negative one and a thin layer of little reactivity followed again by a thick layer of rather strong reactivity. This last layer represents the bulk of the anchoring disc and includes the thin distal portion of the disc (Figs. 64, 65).

The significance of these different layers in the anchoring disc is not known but presumably the anchoring disc me-diates the stimuli for extrusion. Observations of extruded spores reveal that the filament evaginates while rupturing the apical part of the anchoring disc. The medium portion of the disc is then evaginated with the filament and forms a thin sheath upon the proximal part of the evaginated filament. The thin rim of the disc remains within the spore and anchors the filament. Seemingly, no structure attaches this disc to the innermost membrane of the spore shell. Nevertheless, the distal part of the anchoring disc remains in place and securely holds the filament during the extrusion (Vávra, 1972a). The "hinge" in the anchoring disc turns 90° during extrusion and consequently, provides firm evidence that the filament is turned upside down during eversion (Lom, 1972).

D. POSTERIOR VACUOLE

Near the posterior pole of the mature spore there is an area that appears in light optics as an empty vacuole. This so-called posterior vacuole differs in shape and size among various species. It is absent in some species (Vinckier et al., 1970, Canning and Sinden, 1973) and in others it is represented only by a slit-like zone at the posterior pole of the spore. Typically, the vacuole is oval and slightly flattened in the anterior region and is one-fourth to one-third the spore length. Exceptionally, as in *Pleistophora hyphessobryconis*, the posterior vacuole fills about half of the spore volume.

The area occupied by the posterior vacuole is usually not preserved very well during fixation and embedding for electron microscopy. Although no conspicuous changes occur in the vacuole during fixation and initial dehydration steps, some distortion occurs during final dehydration and resin infiltration. The site of the vacuole appears as an empty space with a crenulated outline. Fortunately, there are always some spores that escape this change and our knowledge of the fine structure of the vacuole is based on them. Recent observations confirm that the vacuole is limited by a membrane (Weidner, 1972; Lom, 1972), though some investigators have been unable to resolve any membrane around the vacuole probably due to poor preservation of their material. Ishihara (1968) reported a single membrane around the vacuole but freeze-etched preparations reveal that it is limited by a double membrane. This double membrane has a relatively smooth outer and inner surface. The particles associated with the membrane are coarser than the particles of the nuclear membrane and are thought to be involved in active water transport (Liu and Davies, 1972c).

The content of the posterior vacuole is either flocculent (Weidner, 1972) or irregularly granular (Lom and Corliss, 1967). Often there is a dense "inclusion body" or "posterior body" ("posterosome") surrounded by a fine membrane (Sprague *et al.*, 1968; de Puytorac and Tourret, 1963; Maurand and Vey, 1973; Weiser and Zizka, 1974). The inclusion appears in the maturing sporoblast at the time when the filament is formed as one or several large granules filled with a very dense material similar to that contained in the Golgi cisternae (Walker and Hinsch, 1972). The posterior body has been interpreted as part of the filament material within a Golgi has been interpreted as part of the filament material concentrated or synthesized by the Golgi (Maurand and Vey, 1973). The inclusion body seems identical to the large structure in *Thelohania moenadis* interpreted by Maurand (1973) as a possible mitochondrion. The inclusion body turns somewhat red with Giemsa and stains metachromatically with methylene blue (Vavra, 1962). The posterior body reacts positively with silver methenamine, a stain for complex polysaccharides (Walker and Hinsch, 1972). The posterior body spins vigorously in the vacuole during polar filament extrusion but disappears from the spore precisely when extrusion is completed (Lom and Vavra, unpublished). The behavior of the posterior body during polar tube extrusion strongly suggests that the body may be structurally connected to the filament. One question that arises is whether the posterior body represents the terminal vesicles of the filament.

Although it was hypothesized that the posterior vacuole could
be of nuclear origin (Sprague and Vernick, 1968b; 1969b), it seems
more plausible to interpret the vacuole as a product of the Golgi
zone and as part of the same system as the polaroplast (Sprague
and Vernick, 1969). In fact, the vacuole has the same appearance
as the space occurring within the polaroplast lamellae. Also, in
spores activated for extrusion, the vacuole is infringed by the
laminae of the polaroplast (Sprague et al., 1968).

The relationship between the posterior vacuole and the polar
filament is unclear. Most of the filament is coiled around the
vacuole but separated from it by a membrane. It was reported
that the end of the filament passes into the vacuole but remains
segregated by its own membrane (Weidner, 1972).

Supposedly, the vacuole provides some of the pressure needed for
the polar filament to extrude and for the germ to pass through the
filament. At a certain phase of extrusion the vacuole expands,
and its apical wall pushes in a piston-like manner the spore content into the evaginating filament (Lom and Vávra, 1963b).
Electron micrographs of spores at this state of activation demonstrate that the vacuole expands while remaining transparent. In
those spores that have completely discharged their filament, most
of the inner space is filled by an enormously enlarged posterior
vacuole limited by·a thin highly convoluted membrane. This membrane is distinct and is closely apposed to the severely folded
cytoplasmic membrane that subtends the spore shell; the space
between the two membranes sometimes appears empty or to contain
vesicular cytoplasmic debris (Lom, 1972).

E. ENVELOPE (WALL)

The spore wall is a trilaminar structure consisting of an outer
dense layer, the exospore; an electron transparent middle layer,
the endospore; and a thin mambrane bounding the cytoplasmic content of the spore.

1. Exospore

The exospore varies in thickness among many species but is
usually thin when compared with the endospore. In some species
the exospore is hypertrophied and displays different kinds of
ornamentation on the spore surface (Vavra, 1968a, Fig. 72 D).
The exospore has no apparent substructure but sometimes appears
granular or fibrillar (Vivier and Schrevel, 1973, Szollosi, 1971;
Liu and Davies, 1972b). Some researchers have distinguished
multiple layers in the exospore: three layers in *Pleistophora
hyphessobryconis* (Lom and Corliss, 1967); four or five layers in
Nosema locustae (Huger, 1960) and two dense layers separated by a
transparent one in *Nosema whitei* (Milner, 1972) and *Nosema
spelotremae* (Stanier et al., 1968).

The surface of the exospore is usually finely corrugated. The
surface pattern is best demonstrated in scanning electron

micrographs (Lom and Weiser, 1972; Frost and Nolan, 1972, see
Figs. 68 and 69) or in spore replicas (Vernick *et al.*, 1969).
The surface ornamentation varies from loose and irregularly folded
sheaths (Fig. 68) to ridges or massive ribs. Frequently, filamentous
appendages usually situated at one or both poles of the spore
(e.g. *Caudospora, Weiseria, Mrazekia*) are encountered. These
appendages are visible in the light microscope but their appearance is enhanced by negative staining (Vávra, 1963). Some of the
tubular structures occurring at the surface of the spore can be
observed only in the electron microscope. In *Pleistophora
debaisieuxi*, there are numerous flexible tubules about 100 nm
thick and up to 2 μm long that radiate from the exospore in all
directions (Figs. 29 and 72 G). Smaller tubules originally
described as bristles (Sprague *et al.*, 1968) occur at the surface
of sporoblasts and spores of *Ameson* (syn. *Nosema) michaelis*
(Weidner, 1970). Dwyer and Weidner (1973) have demonstrated that
these bristles have morphological, physical, and chemical properties characteristic to microtubules. The signifcance of these
external microtubules is not known. A layer of mucus ("mucoalyx")
has been observed around spores of some microsporidia from aquatic
hosts (Lom and Vávra, 1961b; 1962b; Komárek and Vávra, 1968;
Weiser, 1963). Negative staining reveals that the mucus layer
consists of a thick coat of long, very fine fibres oriented
perpendicular to the spore surface (Vávra, 1968b, Fig. 31). Nothing
is known about the origin and chemical composition of the mucus
layer but it may be elaborated by the exospore or it may originate
from the pansporoblast cavity and become bound to the exospore.

The origin of the exospore can be traced to the electron dense
membranous complex formed on the outside of the plasma membrane
during the sporogonial part of the life cycle. The exosporal
appendages, various ornamentations, and mucus layers probably
originate from the granulofibrillar material secreted by the
microsporidan cell during development and deposited on the outside
of the cell wall. Some appendages are present at the sporoblast
stage and they may participate in the flow of material to and from
the parasite (Lom and Corliss, 1967; Overstreet and Weidner, 1974).
The flow across the pellicle probably is necessary during sporogenesis for transport of energy material. Also some kinds of
appendages may be important to flotation (Vávra, 1963) or attachment to the substratum (Overstreet and Weidner, 1974) although
no experimental data support these assumptions. Appendages
have been observed only on those microsporidia isolated from aquatic
hosts. Spores from terrestrial hosts have only unconspicuous
wrinkles on their surface.

The exospore appears to be proteinaceous. It is dissolved in
strong alkali (Vávra, 1968a) and 13 amino acids were identified
in alkaline hydrolysates (Vávra, 1964). Maurand and Loubes (1973)
reported sulfur proteins isolated from spore coat.

Fig. 68.   Scanning electron micrograph of spores of *Nosema*
           stricklandi from a black-fly larva. The exospore
           layer is developed in the form of a loose sheath
           folded into irregular ribs. X 10,000.

Fig. 69.   Scanning electron micrograph of *Nosema bombycis* spores.
           The exospore layer is very finely wrinkled. This
           aspect of the spore surface is generally present in
           spores of terrestrial hosts. X 10,000.

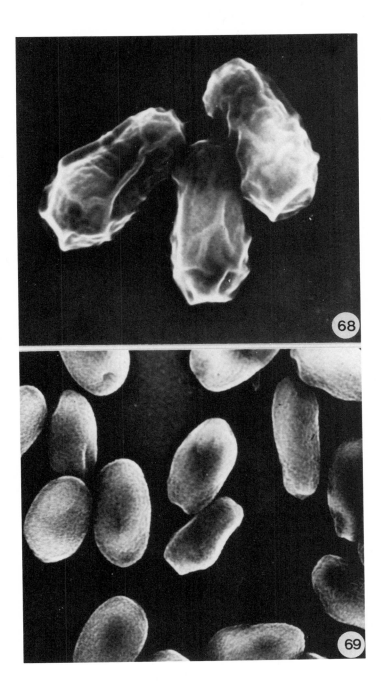

2. Endospore

The endospore is a rather thick, (50–380 nm) electron-transparent layer.   It is very thin in some species (Richards and Sheffield, 1970, Vivier and Schrevel, 1973) and totally absent in others (Sprague, Ormieres and Manier, 1972). Because of its electron transparency, some investigators have erroneously described the endospore as an empty artificial space surrounding the spore (Kudo and Daniels, 1963; Milner, 1972). Liu and Davies (1973a) were unable to distinguish the endospore layer in freeze–etched *Thelohania bracteata* spores. However, their electron micrographs do reveal a fibrillar layer the thickness of which is comparable to the endospore layer observed in thin sections of the same species (Liu and Davies, 1972b).

The dimension of the endospore varies throughout the spore envelope, being considerably thinner at the apical pole of the spore (Fig. 32). This thin area is sometimes called the micropyle but no opening is actually present (Vávra, unpublished observations). Codreanu, *et al.*, (1965) described a spot of dense matter impregnating the apical part of the endospore as a micropyle. Similar darker material was seen in the endospore layer of *Nosema algerae* (Vávra and Undeen, 1970). Lom and Corliss (1967) described in *Pleistophora hyphessobryconis* "a faint indication at the anterior pole of what could be a circular break line ready to be pierced by the thrust of the extruding filament." However, endospores obtained by alkaline hydrolysis and observed in the electron microscope display no specialized part or opening in the layer (Vávra, unpublished). Sometimes the endospore has been resolved by electron microscopy to have a second layer that is thin and slightly electron opaque. It lies immediately adjacent to the plasma membrane and corresponds to the "inner limiting layer of the spore membrane" described by Huger (1960) and to the (innermost spore coat" reported by Liu and Davies (1972b).

The main chemical component of the endospore is chitin. Chitin was believed to be present in microsporidian spores because of the solubility properties of spores (Kudo, 1921), the Van Wysseling's reaction (Koehler, 1921), and the chitosan tests of Campbell (Dissanaike and Canning, 1957). Enzymatic digestion, X-ray diffraction analysis, and infrared absorption spectroscopy of isolated and purified endospores clearly demonstrate the presence of α-chitin (Vávra, 1967 and Vávra, unpublished). Its occurrence also has been confirmed by chromatographic analysis of spore hydrolysates (Erickson and Blanquet, 1970, see Figs. 70 and 71). The chitin occurs in the spore as a protein–chitin complex. In such a complex, both substances are mutually protected against their specific enzymes (Vávra, 1967). Chitin is well known as an extremely nonreactive compound and its presence in the spores renders them very resistant.

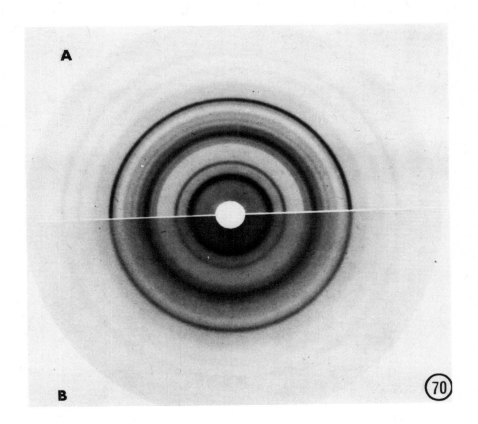

Fig. 70.   X-ray diffractograms of crab chitin (A) and chitin
           isolated from endospores of *Nosema bombycis* (B). The
           photograph was kindly made by Prof. K. M. Rudall,
           University of Leeds, Great Britain. Note that both
           specimens exhibit the same diffraction pattern although
           the microsporidian chitin is less crystalline.

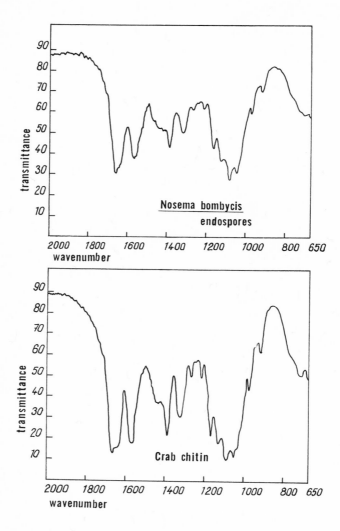

Fig. 71. The comparison of infra-red spectra of *Nosema bombycis*
endospores and of crab chitin. Note the coincidence of
individual absorption peaks confirming the identify of
both materials.

3. *Plasma membrane*

The third and innermost layer is a thin membrane limiting the spore cytoplasm. This membrane is similar to other cytoplasmic membranes. Freeze-etched preparations of *Thelohania bracteata* show that the inner face of the membrane is covered by stud-like projections and granular subunits whereas the outer face bears particles and depressions corresponding to the stud-like projections. Presumably, the projections provide greater friction to prevent the outer spore layers from spinning around during exosporulation (Liu and Davies, 1973a).

The spore wall is differentiated from structural components of the sporoblast cell wall. Several observations indicate that the endospore originates by the progressive thickenning of the transparent interspace between the plasmalemma of the sporoblast and the dark membranous layer (exosporont membrane) situated at its outer surface (Lom and Corliss, 1967; Canning and Sinden, 1973). This mode of spore membrane formation seems to be more probable than the direct transformation of the middle layer of the unit membrane into the chitinous endospore as postulated by Sprague and Vernick (1968b; 1969b; 1974). No experimental data are available on the physical and mechanical properties of the spore wall.

To speculate, the exospore may be involved in the invasion process by determining the physical character of the spore surface and by making the spore more available to the host. The exospore may also provide the spore with additional protection and presumably mediates the stimuli needed for spore activation. The endospore has mainly a protective function. It is also the only layer that is able to provide the spore wall with enough resistance to withstand internal pressure generated during polar filament extrusion. So, the endospore is a pressure vessel of the spore. The cytoplasmic membrane evidently has the same function as any other cell membrane. In spores activated for extrusion, the plasmatic membrane develops numerous deep folds into the spore cytoplasm (Lom, 1972). This phenomenon perhaps can be interpreted as an indication that the cytoplasmic membrane has specific functions during spore germination. Fumidil B, an antibiotic with antimicrosporidian activity, alters the number and distribution of particles found in freeze-etched spore membrane. Because these particles may be important for transport processes, reduction and changes in the number of particles and their distribution may suggest a decrease in functional capacity of the spore membrane (Liu, 1973b).

SUMMARY

The various microsporidian developmental stages represent structurally simple cells that are transformed at the end of the

Fig. 72.   A composite diagram of various spore surfaces in
           microsporidian spores (A-G) and of atypical polar tubes
           (H-K).   A, typical condition where the exospore is finely
           wrinkled; B, exospore with microtubules in *Ameson*
           (syn. *Nosema*) *michaelis*; C, diplospore of *Telomyxa*
           glugeiformis where two spores are contained in a special
           kind of pansporoblast; D, spore of *Caudospora simulii*
           with the exospore hypertrofied into two massive lateral
           ribs, a cauda and two anterior appendages; E, mucous
           layer with filaments in *Gurleya marsoniella*; F, ribs
           with posterior collar in *Weiseria*, G, tubules on the
           surface of spores of *Pleistophora debaisieuxi*; H,
           manubrium with a short polar tube in *Bacillidium*; I,
           polar tube with honeycomb-like outer layer in
           Steinhausia (syn. *Coccospora*) *brachynema*; K, manubrium
           with a short infundibulum-like structure in
           Metchnikovella.

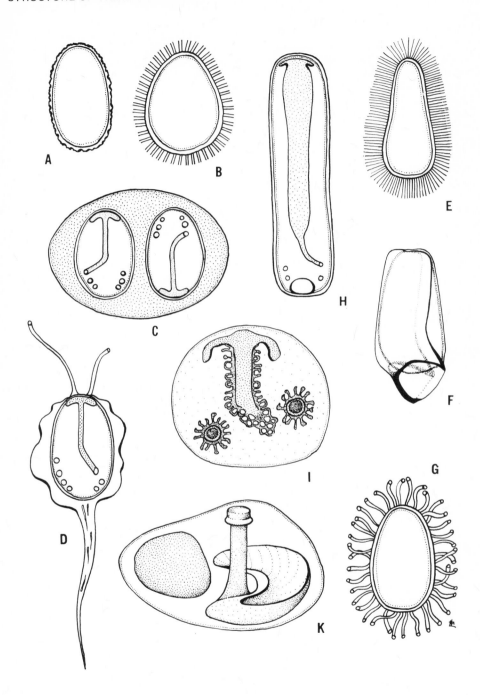

life cycle into structurally complicated spores. The structure of the cell limiting membrane in developmental stages is extremely variable and reflects the intimate relationship of microsporidian parasite to the host cell. The significance of some components associated with the cell limiting membrane during sporogony (pansporoblast membrane, secretion into the pansporoblast cavity, scindosomes) however, remains to be elucidated.

The microsporidian spore is a unicellular entity and all its structural components are formed by endomembranous differentiation of the single cell of the sporoblast. The central role in microsporidian morphogenesis is assumed by the Gogi apparatus, which although atypical and rather inconspicuous in the developmental stages, is greatly hypertrophied in the spore and takes part in the formation of all organelles that belong to the extrusion apparatus. It is very probable that most, if not all, components of the extrusion apparatus represent a continuous membrane system. The microsporidian spore is provided by a multilayered wall in which protein and α-chitin are complexed. The spore content, including the nucleus and the spore cytoplasm, are emptied through the discharging polar tube into the germ vesicle at the distal end of the tube. The spore discharge is a pressure event in which the energy is provided by swelling of the polaroplast and of the posterior vacuole.

REFERENCES

Akao, S. (1969). Studies on the ultrastructure of *Nosema cuniculi*, a microsporidian parasite of rodents. *Jap. J. Parasitol.* **18**, 8–20.

Barker, R. J. (1975). Ultrastructural observations on *Encephalitozoon cuniculi* Levaditi, Nicolau & Schoen 1923, from mouse peritoneal macrophages. *Folia Parasitol.* (Praha) **22**, 1–9.

Burges, H. D., Canning, E. U. and Hulls, I. K. (1974). Ultrastructure of *Nosema oryzaephili* and the taxonomic value of the polar filament. *J. Invert. Pathol.* **23**, 135–139.

Burke, J. M. (1970). A microsporidian in the epidermis of *Eisenia foetida* (Oligochaeta). *J. Invert. Pathol.* **16**, 145–147.

Burnett, R. G. and King, R. C. (1962). Observations on a microsporidian parasite of *Drosophila willistoni* Sturtevant. *J. Insect Pathol.* **4**, 104–112.

Cali, Ann (1971). Morphogenesis in the genus *Nosema*. Proc. Int. Colloq. Insect Pathol., 4th, College Park, Maryland, 1970, pp. 431–438.

Canning, E. U. and Nicholas, J. P. (1974). Light and electron microscope observations on *Unikaryon legeri* (Microsporida, Nosematidae), a parasite of the metacercaria of *Meigymnophallus minutus* in *Cardium edule*. *J. Invert. Pathol.* **23**, 92–100.

Canning, E. U. and Sinden, R. E. (1973). Ultrastructural ob-
    servations on the development of *Nosema algerae* Vavra and
    Undeen (Microsporida, Nosematidae) in the mosquito
    Anopheles stephensi Liston. Protistologica <u>9</u>, 405-415.
Codreanu, R. (1961). Sur la structure bicellulaire des spores
    de *Telomyxa* cf. *glugeiformis* Léger et Hesse, 1910, parasite
    des nymphes d'*Ephemera* (France, Roumanie) et les nouveaux
    sous-ordres des microsporidies Monocytosporea et
    Polycytosporea. C.R. *Acad. Sci.*, Paris, <u>253</u>, 1613-1615.
Codreanu, R. (1964). On the occurrence of spore or sporont
    appendages in the microsporidia and their taxonomic signifi-
    cance. Proc. Int. Cong. Parasitol., 1st, Rome, Italy, 1964.
Codreanu, R., Popa, A. and Voiculescu, R. (1965). Donneés sur
    l'ultrastructure des spores de microsporidies. Bull.
    Apicole, <u>8</u>, 5-16.
Codreanu, R. and Vávra, J. (1970). The structure and ultrastructure
    of the microsporidian *Telomyxa glugeiformis* Léger and Hesse,
    1910, parasite of *Ephemera danica* (Müll) *nymphs. J. Protozool.*
    <u>17</u>, 374-384.
Cossins, A. R. and Bowler, K. (1974). A histological and ultra-
    structural study of *Thelohania contejeani* Henneguy, 1892
    (Nosematidae), microsporidian parasite of the crayfish
    Austropotamobius pallipes Lereboullet. *Parasitology* <u>68</u>,
    81-91.
Coste-Mathiez, F. and Manier, J. F. (1968). *Nosema orthocladii*
    n.sp. (Microsporidie-Nosematidae) parasite des larves
    d'*Orthocladius lignicola* Kieffer (Diptère, Chironomide).
    Bull. Soc. Zool. France. <u>93</u>, 127-133.
Devauchelle, G., Vinckier, D. and Prensier, G. (1970). Origine
    et formation du filament polaire chez *Nosema vivieri.*
    J. Protozool. <u>17</u> (Suppl.), 33.
Dissanaike, A. S. and Canning, E. U. (1957). The mode of emergence
    of the sporoplasm in microspiridia and its relation to the
    structure of the spore. *Parasitology* <u>47</u>, 92-99.
Doby, J. M. and Saguez, F. (1964). *Weiseria*, genre nouveau de
    microsporidies et *Weiseria laurenti* n.sp., parasite de larves
    de *Prosimulium inflatum* Davies, 1957 (Diptères Paranématocères).
    C.R. *Acad. Sci.* Paris, <u>259</u>, 3614-3617.
Doby, J. M., Vávra, J., Weiser, J. and Beaucournu-Saguez, F. (1965).
    Complement a l'étude de la morphologie et du cycle evolutif
    de *Caudospora simulii* Weiser 1947. *Bull. Soc. Zool. France.*
    <u>90</u>, 393-399.
Dwyer, D. M. and Weidner, E. (1973). Microsporidian extrasporular
    microtubules. Ultrastructure, isolation and electrophoretic
    characterization. *Z. Zellforsch.* <u>140</u>, 177-186.
Erickson, B. W. Jr. and Blanquet, R. S. (1969). The occurrence
    of chitin in the spore wall of *Glugea weissenbergi. J. Invert.
    Pathol.* <u>14</u>, 358-364.

Erickson, B. and Sprague, V. (1970). Summary of the contributions of cytochemical reactions to our knowledge of microsporidian spores. SIP Newsletter 2, 11.

Erickson, B. W. Jr., Vernick, S. H. and Sprague, V. (1968). Electron microscope study of the everted polar filament of *Glugea weissenbergi* (Microsporida, Nosematidae). *J. Protozool.* 15, 758-761.

Favard, P. (1969). The Golgi apparatus. *In* "Handbook of Molecular Cytology". (A. Lima-de-Faria, ed.), pp. 1130-1158, North-Holland, Amsterdam, London.

Frost, S. and Nolan, R. A. (1972). The occurrence and morphology of *Caudospora* spp. (Protozoa: Microsporida) in Newfoundland and Labrador blackfly larvae (Diptera:Simuliidae). *Can. J. Zool.* 50, 1363-1366.

Gassouma, M. S. S. and Ellis, D. S. (1973). The ultrastructure of sporogonic stages and spores of *Thelohania* and *Plistophora* (Microsporida, Nosematidae) from *Simulium ornatum* larvae *J. Gen. Microbiol.* 74, 33-43.

Gotz, P. (1974). Homology of the manubrium of *Mrazekia brevicauda* (Microsporida) and the polar filament of *Nosematidae* (Microsporida). Proc. Int. Cong. Parasitol. 3rd, Munchen Germany, 1974.

Hazard, E. I. and Anthony, D. W. (1974). A redescription of the genus *Parathelohania* Codreanu 1966 (Microsporida: Protozoa) with a reexamination of previously described species of *Thelohania* Henneguy 1892 and descriptions of two new species of *Parathelohania* from anopheline mosquitoes. U.S. Dept. Agricul., Agricul. Res. Serv., Washington, D. C., Tech. Bull. No. 1505, 26 pages.

Hazard, E. and Fukuda, T. (1974). *Stempellia milleri* sp.n. (Microsporida: Nosematidae) in the mosquito *Culex pipiens quinquefasciatus*. *J. Protozool.* 21, 497-504.

Hildebrand, H. F. (1974). Observations ultrastructurales sur le stade plasmodial de *Metchnikovella wohlfarthi* Hildebrand et Vivier 1971, microsporidie hyperparasite de la gregarine *Lecudina tuzetae*. *Protistologica* 10, 5-15.

Hildebrand, H. F. and Vivier, E. (1971). Observations ultra-structurales sur le sporoblaste de *Metchnikovella wohlfarthi*, n. sp. (Microsporidies), parasite de la gregarine *Lecudina tuzetae*. *Protistologica* 7, 131-139.

Hollande, A. (1972). Le déroulement de la cryptomitose et les modalités de la ségrégation des chromatides dans quelques groupes de Protozoaires. *Anneé Biologique,* 11, 427-466.

Huger, A. (1960a). Electron microscope study on the cytology of a microsporidian spore by means of ultrathin sectioning. *J. Insect. Pathol.* 2, 84-105.

Huger, A. (1960b). Elektronenmikroskopische Analyse der Innenstruktur von Mikrosporidiensporen. *Naturwiss.* 47, 68.

Huger, A. (1961). Sporentierchen als Insektenfeinde. I. Elektronenmikroskopische Untersuchungen über Bau-und Lebensweise der Mikrosporiden. *Umschau*. 9, 270-272.

Ishihara, R. (1968). Some observations on the fine structure of sporoplasm discharged from spores of a microsporidian, *Nosema bombycis*. *J. Invert. Pathol.* 12, 245-257.

Ishihara, R. (1970). Fine structure of *Nosema bombycis* (Microsporidia, Nosematidae). Developing in the *Silkworm (Bombyx mori)*-L. Bull. Coll. Agr. & Vet. Med. Nihon. Univ. 27, 84-91.

Ishihara, R. and Hayashi, Y. (1968). Some properties of ribosomes from the sporoplasm of *Nosema bombycis*. *J. Invert. Pathol.* 11, 377-385.

Jensen, H. M. and Wellings, S. R. (1970). The formation of the polar filament of a microsporidian parasite. *Anat. Rec.* 166, 324.

Jensen, H. M. and Wellings, S. R. (1972). Development of the polar filament-polaroplast complex in a microsporidian parasite. *J. Protozool.* 19, 297-306.

Jirovec, O. (1932). Ergebnisse der Nuclealfärbung an den Sporen der Mikrosporidien nebst einigen Bemerkungen über *Lymhocystis*. *Arch. Protistenk.* 77, 379-390.

Kahazi-Pakdel. (1970). Ultrastructure des spores de *Nosema melolonthae* Krieg. Proc. Int. Colloq. Insect Pathol. 4th, College Park, Maryland, 1970, pp. 410-414.

Koehler, A. (1921). Ueber die chemische Zusammensetzung der Sporenschale von *Nosema apis*. Zool. Anz. (Leipzig) 53, 85-87.

Komarek, J. and Vavra, J. (1968). In memoriam of *Marsoniella* Lemm. 1900. *Arch. Protistenk.* 111, 12-17.

Kudo, R. (1921). On the nature of structures characteristic of cnidosporidian spores. *Trans. Amer. microsc. Soc.* 40, 59-74.

Kudo, R. (1924). A biologic and taxonomic study of the microsporidia. *Illinois Biol. Monograph* 9, 268 pp.

Kudo, R. R. and Daniels, E. W. (1963). An electron microscope study of the spore of a microsporidian *Thelohania californica*. *J. Protozool.* 10, 112-120.

Krieg, A. (1955). Ueber Infektionskrankheiten bei Engerlingen von *Melolontha* spec. unter besonderer Berücksichtigung einer Mikrosporidien-Erkrankung. Zbl. Bakt., Abt. II 108, 535-538.

Leger, L. (1926). Une microsporidie nouvelle a sporontes épineux. C. R. *Acad. Sci.* Paris 182, 727-729.

Liu, T. P. (1972). A freeze-etching study on the nuclear envelope during development in microsporidian *Thelohania bracteata* (Strickland, 1913). *J. Parasitol.* 58, 1151-1161.

Liu, T. P. (1973a). The fine structure of the frozen etched spore of *Nosema apis* Zander. *Tissue Cell* 5, 315-322.

Liu, T. P. (1973b). Effects of Fumidil B on the spore of *Nosema apis* and on lipids of the host cell as revealed by freeze-etching. *J. Invert. Pathol.* 22, 364-368.

Liu, T. P. and Davies, D. M. (1972a). Fine structure of frozen-etched spores of *Thelohania bracteata* emphasizing the formation of the polaroplast. *Tissue Cell* 4, 1-10.

Liu, T. P. and Davies, D. M. (1972b). Fine structure of developing spores of *Thelohania bracteata* (Strickland, 1913) (Microsporida, Nosematidae) emphasizing polar-filament formation. *J. Protozool.* 19, 461-469.

Liu, T. P. and Davies, D. M. (1972c). Organization of frozen-etched *Thelohania bracteata* (Strickland, 1913) (Microsporida, Nosematidae) emphasizing the fine structure of the posterior vacuole. *Parasitology* 64, 341-345.

Liu, T. P. and Davies, D. M. (1972d). Ultrastructure of the cytoplasm in fat body cells of the black-fly, *Simulium vittatum*, with microsporidian infection; a freeze-etching study. *J. Invert. Pathol.* 19, 208-214.

Liu, T. P. and Davies, D. M. (1973a). Ultrastructural architecture and organization of the spore envelope during development in *Thelohania bracteata* (Strickland, 1913) after freeze-etching. *J. Protozool.* 20, 622-630.

Liu, T. P. and Davies, D. M. (1973b). Ultrastructure of the frozen-etched polar filament in a microsporidan *Thelohania bracteata* (Strickland, 1913). *Can. J. Zool.* 51, 217-219.

Liu, T. P., Darley, J. H. and Davies, D. M. (1971). Preliminary observations on the fine structure of the the pansporoblast of *Thelohania bracteata* (Strickland, 1913) (Microsporida, Nosematidae) as revealed by freeze-etching electron microscopy. *J. Protozool.* 18, 592-596.

Lom, J. (1972). On the structure of the extruded microsporidian polar filament. *Z. Parasitenk.* 38, 200-213.

Lom, J. and Corliss, J. O. (1967). Ultrastructural observations on the development of the microsporidian protozoon *Plistophora hyphessobryconis* Schaperclaus. *J. Protozool.* 14, 141-152.

Lom, J. and Vávra, J. (1961a). Niektoré wyniki badań nad ultrastruktura spor pasoźyta ryb *Plistophora hyphessobryconis* (Microsporidia). *Wiadom. Parazyt.* 7, 828-832.

Lom, J. and Vávra, J. (1961b). Mucous envelope as a taxonomic character in microsporidian spores *J. Protozool.* 8, (Suppl.), 18.

Lom, J. and Vávra, J. (1962a). New facts concerning the extrusion of microsporidian spores. Coll. Int. Pathol. Insects, Paris, 1962, *Entomophaga, Mem. hors série* 2, 101-103.

Lom, J. and Vavra, J. (1962b). Mucous envelopes of spores of the suphylum Cnidospora (Doflein, 1901). *Vest. Čs. Spol. Zool.* 27, 4-6.

Lom, J. and Vavra, J. (1963a). Contribution to the knowledge of microsporidian spore. *In* "Progress in Protozoology" (J. Ludvik, J. Lom, and J. Vavra, eds.) Prague, pp. 487-489, Academia, Praha.

Lom, J. and Vavra, J. (1963b). The mode of sporoplasm extrusion in microsporidian spores. *Acta Protozool.* 1, 81-89.

Lom, J. and Vavra, J. (1963c). Fine morphology of the spore in microsporidia. *Acta Protozool.* 1, 279-283.

Lom, J. and Weiser, J. (1972). Surface pattern of some microsporidian spores as seen in the scanning electron microscope. *Folia Parasitol.* (Praha) 19, 359-363.

Maurand, J. (1966). *Plistophora simulii* (Lutz et Splendore 1904), microsporidie parasite des larves de *Simulium;* cycle, ultrastructure, ses rapports avec *Thelohania bracteata* (Strickland, 1913). *Bull. Soc. Zool. France* 91, 621-630.

Maurand, J. (1973). Recherches biologiques sur les microsporidies des larves de simulies. These, Univ. Tech. du Languedoc, 199 pages.

Maurand, J. and Bouix, G. (1969). Mise en évidence d'un phénomène sécrétoire dans le cycle de *Thelohania fibrata* (Stricklend, 1913), Microsporidie parasite des larves de *Simulium. C. R. Acad. Sci. Paris* 269, 2216-2218.

Maurand, J. and Loubes, C. (1973). Recherches cytochimiques sur quelques microsporidies. *Bull. Soc. Zool. France* 98, 373-383.

Maurand, J. and Manier, F. (1968). Une microsporidie nouvelle pour les larves de simulies. *Protistologica* 3, 445-449.

Maurand, J., Fize, A., Fenwick, B. and Michel, R. (1971). Étude au microscope électronique de *Nosema infirmum* Kudo 1921, microsporidie parasite d'un copépode cyclopoïde; création du genre nouveau *Tuzetia* a propos de cette espèce. *Protistologica* 7, 221-225.

Maurand, J., Fize, A., Michel, R. and Fenwick, B. (1972). Ouelques données sur les microsporidies parasites de copépodes cycloipoïdes des eaux continentales de la région de Montpellier. *Bull. Soc. Zool. France* 97, 707-717.

Maurand, J. and Vey, A. (1973). Etudes histopathologique et ultrastructurale de *Thelohania contejeani* (Microsporida, Nosematidae) parasite de l'ecrevisse *Austropotamobius pallipes Lereboullet. Ann. Parasitol. Hum. Comp.* 48, 411-421.

Milner, R. J. (1972). *Nosema whitei,* a microsporidian pathogen of some species of *Tribolium.* II. Ultrastructure. *J. Invert. Pathol.* 19, 239-247.

Moens, P. B. and Rapport, E. (1971). Spindles, spindle plaques, and meiosis in the yeast *Saccharomyces cerevisiae* (Hansen) *J. Cell Biol.* 50, 344-361.

Morre, J., Mollenhauer, H. H. and Bracker, C. E. (1971). Origin
    and continuity of Golgi apparatus. *In* "Origin and Continuity
    of Cell Organelles: Results and Problems in Cell Differentiation
    (J. Reinert and H. Ursprung, eds.), Vol. 2, pp. 82-126,
    Springer Verlag, Berlin, Heidelberg, and New York.
Ormieres, R. and Sprague, V. (1973). A new family, new genus, and
    new species allied to the microsporida. *J. Invert. Pathol.*
    21, 224-240.
Overstreet, R. M. and Weidner, E. (1974). Differentiation of
    microsporidian spore-tails in *Inodosporus spraguei* gen. et
    sp. n. Z. Parasitenk. **44**, 169-186.
Percy, J. (1973). The intranuclear occurrence and fine structural
    details of schizonts of *Perezia fumiferanae* (Microsporida:
    Nosematidae) in cells of *Choristoneura fumiferana* (Clem.).
    (Lepidoptera: Tortricidae). *Can. J. Zool.* **51**, 553-554.
Petri, M. (1969). Studies on *Nosema cuniculi* found in trans-
    plantable ascites tumours with a survey of microsporidiosis
    in mammals. *Acta. Pathol. Microbiol. Scand. Suppl.* **204**,
    91 pp.
Petri, M. (1974). *Nosema cuniculi.* Some remarkable features of its
    life-cycle. Proc. 3rd Int. Cong. Parasitol., Munchen,
    Germany, 1974.
Petri, M. and Schiodt, T. (1966). On the ultrastructure of *Nosema
    cuniculi* in the cells of the Yoshida rat ascites sarcoma.
    Acta Pathol. Microbiol. Scand. **66**, 437-446.
Puytorac, P. de (1961). L'ultrastructure du filament polaire
    invaginé de la microsporidie *Mrazekia lumbriculi* Jírovec
    1936. *C. R. Acad. Sci. Paris* **253**, 2600-2602.
Puytorac, P. de (1962). Observations sur l'ultrastructure de la
    microsporidie *Mrazekia lumbriculi, Jírovec. J. Microscopie*
    1, 39-46.
Puytorac, P. de and Tourret, M. (1963). Étude de kystes d'origine
    parasitaire (microsporidies ou grégarines) sur la paroi
    interne du corps des vers *Megascolecidae. Ann. Parasitol.
    Hum. Comp.* **38**, 862-874.
Shabanov, M. M. (1973). Studies on the ultrastructure of the
    spores of *Nosema apis* Zander. *C. R. Acad. Bulg. Sci.*
    26, 427-430.
Sheffield, H. G. and Richards, C. S. (1970). Unique host
    relations and ultrastructure of a new microsporidian of the
    genus *Coccospora* infecting *Biomphalaria glabrata.* Proc.
    Int. Colloq. Insect Pathol., 4th, College Park, Maryland,
    pp. 439-452.
Scholtyseck, E. and Danneel, R. (1962). Uber die Feinstruktur
    der Spore von *Nosema apis. Dtsch. Entomol. Z.* **9**, 471-476.
Schubert, G. (1969a). Ultracytologische Untersuchungen an der
    Spore der Mikrosporidienart, *Heterosporis finki, gen. n.,
    sp. n. Z. Parasitenk.* **32**, 59-79.

Schubert, G. (1969b). Elektronenmikroskopische Untersuchungen zur Sporonten-und Sporenentwicklung der Mikrosporidienart *Heterosporis finki*. *Z. Parasitenk.* 32, 80-92.

Sprague, V., Ormiéres, R. and Manier, J. F. (1972). Creation of a new genus and a new family in the microsporida. *J. Invert. Pathol.* 20, 228-231.

Sprague, V. and Vernick, S. H. (1966). Light and electron microscope study of developing stages of *Glugea* sp. (Microsporida) in the stickleback *Apeltes quadracus*. *Amer. Zool.* 6, 555-6.

Sprague, V. and Vernick, S. H. (1967). Transformation of the sporoblast into the microsporidan spore. *J. Protozool.* 14 (Suppl.), 29.

Sprague, V. and Vernick, S. H. (1968a). The Golgi complex of microsporida and its role in spore morphogenesis. *Amer. Zool.* 8, 824.

Sprague, V. and Vernick, S. H. (1968b). Light and electron microscope study of a new species of *Glugea* (Microsporida, Nosematidae) in the 4-spined stickleback *Apeltes quadracus*. *J. Protozool.* 15, 547-571.

Sprague, V. and Vernick, S. H. (1968c). Observations on the spores of *Pleistophora gigantea* (Thelohan, 1895) Swellengrebel 1911, a microsporidan parasite of the fish *Crenilabrus melops*. *J. Protozool.* 15, 662-665.

Sprague, V. and Vernick, S. H. (1969a). Light and electron microscope observations on *Nosema nelsoni* Sprague, 1950 (Microsporida, Nosematidae) with particular reference to its Golgi complex. *J. Protozool.* 16, 264-271.

Sprague, V. and Vernick, S. H. (1969b). Morphogenesis of microsporidan spores. *In* "Progress in Protozoology" (Abstr. 3rd Int. Congr. Protozool.), Nauka, Leningrad.

Sprague, V. and Vernick, S. H. (1971). The ultrastructure of *Encephalitozoon cuniculi* (Microsporida, Nosematidae) and its taxonomic significance. *J. Protozool.* 18, 560-569.

Sprague, V., Vernick, S. H. and Lloyd, B. Jr. (1968). The fine structure of *Nosema* sp. Sprague, 1965 (Microsporida, Nosematidae) with particular reference to stages in sporogony. *J. Invert. Pathol.* 12, 105-117.

Stanier, J. E., Woodhouse, M. A. and Griffin, R. L. (1968). The fine structure of the spore of *Nosema spelotremae*, a microsporidian parasite of a *Spelotrema* metacercaria, encysted in the crab *Carcinus maenas*. *J. Invert. Pathol.* 12, 73-82.

Stempell, W. (1909). Ueber *Nosema bombycis* Nägeli. *Arch. Protistenk.* 16, 281-358.

Stevens, B. J. and André, J. (1969). The nuclear envelope. *In* "Handbook of Molecular Cytology" (A. Lima-de-Faria, ed.), pp. 837-874. North-Holland, Amsterdam and London.

Szollosi, D. G. (1970). Development of a microsporidian spore. *Anat. Rec.* 166, 387.

Szollosi, D. (1971). Development of *Pleistophora* sp. (Microsporidian) in eggs of the polychaete *Armandia brevis*. *J. Invert. Pathol.* 18, 1-15.

Takizawa, H., Vivier, E. and Petiprez, A. (1973). Development intranucleaire de la microsporidie *Nosema bombycis* dans les cellules de Vers à sois après infestation experimentale. *C. R. Acad. Sci. Paris* 277, 1769-1772.

Thelohan, P. (1892). Observations sur les Myxosporidies et essai de classification de ces organismes. Bull. Soc. Philom. 4, 165-178.

Tuzet, O., Maurand, M. J., Fize, A., Michel, R. and Fenwick, B. (1971). Proposition d'un nouveau cadre systématique pour les genres de Microsporidies. *C. R. Acad. Sci. Paris* 272, 1268-1271.

Vávra, J. (1959). Beitrag zur Cytologie einiger Mikrosporidien. *Vest. Cs. Spol. Zool.* 23, 347-350.

Vávra, J. (1962). *Bacillidium cyclopis* n.sp. (Cnidospora, Microsporidia), a new parasite of Copepods. *Vest. Cs. Spol. Zool.* 26, 295-299.

Vávra, J. (1963). Spore projections in Microsporidia. *Acta Protozool.* 1, 153-155.

Vávra, J. (1964). Some recent advances in the study of microsporidian spores. Proc. Intern. Congr. of Parasitol., 1st, Rome, Italy, 1964, pp. 443-444.

Vávra, J. (1965). Étude au microscope electronique de la morphologie et du developpement de quelques microsporidies. *C. R. Acad. Sci. Paris* 261, 3467-3470.

Vávra, J. (1967). Hydrolyse enzymatique des spores de microsporidies. *J. Protozool.* 14 (Suppl.), 205.

Vávra, J. (1968a). Ultrastructural features of *Caudospora simulii* Weiser (Protozoa, Microsporidia.) *Folia Parasitol.* (Praha) 15, 1-9.

Vávra, J. (1968b). The fine structure of the mucus coating of microsporidian spores. *J. Protozool.* 15 (Suppl.), 26.

Vávra, J. (1970). Physiological, morphological, and ecological considerations of some microsporidia and gregarines. *In* "Ecology and Physiology of Parasites" (A. M. Fallis, ed.), University of Toronto Press.

Vávra, J. (1971). Ultrahistochemical detection of carbohydrates in microsporidian spores. *J. Protozool.* 18 (Suppl.), 179.

Vávra, J. (1972a). Detection of polysaccharides in microsporidian spores by means of the periodic acid-thio-semicarbazide-silver proteinate test. *J. Microscopie,* 14, 357-360.

Vávra, J. (1972b). Substructure of the microsporidian polar filament at high resolution. *J. Protozool.,* 19 (Suppl.), 79-80.

Vávra, J. (1973). Morphogenetic events in the developmental cycles of microsporidia. *In* "Progress in Protozoology" 4th Int. Cong. Protozool.), Clermont-Ferrand.

Vavra, J. (1974a). Developmental cycles of protozoa (other than
    Coccidia). *In* "Actualites Protozoologiques" (P. de Puytorac
    and J. Grain, eds.), pp. 99-108, Clermont-Ferrand.
Vavra, J. (1974b). Fine structure as a criterion in the taxonomy
    of microsporidia. Proc. Int. Cong. Parasitol., 3rd
    Munchen, Germany, 1974.
Vavra, J., Joyon, L. and Puytorac, P. de. (1966). Observation
    sur l'ultrastructure du filament polaire des microsporidies.
    Protistologica 2, 109-112.
Vavra, J. and Undeen, A. H. (1970). *Nosema algerae* n.sp.
    (Cnidospora, Microsporida) a pathogen in a laboratory
    colony of *Anopheles stephensi* Liston (Diptera, Culicidae).
    J. Protozool. 17, 240-249.
Vernick, S. H., Sprague, V., Bolivar, J., and Lloyd, J. Jr.
    (1969). Further observations on the fine structure of the
    spores of *Glugea weissenbergi* (Microsporida, Nosematidae).
    J. Protozool. 16, 50-53.
Vernick, S. H., Tousimis, A. and Sprague, V. (1969). Surface
    structure of the spores of *Glugea weissenbergi*. Annu.
    Proc. Electron Micros. Soc. Amer., 27th.
Vey, A. and Vago, C. (1973). Protozoan and fungal diseases of
    Austropotamobius pallipes Lereboullet in France. *In*
    "Freshwater Crayfish" (S. Abrahamson, ed.) pp. 166-179, Lund.
Vinckier, D. (1973). Étude des cycles et de l'ultrastructure de
    Lecudina linei n.sp. (Gregarine parasite de Nemerte) et de
    son parasite, la microsporidie *Nosema vivieri* (V.D. et P.).
    Thèse. Universite des Sci. Tech. de Lille, 52 pages.
Vinckier, D., Devauchelle, G. and Prensier, G. (1971a). *Nosema
    vivieri* n.sp. (Microsporidae, Nosematidae) hyperparasite
    d'une grégarine vivant dans le coelome d'une Némerte.
    C. R. Acad. Sci. Paris 270, 821-823.
Vinckier, D., Devauchelle, G. and Prensier, G. (1971b). Etude
    ultrastructurale du développement de la microsporidie
    Nosema vivieri (V.D. et P. 1970). *Protistologica*
    7, 273-287.
Vivares, C. P. and Tuzet, O. (1974). Ultrastructures comparees
    du développement de trois espèces de Microsporidies parasites
    de Crustacés Décapodes marins. *J. Protozool.* 21, 476.
Vivier, E. (1965). Étude, au microscope électronique, de la
    spore de *Metchnikovella hovassei* n.sp.; appartenance des
    Metchnikovellidae aux Microsporidies. *C. R. Acad. Sci. Paris*
    260, 6982-6984.
Vivier, E. (1965). Présence de microtubules intranucleaires chez
    Metchnikovella hovassei Vivier. *J. Microscopie* 4, 559-562.
Vivier, E. (1966). Observations ultrastructurales sur la
    microsporidie *Metchnikovella hovassei* Vivier. *J. Protozool.*
    13 (Suppl.), 41.
Vivier, E. and Schrevel, J. (1973). Étude en microscopie
    photonique et électronique de différents stades du cycle de
    Metchnikovella hovassei et observations sur la position
    systématique des Metchnikovellidae. *Protistologica* 9, 95-118.

Walker, M. H. and Hinsch, G. W. (1972). Ultrastructural ob-
    servations of a microsporidian protozoan parasite in
    Libinia dubia (Decapoda). *Z. Parasitenk.* 39, 17–26.
Ward, R. T. and Ward, E. (1968). The multiplication of Golgi
    bodies in the oocytes of *Rana pipiens*. *J. Microscopie*
    7, 1007–1020.
Weidner, E. (1970). Ultrastructural study of microsporidian
    development I. *Nosema* sp. Sprague, 1965 in *Callinectes
    sapidus* Rathbun. *Z. Zellforsch.* 105, 33–54.
Weidner, E. (1972). Ultrastructural study of microsporidian
    invasion into cells. *Z. Parasitenk.* 40, 227–242.
Weidner, E. and Trager, W. (1973). Adenosine triphosphate in the
    extracellular survival of an intracellular parasite
    (*Nosema michaelis*, Microsporidia). *J. Cell Biol.* 57,
    586–591.
Weiser, J. (1959). *Nosema laphygmae* n. sp. and the internal
    structure of the microsporidian spore. *J. Insect Pathol.*
    1, 52–59.
Weiser, J. (1961). Die Mikrosporidien als Parasiten der Insekten.
    Monogr. zur Angew. Entomologie 17, 149 pp.
Weiser, J. (1963). Zur Kenntnis der Mikrosporidien aus
    Chironomidenlarven III. *Zool. Anz.* 180, 226–230.
Weiser, J. and Zizka, Z. (1974). Stages in sporogony of
    Pleistophora debaisieuxi (Microsporidia). *J. Protozool.*
    21 (Suppl.), 476.
Wildführ, W. and Fritzsch, W. (1969). Die Feinstruktur der
    Sporen von *Nosema apis*. *Angew. Parasitol.* 10, 39–52.
Youssef, N. N. and Hammond, D. M. (1971). The fine structure of
    the developmental stages of the microsporidian *Nosema
    apis* Zander. *Tissue Cell* 3, 283–294.

ACKNOWLEDGEMENTS

This chapter is dedicated to the memory of my teacher, the late
Professor Otto Jírovec, founder of modern Czechoslovak protozoology
and an eminent microsporidiologist.

Thanks are expressed to Dr. J. Lom, Institute of Parasitology,
Czechoslovak Academy of Sciences, Prague, and Dr. J. Weiser,
Institute of Entomology, Czechoslovak Academy of Sciences, Prague,
for their critical comments and suggestions during the preparation
of the manuscript. Dr. E. Nohynková, Institute of Parasitology,
Czechoslovak Academy of Sciences, Prague, made all hand drawings.

ADDENDUM

After this chapter was written a paper on the fine structure
of *Ichthyosporidium* (another species in which cytoplasmic microtubules occur) by Sprague and Vernick (J. Protozool. 21, 667–677.
1974) appeared, providing additional evidence on several

microsporidian structures. These investigators were unable to observe any clear association of ribosomes with certain membranes in *Ichthyosporidium* probably because of inadequate preservation of the membranous material. Therefore, Sprague and Vernick consider the area of flattened sacs near the nucleus as a component of the Golgi apparatus. It should be pointed out, however, that ribosomes associated with similar flattened sacs have been observed in many microsporidian species. Apparently, this region is rough endoplasmic reticulum and not Golgi. Confusion about the nature of reticulum or Golgi) results from the failure of some fixation procedures to reveal the association between membranes and ribosomes.

Sprague and Vernick (1974) presently reject the idea of the microsporidian Golgi being of a "primitive type." According to them, the microsporidian Golgi has the same components as Golgi described in other organisms. This concept is based on the idea of inclusion into the Golgi of cytoplasmic lamellae thought by other authors to be rough endoplasmic reticulum. The idea that the polar tube proper becomes secondarily invested with membranes that are continuous with some of those in the polaroplast (Sprague and Vernick, 1968a; 1969) has recently been confirmed by the same authors' observations of *Ichthyosporidium*.

Sprague and Vernick believe that the posterior vacuole and its inclusion body originate from Golgi as "inclusion material" that contains a reticulated area bounded by membranes and an amorphous area.

Important data on microsporidian structure from Vinckier, 1973 thesis have recently been published: Vinckier, D. (1975). *Nosemoides* gen. n., *N. vivieri* (Vinckier, Devauchelle & Prensier, 1970) comb. nov. (Microsporidie); étude de la différenciation sporoblastique et genèse des différentes structures de la spore. *J. Protozool*. 22, 170-184.

The occurrence of spirally assembled polyribosomes in sporonts and in spores of *Octosporea* has been elaborated recently in the paper: Ormières, R., Baudoin, J., Brugerolle, G. and Pralavario, R. (1976). Ultrastructure de quelques stades de la Microsporidie *Octosporea muscaedomesticae* Flu 1911, parasite de *Ceratitis capitata* (Wied) (Diptera, Trypetidae). *J. Protozool*., In press.

Paring of the structures (Fig. 4) indicates that these may represent synaptonemal complexes. The occurrence of synaptonemal complexes, which in turn indicate the presence of meiosis and of sexuality in microsporidia, has recently been reported by Loubes, C. Maurand, J., Rousset-Galangau, M. Présence de complexes synaptonématiques dans le cycle biologique de *Gurleya chironomi* Loubès et Maurand, 1975; un argument en faveur d une sexualité chez les Microsporidies? C. R. Acad. Sci. Paris- Sér. D 282: 1025-1027, 1976.

Development of the Microsporidia

JIŘÍ VÁVRA

INSTITUTE OF PARASITOLOGY
CZECHOSLOVAK ACADEMY OF SCIENCES
PRAGUE, CZECHOSLOVAKIA

I. INTRODUCTION

Any student of microsporidia is confronted with two contradictory facts. One is the frustrating smallness of microsporidian developmental stages when seen in the light microscope and the difficulty to resolve some meaningful details in their structure. The second fact is that scientific literature (especially of the beginning of the century, when the art of scientific drawing flourished most) shows many, sometimes very detailed, drawings of complicated microsporidian life cycles.

Anyone coming across this controversy will obviously ask: Are we less competent observers than our scientific predecessors were? Do the microsporidia develop rigidly according to schemes depicted in the literature? What is the present status of knowledge of the microsporidian development? What is the contribution of modern methods such as electron microscopy and tissue culture to the study of microsporidian development? Which problems still remain to be solved in the research of microsporidian life cycles?

The present consideration is rather an essay on the subject with no attempt to analyze individual life cycles described in the past. After all, this would hardly be possible. Despite all attention given to the research of microsporidian development, there are still considerable gaps in our understanding of some life cycle events even in such frequently studied species as *Nosema apis* or *N. bombycis*.

The purpose of this chapter will be fulfilled if the reader is provided with the basic understanding of the microsporidian life cycle and if some of the above-mentioned questions are answered.

The structural aspects of individual stages are treated very briefly as they are the subject of a special chapter in this book. Further data on microsporidian development are available in the monographs by Kudo (1924), Weiser (1961) and in the papers by Vávra (1970, 1974).

II. MICROSPORIDIAN DEVELOPMENT--DEFINITION OF ITS STAGES

Microsporidia are obligatory intracellular parasites, incapable, as far as we know, of active existence outside of the host cell. The life cycle of the microsporidian parasite spans the period between the entrance of the infective germ (sporoplasm) into the cell and the formation of durable spores at the end of the cycle. Both the germ and the spore are unicellular in nature. The microsporidian development consists of several cell cycles in which the parasite grows and divides by schizogony, that includes binary and multiple fission (see Glossary). Binary fission is, however, less frequent because in the microsporidian cell cycle the karyokinesis occurs repeatedly before cytokinesis. Thus, plasmodial stages of various shape and size are formed. These separate later into single cells which change into spores and terminate the development (Fig. 1).

The life cycle has two distinct phases: (*i*) *the vegetative phase or merogony* (commonly called "schizogony"), during which the number of parasites rapidly increases and the infection is spread through the cells, tissues, and organs of the host; and (*ii*) *sporulation*, during which additional multiplication of the parasite occurs and resistant spores are formed. Stages of the merogonial phase of the life cycle (called also vegetative stages or trophozoites) comprise: (a) sporoplasm--the invasive stage; and (b) meront (schizont)--the main multiplicative stage by means of which the infection is spread within the host. The stages of the sporulation phase of the life cycle include: (a) sporont--the initial stage of the additional multiplicative sequence (sporogony) and a stage possibly involved in the autogamic recombination of genes; and (b) sporoblast--a stage undergoing conspicuous morphogenesis when changing into the spore (spore morphogenesis--sporogenesis).

As will be shown elsewhere, the life cycle stages of the merogony and of the sporulation phase are different not only in their structure but also in their relationship to the host cell. The number of parasite generations formed during merogony and during sporogony is different in various microsporidia. In some species the merogony sequence is relatively short and the microsporidian multiplies extensively in the sporogony (*Pleistophora*). In some other forms the vegetative part is the most important, whereas the sporogony is short and the number of spores originating from single sporont is strictly limited (*Nosema, Encephalitozoon, Thelohania,* and others). Cellular condition is supposed to trigger the sporulation (Ishihara, 1969).

Microsporidia are eukaryotic organisms and the structure of all developmental stages is cellular. The stages prior to the spore are structurally simple cells with nuclear component surrounded by cytoplasm with its usual organelles. The nuclear component may be either single nucleus ("monokaryotic state") or two, more or less permanently coupled nuclei--the diplokaryon ("diplokaryotic state"). In some species both types of the nuclear component occur at different phases of the life cycle. In contrast to the developmental stages, the microsporidian spore is a highly differentiated cell (however, its cellular nature is not very obvious), endowed with a protective envelope and possessing a long evaginable tube by which the spore content, including the sporoplasm, is released with explosive force.

III. GENERAL SCHEME OF THE LIFE CYCLE

A. *THE INVASION PROCESS AND THE SPOROPLASM*

The life cycle starts with the injection of the sporoplasm by the evaginating polar tube into a host cell. This event, much discussed in the past (see Lom and Vávra, 1963 for details) is now confirmed beyond any doubt by electron microscope observations (Ishi-

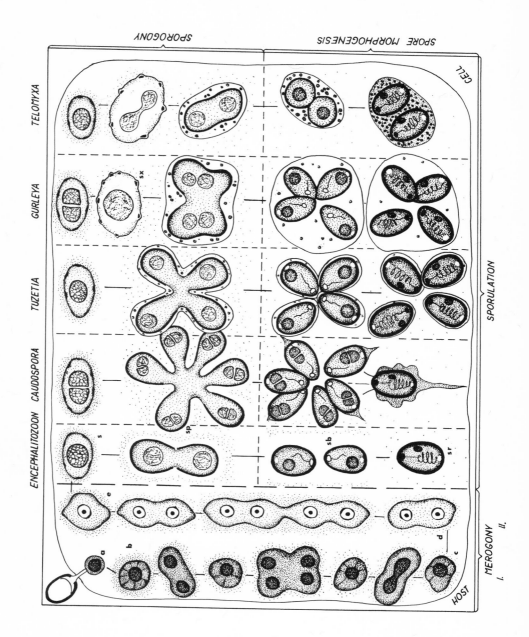

Fig. 1. Schematic representation of the microsporidian life cycle. a, entry of the sporoplasm into the host cell through the polar tube of the spore; b-c, stages of the first merogonial cycle; d-e, stages of the second merogonial cycle; s, sporont; sp, sporogonial plasmodium; sb, sporoblast; sr, spore. The zygote which presumably occurs in some species = sx. The course of sporulation in several microsporidian genera is presented to show various nuclear conditions and various cell membrane differentiations occurring during sporulation. The parasite-host cell interaction and the progressive lysis of the host cytoplasm during sporulation is also shown.

hara, 1968; Weidner, 1972). The freshly injected sporoplasm is a
simple cell with the nuclear component, some cytoplasm without
usual cytoplasmic organelles but with an array of membranes (Ishihara, 1968; Weidner, 1972; Weidner and Trager, 1973). Many authors
in the past (see Kudo, 1924; Weiser, 1961; Steche, 1965) believed
that the sporoplasm is capable of amoeboid movement and penetrates
actively into host cells. None of the more recent observations
confirms that phenomenon. After 15-20 minutes within the host cell
there is nuclear and cytoplasmic rearrangement in the sporoplasm
and the synthesis of the endoplasmic reticulum begins (Weidner,
1972). The sporoplasm changes into the meront by growth and by
differentiation of cytoplasmic organelles.

B. MEROGONY AND THE MERONT

The meront initially is a rounded cell, several microns in size,
with one rather compact nuclear component. The meront grows in
size, its nuclear component divides and small plasmodia are formed.
These separate later into single cells which evidently are able to
start the merogonial cycle again. In some species there seem to
exist two structurally different generations of meronts. Whereas
the first generation is represented by small cells with small compact nuclear component ("micronuclear stages" of Weiser, 1961) and
small, rounded plasmodia, in the second merogonial generation the
parasite grows into long ribbon-like formations with several large
nuclei ("macronuclear stages" of Weiser, 1961) with prominent kary-
osomes arranged in a single row ("Schizontenschlauche"). These entities later cleave into shorter fusiform segments.

The existence of two merogony generations in *N. apis* has recently
been proved beyond any doubt by using the technique of very thin
sections observed in the light microscope (Gray *et al.,* 1969).
Curiously, the electron microscope does not reveal any other difference in meronts than simply quantitative distribution and development of endoplasmic reticulum and of the Golgi apparatus (Youssef
and Hammond, 1971).

An unsolved problem of the merogonial part of the life cycle is
how the meronts are distributed through the tissues of the host.
Kudo (1924) believed that meronts are incapable of active movement.
This opinion is shared by most present investigators. On the other
hand, Ishihara (1969) observed a small binucleate form in *N. bombycis*
that leaves a host cell, migrates freely, and then penetrates another
cell ("secondary infective form"). It is not certain whether this
infective cell is truly a meront because it appears at the time when
spores are already beginning to form. So far, Ishihara's observation
remains isolated and unconfirmed. It has been firmly established
that in some microsporidia meronts are transported by cells with phagocytic activity and are incorporated with them later into specific
tissues (Cali and Briggs, 1967; Weidner, 1970).

Microsporidian meronts are structurally simple cells limited by a unit type membrane. It has been observed in several species that this membrane is involved in endocytosis and that the surface of contact with the host cell cytoplasm is increased due to vesicular or finger-like protrusions interdigitated intimately with the host cell cytoplasm. Besides the nuclear component, there is little cytoplasmic differentiation within the meront: several cisternae of the rough endoplasmic reticulum, some vesicles of the smooth type of reticulum, small amount of freely scattered ribosomes, and one or several areas where dense vesicles are accumulated (Golgi zone).

C. SPORULATION

At a certain period of the life cycle, single cells resulting from merogony enter the second phase called sporulation. Sporulation comprises two distinct periods: (*i*) sporogony, in which the sporont, the initial cell in sporulation, grows and multiplies by binary or multiple fission; and (*ii*) spore morphogenesis, in which sporoblasts, issued from the division of the sporont, transform into spores.

The end of merogony and the onset of sporulation is characterized by structural changes of the parasite and especially of its nuclear component. As will be shown later, the nature of these changes is still poorly understood and the explanation of their significance is a subject of considerable controversy. Research problems of the initial stages of sporulation involve three questions: (*i*) What is the nature of cells entering into the sporulation sequence? (*ii*) How is the sporont characterized? and (*iii*) What is the behavior of parasite nuclear component at the end of merogony and beginning of sporogony?

1. Nature of cells entering sporulation

It seems that in some microsporidia, normal meronts change directly into sporonts due to the influence of environmental factors. Existence of this simple life cycle pattern has been confirmed by recent observations of *Encephalitozoon cuniculi* grown in tissue culture (Vávra *et al.*, 1972) as well as by electron microscopic observations of the same microsporidan developing in mice (Sprague and Vernick, 1971).

According to Weiser (1961), diplokaryotic meronts ("diplokarya") occur at the end of merogony in some species and these undergo nuclear fusion (autogamy), thus changing into sporonts.

In still another microsporidia an additional short merogonial sequence has been described from which binucleate cells with either "daughter" or "cousin" diplokarya originate (Fig. 2; Kudo, 1924). These cells have been named "sporont mother cells" and by fusion of

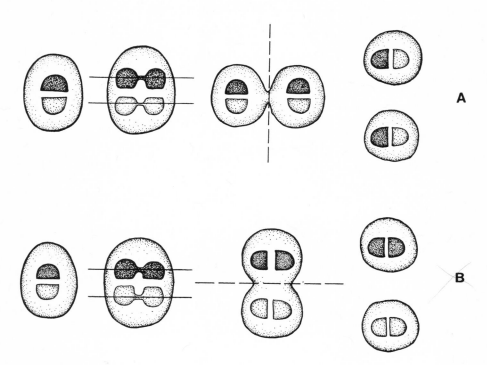

Fig. 2.   Two possible modes of karyo- and cytokinesis in a
          diplokaryotic cell. In A, two cells with "cousin"
          diplokarya originate. In B, two cells with "daughter"
          diplokarya result from the division. Typically, the
          plane of cytoplasmic cleavage (dashed line) is perpen-
          dicular to the plane of the preceeding nuclear separation
          (solid line). The mode shown in B requires a parallel
          alignment of both planes and its existence is doubtful.

their nuclei presumably sporonts arise. The existence of the sporont mother cell remains to be confirmed. The occurrence of "daughter diplokarya" is rather improbable as it would require an unusual
alignment of the nuclear spindle and of the plane along which
daughter cells separate.

According to Mercier (see Kudo, 1924), two meronts fuse to form a
sporont. However, fusion of whole cells at the end of merogony has
never been proved.

2. Characterization of sporont

The generally accepted definition, coined by Debaisieux (see
Glossary), says that sporont is a cell which divides directly into
sporoblasts and is identical with zygote when the latter is present.
This definition, however simple, is difficult to apply. In some
microsporidia the cells which initiate the sporulation are structurally quite similar to meronts and are indistinguishable from them un-
less the electron microscope is used. Another problem is that it is
difficult to be absolutely certain whether a particular cell divides
directly into sporoblasts without any interposed cytoplasmic separation. Electron microscopy is of great assistance in distinguishing
early sporonts from meronts. In an electron micrograph the early
sporont is characterized by appearance of a second membrane around
the cell ("exosporont membrane" of Overstreet and Weidner, 1974) or
the appearance of irregularly spaced patches of dense material deposited on the outside of the sporont limiting membrane(s) (Cali,
1971; Vávra, 1973) or both. Another useful marker is the appearance
of a clear, structureless halo between the parasite and the adjacent
host cell cytoplasm. With the exception of the limiting membrane,
the fine structure of the meront is very similar to that of the
sporont.

3. Microsporidian nucleus at the onset of sporulation

In some microsporidia, cells with relatively large diplokaryon and
with visible chromosomes suddenly appear at the end of merogony.
These cells, because of the prominence of their nuclear component,
have been named "diplokarya" (see Glossary). Their behavior and
fate is undoubtedly the most controversial part of the microsporidian life cycle.

Four types of microsporidian development exist according to the
occurrence of single nucleus or diplokaryon in meronts and sporonts
(Kudo, 1930). In the first type, uninucleate meronts give rise to
uninucleate sporonts. In the second type, uninucleate meronts
change into diplokaryotic meronts; their nuclei later fuse and uninucleate sporonts are produced. In the third type, diplokaryotic
meronts give rise to diplokaryotic sporonts. In the fourth type,

diplokaryotic sporoplasm gives rise to uninucleate meronts which turn into diplokaryotic meronts. Uninucleate sporonts are produced by fusion of nuclei.

The existence of the first and of the third developmental type is exemplified in the life cycles of *E. cuniculi* and *N. bombycis*, respectively, and is well documented by electron microscopic observations (Cali, 1971; Sprague and Vernick, 1971; Youssef and Hammond, 1971).

As for the existence of the second and fourth types, there are microsporidia in which alternation of monokaryotic and diplokaryotic stages has been demonstrated by electron microscopy, e.g., in *Pleistophora debaisieuxi* the meronts are diplokaryotic cells, whereas sporonts and all subsequent stages have single, unpaired nuclei (Vávra, unpublished observations). Another example is that of *Ameson* (syn. *Nosema*) *michaelis* wherein meronts are initially monokaryotic and later become diplokaryotic; the cells are monokaryotic during sporulation (Weidner, 1970). Other examples of alternation of merogonic stages with diplokarya and sporulation stages with single nuclei were pointed out by Maurand and Vey (1973).

It is not exactly understood how the monokaryotic state in the sporont is achieved. One possibility is that both members of the diplokaryon tandem separate at the time that cytoplasmic division splits the originally diplokaryotic cell into two monokaryotic cells. Observations that both nuclei in the diplokaryon of typically diplokaryotic species tend to be less adherent during late merogony and sporulation (Walker and Hinsch, 1972; Ormieres and Sprague, 1973; Youssef and Hammond, 1971) support this explanation. However, the idea that the diplokaryon simply separates into two single nuclei is speculative. Some investigators believe that the monokaryotic condition is achieved in the sporont by fusion of the two nuclei ("pronuclei") of the diplokaryon and that such fusion is a sexual process similar to autogamy (see Kudo, 1924, 1930; Weiser, 1961).

Whether this nuclear fusion exists and for what reason are central questions concerning the microsporidian life cycle. Although karyogamy may be ascertained by direct microscopic observation, it is rather difficult to unequivocally distinguish karyogamy from karyokinesis. Consequently, the electron micrograph of diplokaryon fusion published by Sprague and Vernick (1968) is debatable.

Indirect confirmation of nuclear fusion may also be made from observations of the chromosome cycle. If there is karyogamy, there must be, somewhere later in the cycle, a meiotic division which would restore the number of chromosomes. Due to the smallness of nuclei, the number of chromosomes (usually 6-12; probably N=4, 2N= 8 in *Glugea weissenbergi*) is only approximately known and for a very few microsporidian species (Weiser, 1943, 1961; Sprague and Vernick, 1968). This means that the ploidy of the microsporidian nucleus, either in the monokaryotic or diplokaryotic state, has not been firmly established. So far, it is only known that the presum-

ed zygotic nucleus is relatively large and its chromosomes are easily visible. During succeeding division(s) the chromosomes are arranged in typical mitotic figures ("stages of large mitosis" of
Weiser, 1961). There is only meager evidence that the first division of the presumed zygotic nucleus is meiotic and that chromosome
synapsis immediately follows karyogamy. Thus, it appears that, at
least in some species, the only diploid stage is the zygote (sporont) (Sprague and Vernick, 1968).

To date, there is no solid structural proof of the occurrence of
nuclear fusion in microsporidia. Elucidation of synaptonemal complexes, characteristic of chromosome pairing, would be final proof
for the occurrence of meiosis (and karyogamy) in microsporidia.[1]
Presently, we can only agree with Sprague and Vernick (1968) that
"our present knowledge of sexuality and the chromosome cycle is
quite incomplete and our concepts only vague and tentative".

D.   SPOROGONY

Once the sporont is established, it grows and its nuclear component divides (sporogony) (Figs. 3 and 4). The course of sporogony
is different in various microsporidia; this feature has been exploit-
ed in microsporidian taxonomy (see Sprague, Classification and Phy-
logeny of the Microsporidia, this monograph). The sporont nucleus
divides once or several times. As stated, the first division presumably is meiotic, at least in some species. Further divisions
are evidently mitotic. The first nuclear division may be immediately followed by cytokinesis. In this case, two cells (future
sporoblasts) are issued from a single sporont. Such is the developmental pattern in several genera of microsporidia, e.g. in *Encephalitozoon* and *Nosema*. In some other genera, there are several divisions of the sporont nucleus without subsequent cytoplasmic separation, producing sporogonial plasmodia of various sizes. Later, by
constriction of the cell membrane of the plasmodium, unicellular
buds (future sporoblasts) are pinched off. In this way, variable
numbers of sporoblasts (and of spores) are formed from each sporont.
This number is highly regular in some species, but rather variable
in others. As will be discussed later, environmental conditions
may influence the course of sporogony in many microsporidian species.
Supposedly, sporonts are non-motile cells, but a cytoplasmic protuberance "suggestive of a locomotory organelle" has been found in
sporonts of *Unikaryon legeri* (Canning and Nicholas, 1974). This
protuberance, however, seems to be a protrusion left behind after
the cleavage of a ribbon-like plasmodium.

In some microsporidia, the sporogonial stages are enveloped only
by a thick membrane complex (cell "wall") homologous to the original
membrane of the sporont (suborders Diplokaryonina and Monokaryonina)
whereas in others an additional thin membrane (pansporoblastic membrane) is differentiated around the sporogonial plasmodium. This

Fig. 3.   Sporulation stages in *Pleistophora debaisieuxi*. a,
          diplokaryotic meronts entering the sporulation sequence
          (chromosomes are visible as irregular coils); b,
          monokaryotic sporonts with very large nuclei (xygote?);
          c, the same stage as in b, but showing intranuclear
          spindle of the first sporogonial division; d, further
          progress of the first sporogonial division; e, second
          sporogonial division, the cytoplasm starts to cleave
          along the plane perpendicular to the plane of the first
          karyokinesis; f, sporogonial plasmodium more advanced
          in the second sporogonial karyokinesis; g, a similar
          stage like in f but the cytoplasmic separation is more
          advanced; h, last sporogonial karyokinesis. The cyto-
          plasmic cleavage of the sporogonial plasmodium has pro-
          gressed to such extent that individual cells are
          connected only by narrow isthmus. Single cells formed
          at the end of this division are the sporoblasts. i,
          cluster of young spores. Arrows point to active spindle
          plaques at poles of the intranuclear spindle; arrowheads
          indicate structures occurring regularly near the isthmus
          of dividing nuclei, presumably "dormant" spindle plaques
          of the next nuclear division. Line=5 μm. "In vivo",
          phase contrast.

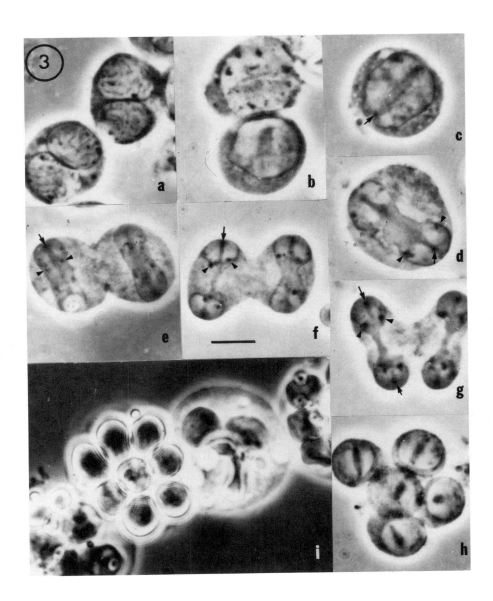

Fig. 4.   Sporogonial plasmodia of *Pleistophora simulii*.   a,
          plasmodium in which cytoplasmic cleavage has not yet
          started; b, plasmodium cleaving into sporoblasts. ps,
          membrane of the pansporoblast; s, "secretion"; sp,
          body of the sporogonial plasmodium. Line=5 µm.
          "In vivo", phase contrast.

Fig. 5.   Sporulation stages of *Nosema algerae*. Note the increase
          in the size of the nucleus between a and c and again the
          condensation of the nuclear volume between d and h.
          Giemsa stain. Line=5 µm (From Vávra and Undeen, 1970).

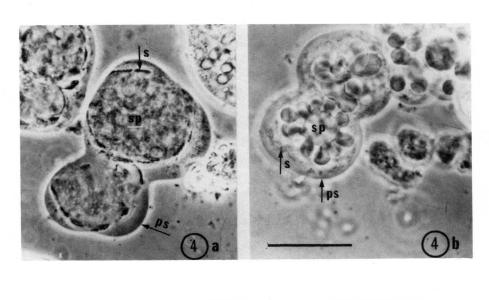

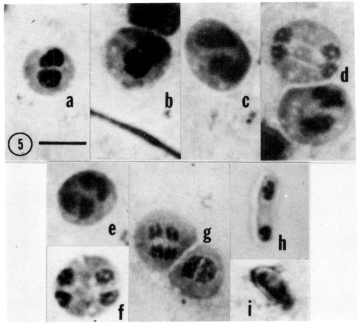

membrane then envelopes, much like a sachet, the sporoblasts originating from one sporont (suborder Pansporoblastina). In the family
Tuzetiidae the pansporoblast membrane is somewhat closely applied
to the wall of sporogonial plasmodium and remains so during division. In this family, each sporoblast has its own pansporoblast
sachet.

According to Weiser (1961), each sporont is provided with two
regulating mechanisms. The first regulates the number of divisions
of the sporont; the second controls proportionality and size of the
cells in the sporogonial cycle. Weiser believes that the first
mechanism functions properly up to the 5th or 6th division of the
sporont nucleus. This is why the number of nuclei in plasmodia
with 2, 4, 8, 16 or 32 nuclei is usually more regular than in large
plasmodia with 64, 128 or more nuclei.

Whereas a sporont is structurally similar to a meront, the structure of more advanced sporogonial stages is clearly different. The
cell membrane is thicker and the electron microscope reveals it
represented by one or two unit membranes covered by a thick electron-dense coat. The density of the cytoplasm also is increased.
There are more ribosomes and endoplasmic reticulum in the later
sporogonial stages. Further, there is a conspicuously greater
abundance of vesicular profiles of smooth membranes as well as
larger Golgi zones with more opaque vesicles. And additional
membrane (pansporoblastic membrane) differentiates at the
surface of the sporont or sporogonial plasmodium in many species.
In the space between the pansporoblast membrane and the membrane
of the sporont or sporogonial plasmodium ("pansporoblast cavity"--
or "pansporoblast determinate area" as Overstreet and Weidner, 1974,
call it) there appear dense inclusions which are apparently secreted from the microsporidian cell. The significance of these entities are discussed later.

E. THE SPOROBLAST

Single cells resulting from the division of the sporont or of
the sporogonial plasmodium are the sporoblasts. The sporoblast is
a rather clearly defined stage that immediately preceeds the spore.
It is the stage at which spore organelles start to form and the
microsporidian cell, for the first time, acquires definite polarity.
Through light optics, the sporoblast is recognizable by its dense
cytoplasm limited by a thick cell wall. The cytoplasm of the sporoblast is rather dense, which may be partially explained by the condensation of the cell volume. Condensation begins in the sporoblast stage and proceeds during early spore development.

F. SPORE MORPHOGENESIS

The final event of the microsporidian life cycle is gradual transformation of the sporoblast to the spore. Electron microscopic observations of this part of the life cycle demonstrate that polar filament and polar sac are usually differentiated first, followed by the polaroplast and posterior vacuole. The last event is formation of the thick endospore layer of the spore wall. However complicated the spore morphogenesis may seem to be, it is a rather fast process; generally, not many transforming sporoblasts are encountered in ultrathin sections.

IV. MICROSPORIDIAN DEVELOPMENT--PROBLEMS AND COMMENTS

Earlier literature abounds with excellent drawings of life cycles of individual microsporidia. One must realize that these schemes were constructed to some degree from individual interpretation and may not be accurate. Inaccuracies result from: (*i*) smallness of the various life stages, the structural details of which approach the limits of resolution attainable by light optics; (*ii*) presence of artifacts which, due to limited understanding of microsporidian structure, has in the past not been recognized; (*iii*) difficulty to arrange individual stages in proper sequence; (*iv*) inability to observe the full range of developmental stages in a single host animal; and (*v*) failure to recognize the adaptability of the microsporidians to environmental conditions.

A. ENVIRONMENTAL INFLUENCE ON THE LIFE CYCLE

Recent observations reveal that the microsporidian life cycle is not a rigid scheme unaffected by various environmental conditions. This situation is exemplified by the temperature-dependent development of *N. necatrix* which at higher temperatures produces *Nosema*-like spores and at lower temperatures produces *Thelohania*-like pansporoblasts (Maddox, unpublished results; Fowler and Reeves, 1974). Hazard and Weiser (1968) found that one species of *Parathelohania* may have two completely different types of development; one corresponding to the genus *Nosema* and the other to the genus *Thelohania*; the kind of development depends on whether the host is a larval or adult mosquito. This duality in life cycle has recently been found in several other microsporidian species that inhabit mosquitoes (Hazard and Anthony, 1974) and it may be that inclement temperature of the mosquitoes is also a morphogenetic determinant.

Temperature and physiological condition of the host have profound influence on the life cycle of *N. apis*. In summer bees, the parasite develops through a relatively simple life cycle that does not include karyogamy. In winter bees, the life cycle is more compli-

cated and includes nuclear fusion (Steche, 1965). Electron microscopic observations by Youssef and Hammond (1971) confirm that there
are structural differences in some stages depending on whether the
hosts are winter or summer bees.

Striking examples of the influence of environmental factors upon
development are provided by other microsporidia living in mosquitoes.
In some particular host-parasite combinations, sporogony is suppres-
sed in females (Kellen *et al*., 1965). In hybrid mosquitoes where
one of the parents is an unsuitable host, the development seems to
proceed normally during merogony and early sporulation, whereas
spore morphogenesis proceeds abnormally and results in aberant spores
(Kellen *et al*., 1966). Remarkably, in both examples the sporulation
phase is more sensitive. This phenomenon seems to be characteristic
of microsporidian cycles; irregularities in the sporulation phase are
evoked by unknown stimuli and spores of various size (macrospores and
microspores) and sometimes of various shape are produced. It has
been suggested, although not confirmed, that spores of different size
occurring in a single species, serve different functions--either in
a propagation of the parasite within or outside the original host
animal (see Kudo, 1930).

It has also been reported that there are two different kinds of
life cycles within the same tissue of a single host. Meronts of
Stempellia milleri develop in haemocytes, whereas sporogony takes
place in the fat body. One aspect of the cycle involves diplokaryotic meronts that give rise to diplokaryotic sporoblasts and to diplokaryotic thick-walled spores. In another aspect, there is a fusion
of diplokaryon nuclei in the sporont. Subsequently, the sporont
grows into sporogonial plasmodia with 2-16 nuclei that cleave into
monokaryotic sporoblasts and thin-walled spores containing one nucleus (Hazard and Fukuda, 1974). An explanation for this dichotomy of
life cycle remains elusive. Another species of the genus *Stempellia*,
S. simulii, is reported having two types of sporogonial plasmodia
(pansporoblasts). In one type, either eight or sixteen spores are
produced whereas in the other, twelve spores invariably occur (Maur-
and and Manier, 1968).

B. PROBLEMS RELATED TO THE MICROSPORIDIAN NUCLEUS

The nuclei are very small and compact in merogony whereas in sporogony (especially at the beginning) they are relatively large and
exhibit characteristic chromosome profiles during mitosis. Later,
in advanced sporogony, the nucleus decreases in size with each successive division (Figs. 3-5).

Size fluctuation of the nucleus and the sudden appearance of chromosomes raises another unresolved question. Does the change in the
structure of the nucleus merely reflect an alteration in the extent
of nuclear condensation or does it indicate a variation in the number
of chromosomes, or both?

Nuclear division in the meront has been described as "amitosis" (see Kudo, 1924; Gingrich, 1965), the size of the sporont nucleus being considered the result of nuclear fusion. Weiser (1961) speaks about "grain-like" chromosomes in the dividing meront nuclei and the chromosomes in sporogonial stages as "thin and hook-like". The occurrence of amitosis in cells which carry the genetic information to the progeny is highly improbable. Furthermore, the size and structure of chromosomes of a given species theoretically is constant in each cell cycle. Nuclear fusion at the onset of sporogony has not been established and there is no information about the DNA content of the microsporidian nucleus during any of the life cycle stages. In the absence of more complete data, it is presumed that the microsporidian nucleus divides by mitosis throughout the entire cycle (indeed there is some e.m. evidence in this sense). Although electron micrographs depict such division, the chromosomes are so tightly packed during merogony that they cannot be individually resolved. Their sudden appearance at the sporont stage could be merely an optical effect because of the increase in the total volume of the nucleus.

C. PLASTICITY OF THE LIFE CYCLE

It is during the life cycle that the parasite multiplies inside its host and assures successful transmission of itself to other receptive hosts. Development of the various life cycle stages must be done so as to not seriously damage the host organism until at least spores have been formed. The parasite, completely dependent on the host for food supply, must sporulate before the infected cell collapses. Obviously, the microsporidian has to maintain an equilibrium with its host in order to successfully reach the spore stage. Ishihara (1969) believes that a certain cellular condition triggers microsporidian sporulation.

That host cell condition is important in regulating the microsporidian life cycle has been inferred from gradients of various developmental stages observed within infected cells (Maurand, 1966; Sprague and Vernick, 1966, 1971). In the egg condition, microsporidian development is arrested for a considerable time until embryo formation has begun (see Weiser, 1961). Obviously, the parasite must be plastic enough to respond quickly to stimuli that may induce or delay sporulation.

The microsporidian life cycle can be relatively short. A generation time of 24 hours has been reported (see Milner, 1972). Ishihara (1970) confirmed by electron microscopy that spore formation in N. bombycis begins as early as 48 hours after infection. Although there is some synchrony of the life cycle within a single host, there are always some prespore developmental forms that remain throughout the cycle and probably serve as a reserve for possible additional multiplication. The possibility that differentiated sporoblasts may revert to earlier stages has been suggested (Maurand, 1966), though such a phenomenon is unlikely.

SUMMARY

Sporoplasm injected into a host cell by the polar tube undergoes several cell cycles in which cytoplasmic separation is usually delayed relevant to nuclear division. All development occurs intracellularly, either in the cell of original entry or in a cell to which the infection was secondarily disseminated. The modes of dissemination are not well known.

In the merogonial sequence, the parasite is limited by a single unit membrane and is in immediate contact with the host cell cytoplasm. In the sporulation phase, the parasite develops a complicated cell wall and an "empty" zone appears around it.

Some species have single, unpaired nuclei throughout the whole life cycle; other species are diplokaryotic. There is no explanation for this difference. Some species alternate diplokaryotic stages (typically in merogony) with monokaryotic stages in sporogony. It is not well known how the monokaryotic condition is achieved, but it is supposed that karyogamy occurs in the sporont. The number of chromosomes in the microsporidian nucleus and their behaviour are not well known.

In many species the pattern of life stages is significantly influenced by host cell condition, suggesting that microsporidian development is adaptable.

REFERENCES

Cali, A. (1971). Morphogenesis in the genus *Nosema*. *Proc. Int. Colloq. Insect Pathol.*, *4th*, College Park, Maryland, 1970, pp. 431-438.

Cali, A. and Briggs, J. D. (1967). The biology and life history of *Nosema tracheophila* sp.n. (Protozoa: Cnidospora: Microsporidea) found in *Coccinella septempunctata* Linnaeus (Coleoptera: Coccinellidae). *J. Invert. Pathol.* 9, 515-522.

Canning, E. U. and Nicholas, J. P. (1974). Light and electron microscope observations on *Unikaryon legeri* (Microsporida, Nosematidae), a parasite of the metacercaria of *Meigymnophallus minutus* in *Cardium edule*. *J. Invert. Pathol.* 23, 92-100.

Fowler, J. L. and Reeves, E. L. (1974). Spore dimorphism in a microsporidian isolate. *J. Protozool.* 21, 538-542.

Gingrich, R. E. (1965). *Thelohania tabani* sp.n., a microsporidian from larvae of the black horse fly, *Tabanus atratus* Fabricius. *J. Invert. Pathol.* 7, 236-240.

Gray, F. H., Cali, A. and Briggs, J. D. (1969). Intracellular stages in the life cycle of the microsporidian *Nosema apis*. *J. Invert. Pathol.* 14, 391-394.

Hazard, E. and Anthony, D. (1974). A redescription of the genus *Parathelohania* Codreanu 1966 (Microsporida: Protozoa) with a reexamination of previously described species of *Thelohania* Henneguy 1892 and descriptions of two new species of *Parathelohania* from anopheline mosquitoes. U.S. Dept. Agricul., Agricul. Res. Serv., Washington, D.C., Tech. Bull. No. 1505, 26 pages.

Hazard, E. and Fukuda, T. (1974). *Stempellia milleri* sp.n. (Microsporida: Nosematidae) in the mosquito *Culex pipiens quinquefasciatus* Say. *J. Protozool.* 21, 497-504.

Hazard, E. and Weiser, J. (1968). Spores of *Thelohania* in adult female *Anopheles*: development and transovarial transmission and redescription of *T. legeri* Hesse and *T. obesa* Kudo. *J. Protozool.* 15, 817-823.

Ishihara, R. (1968). Some observations on the fine structure of sporoplasm discharged from spores of a microsporidian, *Nosema bombycis*. *J. Invert. Pathol.* 12, 245-258.

Ishihara, R. (1969). The life cycle of *Nosema bombycis* as revealed in tissue culture cells of *Bombyx mori*. *J. Invert. Pathol.* 14, 316-320.

Ishihara, R. (1970). Fine structure of *Nosema bombycis* (Microsporidia, Nosematidae) developing in the silkworm (*Bombyx mori*) - I. Bull. Coll. Agricul. Vet. Med., Nihon Univ., No. 27, 84-91.

Kellen, W. R., Chapman, H. C., Clark, T. B. and Lindegren, J. E. (1965). Host-parasite relationship of some *Thelohania* from mosquitoes (Nosematidae: Microsporidia). *J. Invert. Pathol.* 7, 161-166.

Kellen, W. R., Clark, T. B., Lindegren, J. E. and Sanders, R. D. (1966). Development of *Thelohania californica* in two hybrid mosquitoes. *Exp. Parasitol.* 18, 251-254.

Kudo, R. (1924). A biologic and taxonomic study of the microsporidia. *Illinois Biol. Monogr.* 9, 1-268.

Kudo, R. (1930). Microsporidia. *In* "Problems and Methods of Research in Protozoology" (R. Hegner and J. Andrews, eds.), pp. 325-347, Macmillan Co., New York.

Lom, J. and Vávra, J. (1963). The mode of sporoplasm extrusion in microsporidian spores. *Acta Protozool.* 1, 81-89.

Maurand, J. (1966). *Plistophora simulii* (Lutz et Splendore, 1904), Microsporidie parasite des larves de Simulies: cycle, ultrastructure, ses rapports avec *Thelohania bracteata* (Strickland, 1913). *Bull. Soc. Zool.* 91, 621-629.

Maurand, J. (1973). Recherches biologiques sur les Microsporidies des larves de Simulies. Thèse, Univ. Sci. Tech. Languedoc, 199 pages.

Maurand, J. and Manier, J.-F. (1968). Une Microsporidie nouvelle pour les larves de Simulies. *Protistologica* 3, 445-449.

Maurand, J. and Vey, A. (1973). Etudes histopathologique et ultrastructurale de *Thelohania contejeani* (Microsporida, Nosematidae) parasite de l'Ecrevisse *Austropotamobius pallipes* Lereboullet. *Ann. Parasitol. Hum. Comp.* 48, 411-421.

Milner, R. J. (1972). *Nosema whitei,* a microsporidan pathogen of some species of *Tribolium.* I. Morphology, life cycle and generation time. *J. Invert. Pathol.* 19, 231-238.

Ormières, R. and Sprague, V. (1973). A new family, new genus and new species allied to the Microsporida. *J. Invert. Pathol.* 21, 224-240.

Sprague, V. and Vernick, S. H. (1966). Light and electron microscope study of developing stages of *Glugea* sp. (Microsporida) in the stickleback *Apeltes quadracus.* *Amer. Zool.* 6, 555-556.

Sprague, V. and Vernick, S. H. (1968). Light and electron microscope study of a new species of *Glugea* (Microsporidia, Nosematidae) in the 4-spored stickleback *Apeltes quadracus.* *J. Protozool.* 15, 547-571.

Sprague, V. and Vernick, S. H. (1971). The ultrastructure of *Encephalitozoon cuniculi* (Microsporida-Nosematidae) and its taxonomic significance. *J. Protozool.* 18, 560-569.

Steche, W. (1965). Zur Ontologie von *Nosema apis* Zander in Mitteldarm der Arbeitsbiene. *Bull. Apicole* 8, 181-212.

Vávra, J. (1970). Physiological, morphological, and ecological considerations of some microsporidia and gregarines. *In* "Ecology and Physiology of Parasites" (A. M. Fallis, Ed.), Symposium, Univ. Toronto, pp. 92-103. University of Toronto Press.

Vávra, J. (1974). Developmental cycles of Protozoa (other than Coccidia). *In* "Actualités Protozoologiques" (P. de Puytorac et J. Grain, eds.), Rés. Discuss. 4e Congr. Intern. Protozool. 1, pp. 99-108. Clermont-Ferrand, Université de Clermont.

Vávra, J., Bedrník, P. and Činátl, J. (1972). Isolation and in vitro cultivation of the mammalian microsporidian *Encephalitozoon cuniculi.* *Folia Parasitol.* *(Praha)* 19, 349-354.

Vávra, J. and Undeen, A. (1970). *Nosema algerae* n.sp. (Cnidospora, Microsporida) a pathogen in a laboratory colony of *Anopheles stephensi* Liston (Diptera, Culicidae). *J. Protozool.* 17, 240-249.

Walker, M. H. and Hinsch, G. W. (1972). Ultrastructural observations of a microsporidian protozoan parasite in *Libinia dubia* (Decapoda). I. Early spore development. *Z. Parasitenk.* 39, 17-26.

Weidner, E. (1970). Ultrastructural study of microsporidian development. I. *Nosema* sp. Sprague 1965 in *Callinectes sapidus* Rathbun. *Z. Zellforsch.* 105, 33-54.

Weidner, E. (1972). Ultrastructural study of microsporidian invasion into cells. *Z. Parasitenk.* 40, 227-242.

Weidner, E. and Trager, W. (1973). Adenosine triphosphate in the extracellular survival of an intracellular parasite (*Nosema michaelis,* Microsporidia). *J. Cell Biol.* 57, 586-591.

Weiser, J. (1943). Zur Kenntnis der Mikrosporidien aus Chironomiden-Larven II. *Zool. Anz.* 141, 255-264.

Weiser, J. (1961). Die Mikrosporidien als Parasiten der Insekten. *Monographien zur Angew. Entomol.* 17, 1-149.

Youssef, N. N. and Hammond, D. M. (1971). The fine structure of the developmental stages of the microsporidian *Nosema apis* Zander. *Tissue Cell* <u>3</u>, 283-294.

FOOTNOTE ADDED IN PROOF

[1]Structures which may represent synaptonemal complexes are shown in Fig. 4 in the chapter *Structure of the Microsporidia*, this Volume. Their identity is confirmed by the recent report of synaptonemal complexes occurring during the first division of the nucleus of the sporont in *Gurleya chironomi*: Loubès, C., Maurand, J., Rousset-Galangau, M.: Présence de complexes synaptonématiques dans le cycle biologique de *Gurleya chironomi* Loubès et Maurand, 1975; un argument en faveur d une sexualité chez les Microsporidies? C. R. Acad. Sci. Paris- Sér. D. 282: 1025-1027, 1976.

Some Aspects of Microsporidian Physiology

EARL WEIDNER

DEPARTMENT OF ZOOLOGY
LOUISIANA STATE UNIVERSITY
BATON ROUGE, LOUISIANA

Biochemical and physiological studies of microsporidians that have been accomplished in the past few years are due, in large part, to their recent availability and to methods for cultivation and maintenance of these organisms in the laboratory. New experimental techniques have facilitated obtaining basic insight of some of the general features of this group of parasites.

I. ENERGY CONDITIONS IN THE SPORE STAGE

The energy turnover in spores is usually low. Ohshima (1964) reported that *Nosema bombycis* spores remain viable up to ten years in distilled water. The free amino acid pool in spores is small but qualitatively similar among various microsporidian spores (see

Table I). Vandermeer and Gochnauer (1969) maintained *N. apis* in water above 45°C and recovered amino acids and carbohydrates without destroying spore viability.

There is some evidence that spore walls are selectively permeable to certain ions or molecules that may effectively trigger the extrusion. *Nosema lophii*, *Encephlitozoon cuniculi* and *N. bombycis* resist noxious concentrations of NaOH and HCl; however, these species often hatch when exposed to certain osmotic and ionic shifts.

The carbohydrate pool is substantial in spores as is shown by the strong reactivity of the spore matrix to the periodic acid-silver methenamine reagent used by Rambourg (1967). Such reactivity, as well as electron opacity of the spore matrix, is lost during collapse of the aperture barrier (see Weidner, 1972). Presumably the carbohydrate is hydrolyzed upon aperture collapse. Vandermeer and Gochnauer (1971) reported that trehalose is an important carbohydrate in *N. apis* spores. When this disaccharide is released from disrupted spores, it is split by native trehalase into two glucose molecules.

II. ENERGY CONDITIONS DURING SPORE DISCHARGE, SPOROPLASM EXTRUSION, AND HOST INVASION

The energy release associated with spore extrusion is due to an osmotic shift. Presumably, the collapse of the spore aperture allows an inflow of water, producing a sudden buildup in hydrostatic pressure within the spore. Discharge intensity is directly proportional to the osmotic condition or the viscosity of the medium exterior to the spore (Lom and Vávra, 1963). A slight glutaraldehyde cross-linking of the polar tube protein prior to discharge slows extrusion. Under optimum conditions, the intensity of discharge allows the tube to penetrate formidable barriers such as other spores in the path of the force.

Spore extrusion can produce discharge tubes with different structural arrangements. Drying *N. lophii* spores pre-treated in distilled water frequently causes extrusion of discharge tubes in directions other than through the aperture; in such an instance, the tube remains structurally arranged in a manner resembling the predischarged condition. In contrast, when natural discharge occurs through a collapsing aperture barrier, a polar tube protein (PTP) is forced out and assembles as an exterior sheath surrounding the discharged tube (Fig. 1). This PTP sheath is insoluble in sodium dodecyl sulfate (SDS) and, therefore, is easy to isolate from other discharged constituents that are SDS-soluble (Fig. 2). PTP is insoluble contained within disrupted, undischarged spores previously treated with 1% SDS and exposed to 100°C; the undischarged polar tube is soluble (except for the PTP core component) in SDS (Weidner, 1972). Discharged sheath PTP can be reduced with 2-mercaptoethanol; and with polyacrylamide disc gel systems, it migrates as a single band in

Table 1. Free Amino Acid Pool (u moles/mg sample) in Microsporidian Spores.

	Glugea hertwigi (from smelt)	*Glugea stephani* (from winter flounder)	*Inodosporus spraguei* (from grass shrimp)
Lysine	trace	trace	trace
Aspartic acid	0.001	0.0039	0.0025
Threonine	trace	trace	0.0008
Serine	0.0028	0.0031	0.0016
Glutamic acid	trace	0.002	0.0017
Proline	trace	trace	trace
Glycine	0.0018	0.0026	0.004
Alanine	0.002	0.0045	0.0023
Valine	trace	trace	trace

Fig. 1. Negatively stained, partially extruded *Nosema michaelis*
         spore. Discharging tube retains a uniform dimension
         until sporoplasm passes out. Note PTP sheath (arrows)
         protein in an assembled condition at the distal end
         of discharging tube. X 30,000.

Fig. 2. SDS insoluble PTP sheaths of extruded *N. michaelis*
         discharge tubes. Treatment of this pellet preparation
         with 2-mercaptoethanol solubilizes the PTP sheaths.
         X 60,000.

Figs. 3
 and 4. Newly extruded sporoplasms of *N. michaelis*. Fig. 3
         shows sporoplasm separated from external PTP sheath
         (arrows) by an unusual space. The natural condition of
         PTP sheath is illustrated by Fig. 4. PTPS, polar tube
         protein sheath. X 35,000.

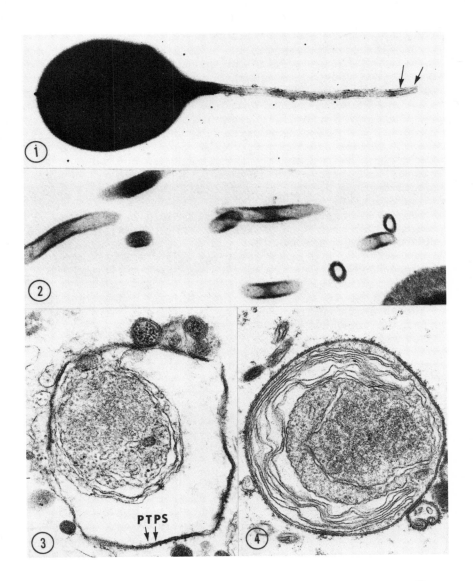

PTPS

polyacrylamide gels and has a molecular weight of approximately 23,000 (Weidner, unpublished data). Initially, it was thought that PTP might be actin because of the cinematographic resemblance of microsporidian discharge to actin release during acrosomal discharge from certain echinoderm sperm (Tilney *et al.*, 1973); however, PTP appears chemically and physically different from actin. It is believed that PTP serves as a platform during tube discharge and almost simultaneously disassembles and reassembles as a sheath on the exterior of the extruding membranous tube.

There is some question as to whether the sporoplasm is contained within a plasma membrane before extrusion from the spore. During extrusion, the plasma membrane within the spore does not discharge to the exterior. Various microsporidian species such as *N. Lophii*, *N. michaelis*, and *Inodosporus spraguei* contain uncompartmentalized sporoplasms prior to extrusion. Based on my experience with *N. michaelis*, I believe that the plasma membrane may have origins with the extrusion apparatus; in any event, a rapid shift is made on the functional demands of this membrane once the sporoplasm is established in the host cytoplasm.

The sporoplasm has few distinguishable organelles that perform some urgent functions after discharge (Figs. 3, 4). Perhaps the PTP sheath, which envelopes the sporoplasm and the discharge tube of *N. michaelis*, serves as a temporary osmotic cover until the sporoplasm begins to regulate metabolic traffic between the parasite and the host cytoplasm.

The invading sporoplasm of *N. michaelis* has a small free amino acid pool, a small undifferentiated cytoplasmic matrix, and no mitochondria. Our observations indicate that after discharge, sporoplasms are partially dependent on external energy. Newly hatched *N. michaelis* sporoplasms disintegrate in Medium 199 alone, with ADP, or with 5' adenylic acid supplement. In contrast, sporoplasms maintain their structural integrity for at least 4-6 hours in the presence of exogenous ATP (Weidner and Trager, 1973).

III. ENERGY CONDITIONS IN THE VEGETATIVE STAGE

Energy conditions of vegetative cells may vary depending on the different associations with host cytoplasm. Many microsporidian species grow freely suspended within host cytoplasm (Figs. 5, 6); in other instances, schizonts situate within cisternae of the endoplasmic reticulum (Szollosi, 1971). Short, slender filopods are often observed when *N. michaelis* schizonts are suspended within host cytoplasm (Figs. 5, 6). These extensions are suspected of imposing ion gradients against host cytoplasm to facilitate transport from host to parasite. Ultrastructural examinations, combined with predictable cytochemical procedures, indicate an absence of deleterious secretory activity imposed by vegetative parasites on host cytoplasm.

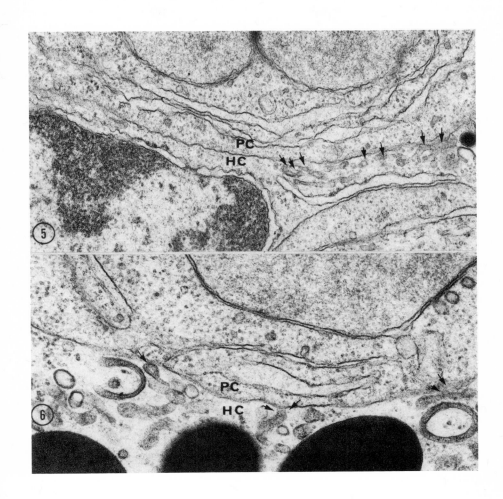

Figs. 5
and 6.   Vegetative *N. michaelis* freely suspended within host
         cytoplasm. Note clender filopods (see arrows) which
         extend from parasite into host cytoplasm. PC, parasite's
         cytoplasm; HC, host cytoplasm.

Vegetative schizonts of *E. cuniculi* grow within ever-increasing
parasitophorous vacuoles (PV) in mammalian cells (Vávra *et al.*,
1972; Petri, 1969). The host cells lose cytoplasmic mass during
this PV growth; furthermore, the rate of cytoplasmic loss is closely
proportional to the number of vegetative parasites within the PV.
The PV membrane boundary conforms to a rich canopy of blebs extending into PV space (Fig. 7); in addition, numerous but similar unat-
tached vesicles locate within the PV space. Using a marking procedure developed by Martin and Spicer (1974), I found Concanavalin A-
iron dextran bound to Con A receptors on the boundary blebs and on
free vesicles within PV space (Weidner, unpublished data). Because
the iron marker did not appear on other membranous structures within
the PV, the vesicles were suspected of originating from the blebs.
These results, combined with observations that the PV grows at the
expense of the host cytoplasm, implicate the PV membrane boundary
of interiorizing by a pinocytic mechanism. Edelson and Cohn (1974)
recently showed that Con A causes the pinocytic mechanism on plasma
membranes of macrophages. These workers showed that Con A vesicles
fuse only with other Con A vesicles until a large Con A pinosome
develops. The Con A-lined pinosome displays blebs; furthermore,
lysosomes failed to fuse with these pinosomes as long as the Con A
remained bound to the surface. This phenomenon closely resembles
the behavior of parasitophorous vacuoles with vegetative *E. cuniculi.*

Xenoma parasitism is one of the most intriguing microsporidian
associations. Weissenberg (1968) described the xenoma as a cell
tumor induced by repetitive host nuclear amitosis accompanied by
extensive cytoplasmic growth. This growth is attributed, in part,
to the simultaneous multiplication and development of vegetative
microsporidian parasites. Xenomas commonly have millimeter dimensions (Sprague and Vernick, 1968). Curiously, during the rapid
growth of vegetative parasites, the surrounding host cytoplasm displays little or no degeneration; to the contrary, the host cytoplasm
continues synthesis (Figs. 8, 9).

Nosema and structurally related species often show obvious effects
on host cytoplasm during spore formation. For example, infected
muscle tissue of *Callinectes sapidus* tends to undergo actin and myo-
sin filament disassembly in the presence of *N. michaelis* sporoblasts
(Weidner, 1970). These sporoblasts have microtubules situated as
ports within the developing spore wall (Dwyer and Weidner, 1973).
In another microsporidian species, pansporoblast-forming *I. spraguei*
has adenosine triphosphatase activity on microtubule-studded pansporoblast envelopes; in addition, *I. spraguei* has an extensive
glycocalyx which coats the channels extending from the pansporoblast
envelope to the sporoblasts inside (Overstreet and Weidner, 1974).

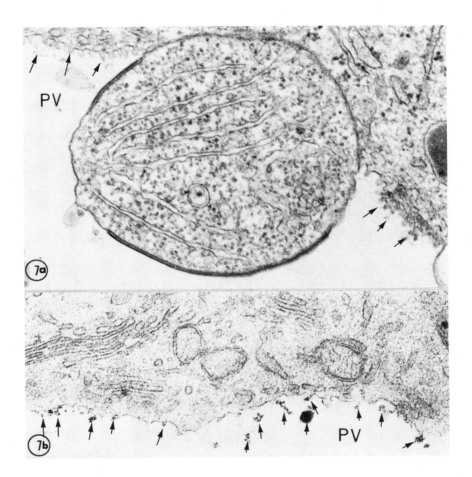

Fig. 7. a, *Encephalitozoon cuniculi* vegetative cell with tight-
junction-like attachment to membrane boundary of parasitophorous vacuole (PV) within mouse peritoneal macrophage. Note free PV boundary conforms to rich canopy of
blebs (see arrows); b, Parasitophorous vacuole (PV) with
Con A-iron dextran marker on blebs and free vesicles
(arrows). This marker did not attach to other structures
within PV. X 50,000.

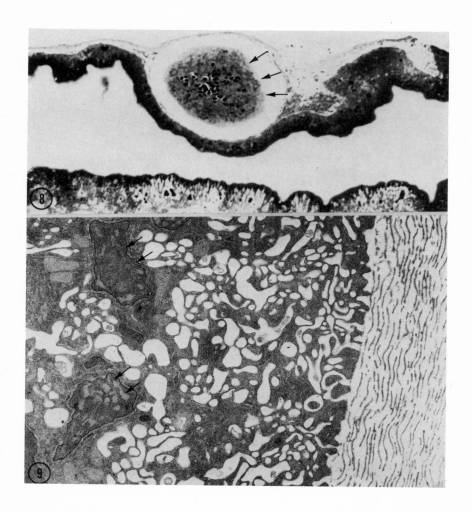

Fig. 8. Low power view of intestine of winter flounder with xenoma
         infection of *Glugea stephani*, Arrow indicates xenoma.
         X 1,000.

Fig. 9. Blowup of perimeter of xenoma. Vegetative parasites (see
         arrows) are distributed throughout host cytoplasm, which
         displays little or no degeneration. X 10,000.

IV. INTERACTIONS BETWEEN MICROSPORIDIAN STAGES AND HOST CYTOPLASM

Spore discharge and host invasion. Microsporidian invasion
characteristically begins with a piercing action of the spore discharge tube across the plasma membrane of the host. *Nosema michaelis*
and *Glugea stephani* spores explosively discharge a tube. The physical profile of *N. michaelis* tubes is such that the host cell plasma
membrane tends to flow with capillarity up the tube. On the other
hand, discharging spores of *E. cuniculi* appear to lack a piercing
capacity; these sporoplasms have been observed moving out almost
simultaneously with the discharge tube. Conceivably, the latter
condition enables cells such as macrophages to phagocytize the invading *E. cuniculi* sporoplasms.

During spore extrusion, *N. michaelis* sporoplasms and discharge
tubes are surrounded by the PTP sheath. When the coated sporoplasms
are inserted into the cytoplasmic milieu of ascites leukemia EL4
and ascites neuroblastoma C1300, a corona of fibrous material ac-
cumulates around the sporoplasm. This material is believed to be
host cell reaction binding to the PTP sheath since it is not observed
around sporoplasms extruded into free culture medium or within red
blood cells (Weidner, 1972).

Prevention of lysosomal fusion with parasitophorous vacuoles.
Lysosomes fail to deliver to macrophage parasitophorous vacuoles
(PV) containing *E. cuniculi* schizonts (Weidner, unpublished results). Ferritin-labeling of lysosomes and pinocytic vesicles was
performed by using the procedure of Jones and Hirsch (1972). After
ferritin incubations of up to 18 hours, marker was located in secondary lysosomes, phagocytic vacuoles, and pinocytic vesicles (Figs. 10,
11). Ferritin readily delivered to secondary lysosomes and to phagocytic vacuoles containing hatched *E. cuniculi* spores; however,
ferritin was always excluded from the PV. The absence of lysosomal
fusion with parasitophorous vacuoles is probably a general phenomenon induced by many intracellular parasites; this mechanism seems
to operate in macrophages infected with tubercle bacilli, with
Chlamydia species in fibroblasts, and with *Toxoplasma gondii* in
peritoneal macrophages (see Jones and Hirsch, 1972).

V. PROCEDURES FOR ISOLATING STAGES OF MICROSPORIDIANS

A. SPORES

The resistant nature of the spore wall enables easy isolation of
this stage from host cells. Sodium hydroxide (0.1-0.2N) is effective in breaking host cells. Subsequent treatment in a Waring
blender with repeated washings and centrifugations eventually produce a pure white pellet of spores. Undeen and Alger (1971) recommend a density gradient method for fractionating spores from host

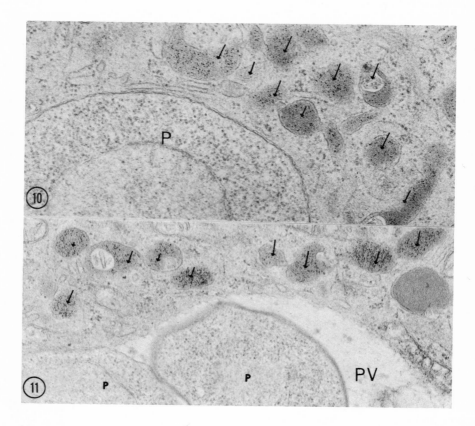

Figs. 10
and 11.   Two views of peritoneal macrophages exposed for 2 hrs
          to ferritin at 37°C. Note ferritin in presumptive
          secondary lysosomes (arrows). Ferritin was never
          observed within intact parasitophorous vacuoles
          containing viable *E. cuniculi* vegetative parasites.
          P, parasite; PV, parasitophorous vacuole.

material. Spore clusters recovered from mature fish xenomas have such a high spore population density that only three or four washings and centrifugations are necessary to obtain a pure spore pellet.

Spore disruption for biochemical analysis has proven more difficult than purifying spores. Sonication and French pressure treatment have not been particularly successful. Vandermeer and Gochnauer (1971) reported that *N. apis* spores are disrupted by a shearing action in liquid nitrogen. The Braun Model MSK (Will Scientific, Inc.) has been a useful homogenizer that also applies a shearing action produced by a rapid circular agitation with glass beads.

Chemical treatment of spores with 3% sodium hypochlorite (Chlorox®) for 5-10 minutes, followed by soaking in 1-2% 2-mercaptoethanol, produces leaky spores. Treatment of spores with sodium hypochlorite, followed by mechanical homogenization can increase the yield of collapsed spores. This procedure may be followed by the Undeen and Alger fractionating method (1971) applied to sort spore components.

B. SPOROPLASMS

The uncompartmentalized condition of sporoplasms within the spore requires extrusion for recovering viable sporoplasms. Unfortunately, no universal method is available for inducing spore hatching and viable sporoplasm release in the many microsporidian species. When such a method becomes available, the doors will be open for obtaining the much needed information about the physiological qualifications and adaptabilities of this stage; the sporoplasm injection phenomenon may also be useful in acquiring knowledge about the interaction capacities of known host cell lines *in vitro*.

Nosema michaelis has been useful since large numbers of spores can be accumulated from infected blue crabs. Spore hatching can be predictably induced in culture medium and viable sporoplasms harvested (Weidner and Trager, 1973). *Nosema bombycis* has been useful since the spores readily hatch and the sporoplasms will grow and differentiate in a variety of cells (Ishihara and Sohi, 1966).

C. VEGETATIVE CELLS

Young xenomas are a good source of vegetative parasites. These parasite colonies are big enough to be identified in infected fish such as winter flounder (see Stunkard and Lux, 1965). Schizonts tend to be freely suspended within xenoma cytoplasm. By disrupting host cytoplasm, the vegetative parasites sort from the host material during buffer washes and centrifugations.

Several laboratories have reported developing routinely high level *E. cuniculi* infections of rabbit choroid plexus cells in tissue culture (Shadduck, 1969; Vávra *et al.*, 1972). Since *E. cuniculi* tends

to grow in large parasitophorous vacuoles, there has been some
measured success in separating these parasites from the host.
Currently, we are working with a new method successfully used by A.
Larson and L. T. Hart (unpublished) for isolating pure populations
of infective *Anaplasma marginale* from red blood cells. These workers have isolated a heat stable lysin which is secreted into broth
culture medium by *Pseudomonas aeruginosa*. The lysin readily attacks
cell membranes; however, it has a sensitivity that can be manipulated
so that infective viable intracellular parasites can be recovered.
Trager *et al.* (1972) applied a variety of isolating procedures and
reported on the structural and physiological condition of isolated
malaria parasites.

D. SPOROBLASTS

Nosema michaelis undergoes sporogenesis in the muscle tissue of
blue crab, *C. sapidus*. Growth may be so extensive that large numbers of sporoblasts can be recovered from a single animal. Isolation of sporoblasts has been achieved by gently homogenizing infected
tissue with a Waring blender at low speed for 30 seconds and diluting
the homogenate with phosphate buffer (10–15 volumes) in the presence
of 0.1–0.2% trypsin solution for 15–30 minutes. The sporoblasts tend
to resist trypsin and subsequent isolation has been achieved with
washings and low-speed centrifugations.
  Pure populations of pansporoblastic *I. spraguei* (see Overstreet
and Weidner, 1974) have been isolated with intact pansporoblasts.
Host tissue was roughly homogenized and after repeated washings with
phosphate buffer or Kreb's Ringers, the 8–10 μm sacs readily segre-
gate from the host material upon low-speed centrifugation.

REFERENCES

Dwyer, D. M., and E. Weidner (1973). Microsporidian extrasporular
    microtubules: Ultrastructure, isolation and electrophoretic
    characterization. *Z. Zellforsch.* **140**, 170–186.
Edelson, P. J. and Z. A. Cohn (1974). Effects of Concanavalin A
    on mouse peritoneal macraphages. *J. Exp. Med.* **140**, 1364–1386.
Ishihara, R. and S. Sohi (1966). Infection of ovarian tissue
    culture of *Bombyx mori* by *Nosema bombycis* spores. *J. Invert.
    Path.* **8**, 538–540.
Jones, T. C. and J. G. Hirsch (1972). The interaction of
    Toxoplasma gondii and mammalian cells. II. The absence of
    lysosomal fusion with phagocytic vacuoles containing living
    parasites. *J. Exp. Med.* **136**, 1173–1194.
Lom, J. and J. Vavra (1963). The mode of sporoplasm extrusion in
    microsporidian spores. *Acta Protozool.* **1**, 81–89.

Martin, B. J. and S. S. Spicer (1974). Concanavalin A-iron dextram technique for staining cell surface mucosubstances. *J. Histochem and Cytochem* 22, 206-207.

Ohshima, K. (1964). Method of gathering and purifying active spores of *Nosema bombycis* and preserving them in good condition. *Annotnes Zool. Jap.* 37, 94-101.

Overstreet, R. M. and E. Weidner (1974). Differentiation of microsporidian spore tails in *Inodosporus spraguei* Gen et Sp. N. *Z. Parasitenkunde* 44, 169-186.

Petri, M. (1969). Studies on *Nosema cuniculi* found in transplantable ascites tumours with a survey of microsporidiosis in mammals. *Acta Path. Microbiol. Scand. Suppl.* 204, 1-92.

Rambourg, A. (1967). An improved silver methenamine technique for the detection of periodic acid reactive complex carbohydrates with the electron microscope. *J. Histochem. Cytochem.* 15, 409-412.

Sprague, V. and S. H. Vernick (1968). Light and electron microscope study of a new species of Glugea (Microsporida, Nosematidae) in the 4-spined stickleback *Apeltes quadracus*. *J. Protozool.* 15, 547-571.

Stunkard, H. W. and F. E. Lux (1965). A microsporidian infection of the digestive tract of the winter flounder, *Pseudopleuronectes americanus*. *Biol. Bull.* 129, 371-387.

Szollosi, D. (1971). Development of *Pleistophora* sp. (microsporidian) in eggs of the polychaete Armandia brevis. *J. Invert. Pathol.* 18, 1-15.

Tilney, L. G., S. Hatano, H. Ishikawa and M. S. Mooseker (1973). The polymerization of actin: its role in the generation of the acrosomal process of certain echinoderm sperm. *J. Cell Biol.* 59, 109-126.

Trager, W., S. G. Langreth and E. G. Platzer (1972). Viability and fine structure of extracellular Plasmodium lophurae prepared by different methods. *Proc. Helminth Soc. Wash.* 39, 220-230.

Undeen, A. H. and N. E. Alger (1971). A density gradient method for fractionating microsporidian spores. *J. Invert. Pathol.* 18, 419-420.

Vandermeer, J. W. and T. A. Gochnauer (1969). Some effects of sublethal heat on spores of *Nosema apis*. *J. Invert. Pathol.* 13, 442-446.

Vandermeer, J. W. and T. A. Gochnauer (1971). Trehalase activity associated with spores of *Nosema apis*. *J. Invert. Pathol.* 17, 38-41.

Vavra, J., P. Bedrnik, and J. Cinatl (1972). Isolation and in vitro cultivation of the mammalian microsporidian *Encephalitozoon cuniculi*. *Folia Parasitologica* (Praha) 19, 349.

Weidner, E. (1970). Ultrastructural study of microsporidian development. *Z. Zellforsch.* 105, 33-54.

Weidner, E. (1972). Ultrastructural study of microsporidian invasion into cells. *Z. Parasitenk.* 40, 227–242.

Weidner, E. and W. Trager (1973). Adenosine triphosphate in the extracellular survival of an intracellular parasite *(Nosema michaelis,* Microsporidia). *J. Cell Biol.* 57, 586–591.

Weissenberg, R. (1968). Intracellular development of the microsporidian *Glugea anomala* Moniez in hypertrophying migratory cells of the fish *Gasterosteus aculeatus* L., and example of the formation of "Xenoma" tumors. *J. Protozool.* 15, 44–57.

The Extra-Corporeal Ecology of Microsporidia

JOHN PAUL KRAMER

DEPARTMENT OF ENTOMOLOGY
CORNELL UNIVERSITY
ITHACA, NEW YORK

I. INTRODUCTION

The two environments of microsporidians are: *(i)* the intra-corporeal, formed by the tissues of the host in which these parasites grow and multiply; and *(ii)* the extra-corporeal, formed by all that surrounds these tissues. Whereas these two environments are intimately related and at times inseparable, I have attempted to separate them for the purpose of discussion. It would not be profitable nor even practicable to attempt to catalog all the known information that treats some aspect of the extra-corporeal ecology of microsporidians. Therefore, I have attempted to present a cohesive overview of the subject with some examples that illustrate specific points. To provide the reader with a sense of continuity, the discussion first centers around the process of dissemination and this is followed by a commentary on other facets of microsporidian life in the extra-corporeal environment. Recent reviews that relate in part to the topic at hand are those by Canning (1970) and Maddox (1973). Reviews by Putz and McLaughlin (1970) and Sindermann (1970) also contain some information that bears upon the extra-corporeal experience of spores.

II. DISSEMINATION OF MICROSPORIDIANS

Dissemination involves transport of the microsporidian from an original host to a new host where it finds a niche suitable for the continuance of its life cycle. Nonsporulated forms as well as spores are disseminated but the latter are of greater importance in this process if one views the microsporidians as a whole. Most species of microsporidians do not solve the problems associated with dissemination in a single way and the examples given in the following discussion serve only to illustrate the diverse strategies employed by the microsporidians as a group. For purposes of orderly treatment, the sequential steps in the process of dissemination are considered as escape, conveyance and entry.

A. ESCAPE

A variety of discharges provide spores with avenues of escape. The most conspicuous of these are the feces, but urine, vomitus, secretions of specialized glands, and fluids from tumorous cysts may also supply avenues of escape. In each case the discharge corresponds to the niche where the spore was formed. Thus, spores of enteric microsporidians of insects are always found in the feces of the host (see Weiser, 1961a) and spores of renal microsporidians of mammals are always present in the urine of the host (see Canning, 1970). Regurgitations of lepidopteran larvae provide one avenue of escape for spores of some species (Thomson, 1958). The capsular spermatophore produced in the adult male insect provides another (Thomson, 1958; see Kellen and Lindegren, 1971). The egg-cementing fluids from accessory glands of female moths provide still another (Kramer, 1959). The exudates from integumental cysts and bulges furnish spores of pisciphilic species with a passage for exit (see Putz and McLaughlin, 1970).

The degradative action of physical forces and microbiotic agents commonly provide an avenue of escape for species whose spores are locked within the dead body of the host. This is best illustrated by the liberation of spores of species occurring in the larvae of aquatic insects. The tattering of the delicate corpse of a black-fly larva by fast-moving waters liberates spores from its fat body. In a quiet pool saprophytic bacteria and fungi eventually disrupt the body wall of the dead mosquito larva and thereby release the microsporidian spores previously trapped within its tissues.

Another less common avenue of escape is the blood stream. For example, the exit of some lepidopterophilic species is engineered by parasitoidal wasps whose ovipositors become tainted with spores in the course of egg laying (see Weiser, 1961a). The blood stream probably provides an avenue of escape for the murine microsporidian *Nosema muris* as it passes from the female mouse to her offspring via the placenta (Weiser, 1965a).

Spores, having escaped via discharges or by other means, are deposited in environments of many types that encompass the habitats of host species. Striking qualitative differences found among these environments are illustrated in the following examples which have been extrapolated in part from the literature. Spores of *Nosema michaelis* from the blue crab *Callinectes sapidus* are found in marine waters (see Sprague, 1970) whereas spores of *Pleistophora ovariae* from the minnow *Notemigonus crysoleucas* are found in fresh waters (Summerfelt and Warner, 1970). Spores of *Nosema termitis* repose on the inner surfaces of the dark and humid tunnels built and inhabited by its termite host *Reticulitermes flavipes* (see Kudo, 1943). Spores of *Nosema juli* rest upon the moist, microbe-rich soil surfaces frequented by its millipede host *Diploiulus londinensis caeruleocinctus* (see Wilson, 1971). Spores of *Nosema oryzaephili* from the saw-toothed grain beetle *Oryzaephilus surinamensis* rest among particles of dry flour (see Burges *et al.*, 1971). The mechanisms that assure the survival of spores in each of these grossly different extra-corporeal environments must reflect some special features of its host's habitat; the precise nature of these mechanisms awaits discovery.

B. CONVEYANCE

Having escaped from the host of origin, the microsporidian is faced with the problem of reaching a new susceptible host, that is, conveyance. Conveyance may be effected in two ways: by direct contact or by indirect contact. In the former case the microsporidian is transferred directly from the original host to the new susceptible host. In the latter case microsporidian spores are dispersed by physical agents or they are carried by a vector.

Transfer of a microsporidian from a parent to its offspring during the process of reproduction best exemplifies conveyance by direct contact. In such a manner, nonsporulated forms and possibly spores of *Nosema notabilis* are transferred during plasmotomy of the trophozoites of its myxosporidian host *Sphaerospora polymorpha* (Kudo, 1944). Nonsporulated forms and spores are often incorporated into developing eggs within the microsporidian-containing tissues of female invertebrates of many species. Some examples are found among microsporidians from lepidopterons (see Weiser, 1961a and Tanada, 1963), coleopterons (Weiser, 1958), culicids (Kellen and Wills, 1962; see Canning, 1970), parasitoidal hymenopterons (see Brooks, 1973), aquatic crustaceans (see Bulnheim and Vávra, 1968), and coelenterates (Spangenberg and Claybrook, 1961). This phenomenon also occurs among microsporidians of the teleost fishes (see Weiser, 1949). Transference of *N. muris* by way of the placenta in the mouse is another variation on the same theme (see Weiser, 1965a and Canning, 1970). Cannibalism probably occurs in nearly all major groups of animals that serve as hosts for microsporidians and it constitutes

another example of conveyance by direct contact. For instance,
spores of *Nosema plodiae* may be transferred directly from a dead
or dying larva of the Indian meal moth *Plodia interpunctella* to a
healthy one as a result of the latter devouring the former (see
Kellen and Lindegren, 1968).

Physical agents that facilitate the conveyance of microsporidian
spores consist primarily of gravity and pressure, sudden jars that
provide mechanical disturbances, and currents of air and of water.
Microsporidian spores have not evolved special mechanisms to facilitate dispersal of spores in air. Instead, mechanical disturbances
probably carry particles of soil, excreta, and the like, into the
air along with clumps of spores. How interacting forces such as
gravitation, velocity of fall, horizontal air movement, and atmos-
pheric turbulence influence the dispersal of microsporidian spores
has not been investigated. Spores discharged or liberated from
aquatic hosts may be conveyed by currents within streams, lakes,
or oceans. Oval or spherical spores with smooth walls tend to
settle to the bottom of slow-moving waters rather quickly, whereas
those bearing long appendages or gelatinous envelopes or both are
probably carried for long distances (see Lom and Vávra, 1963;
Vávra, 1963).

Most vectors of microsporidians consume the spore-filled tissues
of the host and the unchanged spores are eventually discharged with
their feces. Mechanical vectors of this type are predators or
scavengers. For example, ground beetles (*Calosoma sycophanta*) and
ants (*Formica rufa*) acquire and shed spores of the lepidopterophilic species *Thelohania hyphantriae* in the foregoing manner
(Weiser, 1957); staphylinid beetles do the same with spores of
Nosema curvidentis from the corpses of the bark beetle *Pityokteines
curvidens* (Weiser, 1961b). Insectivorous birds may also serve as
vectors in this manner for other entomophilic microsporidans (see
Günther, 1959). Other vectors that feed within the remains of
spore-filled hosts are contaminated with spores both externally and
internally; these vectors are then eaten by a new susceptible host.
Pleistophora myotrophica of toads (*Bufo bufo*) is probably transmitted in this manner by insects, slugs or earthworms (Canning, 1966).
Glugea anomala of the freshwater stickleback *Gasterosteus aculeatus*
is vectored in a similar manner by the ingestion of spore-contain-
ing species of *Cyclops* and *Daphnia* (see Stunkard, 1969). Spores of
some helminthophilic microsporidians are accidentally ingested by
grazing helminth-infected animals and thereby these hyperparasitic
species reach their hosts (see Joe and Nasemary, 1973). Spores of
several lepidopterophilic species are carried from the caterpillar
host of origin to another caterpillar on the ovipositor of parasitoidal hymenopterons (see Brooks, 1973). Some species producing
sticky, mucus-covered spores and parasitizing aquatic invertebrates
are probably vectored on the feathers of water fowl (Weiser, 1965b).

C. ENTRY

   Three natural portals of entry provide microsporidians with access
to host tissues in which they can reside and multiply: the oral
portal, the cuticular portal, and the ovarial portal. Entry via
the oral portal involves the ingestion of spores lodged in the food
or drink of the recipient host; typically such spores have been excreted in the feces of the host of origin. Entry via the cuticular
portal involves the injection of spores through the originally intact integument by a parasitoidal wasp engaged in oviposition; to
date this phenomenon is recognized only among microsporidians associated with insects and their parasitoids. Entry via the ovarial
portal involves the incorporation of spores and nonsporulated forms
into developing ova or embryos within the female reproductive tract;
this phenomenon is best known among microsporidians of invertebrates
but it also occurs among species found in the vertebrates. Micro-
sporidans such as *Nosema apis* of the honey bee utilize only the oral
portal (see Bailey, 1963), whereas others such as *T. campbelli* of
the mosquito *Culiseta incidens* use both the oral and ovarial portals
(Kellen *et al.*, 1965); still others like *Nosema heliothidis* of lepidopterons (*Heliothis zea* and *H. virescens*) employ all three portals (see Brooks, 1973).

III. SPORES IN THE EXTRA-CORPOREAL ENVIRONMENT

   The period of time a microsporidian spends in its extra-corporeal
environment is closely related to its portal of entry. If the
ovarial portal is used, no such time period really exists; the same
may be said of spores conveyed by the cannibalistic actions of their
hosts. When the cuticular portal is used for the mechanical transfer of spores, this time period probably does not exceed a few days.
For spores cast into the general environment and using the oral portal of entry, this time period is extremely variable, ranging from
a matter of seconds to several days or much longer. The problem of
survival assumes great proportions for spores in this latter group.
To date, there is no data pertaining to spore life in the extra-
corporeal environment for more than 90% of the known species of
microsporidians. In fact, published accounts concerning the longevity and survival of spores and related topics are very nearly limited to laboratory investigations of species whose hosts are economi-
cally important terrestrial insects.
   The longevity of spores from terrestrial insects in the extra-
corporeal environment stems from an ability to survive in the face
of a large number of interacting challenges provided by meteorolo-
gical elements such as temperature, moisture, and solar radiation.
The nature of the substrate supporting the spores also influences
longevity. The bits and pieces of information pertaining to this
subject were reviewed by Kramer (1970) and the data he presented

suggests that: (i) the ability to survive varies from species to species; (ii) spores of some species bound in dried feces or in dried cadavers remain viable for one year or somewhat longer under room conditions; longevity of other species under these conditions may be three months or less; (iii) longevity of naked dried spores under room conditions generally does not exceed four months; and (iv) some naked spores in a cold clean aqueous medium may survive for seven to ten years. Maddox (1973) aptly notes that the viability of any spore population decreases over a period of time and expressions of spore longevity in absolute terms tend to oversimplify the question of spore persistance in the extra-corporeal environment. He concludes that: (i) spores of most species do not persist in the general environment for more than one year; (ii) temperatures above 35°C greatly reduce the viability of spore populations; and (iii) naked spores cannot withstand exposure to direct sunlight for more than a few days.

The principal threat to the survival of microsporidian spores is probably slow dehydration which may be brought about by low humidities at moderate to high temperatures or by freezing, water being lost from the spore through the thinner portion of the spore shell at the apical pole. Debilitating intoxication is another threat to the welfare of the spore and its contents. Toxins from various sources may kill the sporoplasm or severely damage the polar filament within the intact spore or both (see Ohshima, 1973). Perhaps the rather rapid deactivation of spores found in water with putrefying debris results from the entry of bacterial toxins through the thinner portion of the spore shell. Perhaps spores from some marine hosts are sensitive to variations in osmotic pressure and cannot withstand for extended periods the stress imposed by sea water. Prolonged exposure to direct sunlight menaces spores from terrestrial hosts. Whereas spore deactivation under such conditions is partly due to dehydration, solar radiation is also a factor (see Wilson, 1974). Daubs of fecal material or other substances that fortuitously cover spores and mucus envelopes, mentioned previously, tend to protect some spores from the foregoing threats. The tentative character of this discussion reflects the primitive state of our knowledge concerning spore life in the extra-corporeal environment.

REFERENCES

Bailey, L. (1963). *Nosema apis* Zander. *In* "Infectious Diseases of the Honey-bee," pp. 39-48. Land Books Ltd., London.
Brooks, W. M. (1973). Protozoa: host-parasite-pathogen interrelationships. *Misc. Publs. Entomol. Soc. Amer.* 9, 105-111.
Bulnheim, H.-P. and Vávra, J. (1968). Infection by the microsporidian *Octosporea effeminans* sp.n. and its sex determining influence in the amphipod *Gammaris duebeni*. *J. Parasitol.* 54, 241-248.

Burges, H. D., Canning, E. U., and Hurst, J. A. (1971). Morphology, development, and pathogenicity of *Nosema oryzaephili* n.sp. in *Oryzaephilus surinamensis* and its host range among granivorous insects. *J. Invert. Pathol.* 17, 419-432.

Canning, E. U. (1966). The transmission of *Plistophora myotrophica*, a microsporidian infecting the voluntary muscles of the common toad. *Proc. Int. Cong. Parasitol.*, 1st, Roma, 1964 (A. Corradeti, ed.), pp. 446-447.

Canning, E. U. (1970). Transmission of microsporida. *Proc. Int. Colloq. Insect Pathol.*, 4th, 1970, pp. 415-424.

Günther, S. (1959). Über die Auswirkung auf die Infektiosität bei der Passage insektenpathogener Mikrosporidien durch den Darm von Vögeln und Insekten. *Nachrichtenblatt für den Deutschen Pflanzenschutzdienst.* 13, 19-21.

Joe, L. K. and Nasemary, M. (1973). Transmission of *Nosema eurytremae* (Microsporida: Nosematidae) to various trematode larvae. *Zeitschr. Parasitenk.* 41, 109-117.

Kellen, W. R., Chapman, H. C., Clark, T. B. and Lindegren, J. E. (1965). Host-parasite relationships of some *Thelohania* from mosquitoes (Nosematidae: Microsporidia). *J. Invert. Pathol.* 7, 161-166.

Kellen, W. R. and Lindegren, J. E. (1968). Biology of *Nosema plodiae* sp.n., a microsporidian pathogen of the Indian meal moth, *Plodia interpunctella* (Hübner), (Lepidoptera: Phycitidae). *J. Invert. Pathol.* 11, 104-111.

Kellen, W. R. and Lindegren, J. E. (1971). Modes of transmission of *Nosema plodiae* Kellen and Lindegren, a pathogen of *Plodia interpunctella* (Hübner). *J. Stored Products Res.* 7, 31-34.

Kellen, W. R. and Wills, W. (1962). The transovarian transmission of *Thelohania californica* Kellen and Lipa in *Culex tarsalis* Coquillet. *J. Insect Pathol.* 4, 321-326.

Kramer, J. P. (1959). Some relationships between *Perezia pyraustae* Paillot (Sporozoa, Nosematidae) and *Pyrausta nubilalis* (Hübner) (Lepidoptera, Pyralidae). *J. Insect Pathol.* 1, 25-33.

Kramer, J. P. (1970). Longevity of microsporidian spores with special reference to *Octosporea muscaedomesticae* Flu. *Acta Protozool.* 15, 217-224.

Kudo, R. R. (1943). *Nosema termitis* n.sp., parasitic in *Reticulitermes flavipes*. *J. Morphol.* 73, 265-279.

Kudo, R. R. (1944). Morphology and development of *Nosema notabilis* Kudo, parasitic in *Sphaerospora polymorpha* Davis, a parasite of *Opsanus tau* and *O. beta*. *Illinois Biol. Monogr.* 20, 1-83.

Lom, J. and Vávra, J. (1963). Mucous envelopes of spores of the Subphylum Cnidospora (Doflein, 1901). *Vest. Ceskolovenské Spole. Zool.* 27, 4-6.

Maddox, J. V. (1973). The persistence of the microsporida in the environment. *Misc. Publs. Entomol. Soc. Amer.* 9, 99-104.

Ohshima, K. (1973). Change of relation between infectivity and filament evagination of debilitated spores of *Nosema bombycis*. *Annotationes Zool. Japonenses* 46, 188-198.

Putz, R. E. and McLaughlin, J. J. A. (1970). Biology of Nosemati-
    dae (Microsporida) from freshwater and euryhaline fishes. *In*
    "A Symposium on Diseases of Fishes and Shellfishes" (S. F.
    Snieszko, ed.), Spec. Publ., 5, pp. 124-132, Amer. Fish. Soc.,
    Washington, D.C.
Sindermann, C. J. (1970). "Principal Diseases of Marine Fish and
    Shellfish." Academic Press, New York and London.
Sprague, V. (1970). Some protozoan parasites and hyperparasites
    in marine decapod crustacea. *In* "A Symposium on Diseases of
    Fishes and Shellfishes" (S. F. Snieszko, ed.), Spec. Publ.,
    5, pp. 416-430, Amer. Fish. Soc., Washington, D.C.
Spangenberg, D. B. and Claybrook, D. L. (1961). Infection of
    hydra by microsporidia. *J. Protozool.* 8, 151-152.
Stunkard, H. W. (1969). The sporozoa: with particular reference
    to infections in fishes. *J. Fish. Res. Board Canada* 26, 725-
    739.
Summerfelt, R. C. and Warner, M. C. (1970). Geographical distri-
    bution and host-parasite relationships of *Plistophora ovariae*
    (Microsporida, Nosematidae) in *Notemigonus crysoleucas*. *J.
    Wildlife Diseases* 6, 457-465.
Tanada, Y. (1963). Epizootiology of infectious diseases. *In* "In-
    sect Pathology, an Advanced Treatise" (E. A. Steinhaus, ed.)
    2, pp. 423-475. Academic Press, New York and London.
Thomson, H. M. (1958). Some aspects of the epidemiology of a
    microsporidian parasite of the spruce budworm, *Choristoneura
    fumiferana* (Clem.). *Canad. J. Zool.* 36, 309-316.
Vávra, J. (1963). Spore projections in Microsporidia. *Acta Pro-
    tozool.* 1, 153-155.
Weiser, J. (1949). Studies on some parasites of fishes. *Parasi-
    tology* 39, 164-166.
Weiser, J. (1957). Moznosti biologického boje s prástevnickem
    americkým (*Hyphantria cunea* Drury) III. *Ceskoslov. Parasitol.*
    4, 359-367.
Weiser, J. (1958). Transovariale Übertragung der *Nosema otiorrhyn-
    chi* W. *Vest. Ceskolovenské. Spole. Zool.* 22, 10-12.
Weiser, J. (1961a). Die Mikrosporidien als Parasiten der Insekten.
    Monogr. Angew. Entomol. 17, 1-149.
Weiser, J. (1961b). A new microsporidian from the bark beetle
    Pityokteines curvidens Germar (*Coleoptera*, Scolytidae) in
    Czechoslovakia. *J. Insect Pathol.* 3, 324-329.
Weiser, J. (1965a). *Nosema muris* n.sp., a new microsporidian
    parasite of the white mouse (*Mus musculus* L.). *J. Protozool.*
    12, 78-83.
Weiser, J. (1965b). Influence of environmental factors on proto-
    zoan diseases of insects. *Proc. Int. Cong. Entomol.*, *12th*,
    London, 1964. p. 726.
Wilson, G. G. (1971). *Nosema juli* n.sp., a microsporidian para-
    site in the millipede *Diploiulus londinensis caeruleocinctus*
    (Wood) (Diplopoda: Julidae). *Canad. J. Zool.* 49, 1279-1282.

Wilson, G. G. (1974). The effects of temperature and ultraviolet radiation on the infection of *Choristoneura fumiferana* and *Malacosoma pluviale* by a microsporidian parasite, *Nosema (Perezia) fumiferanae* (Thom.). *Canad. J. Zool.* <u>52</u>, 59-63.

Microsporidia in Vertebrates: Host-Parasite Relations at the Organismal Level

ELIZABETH U. CANNING

DEPARTMENT OF ZOOLOGY
IMPERIAL COLLEGE
LONDON, ENGLAND

I. INTRODUCTION

Most of the species of microsporidia and their pathological effects on vertebrates have been described from naturally occurring infections. Few of these parasites have been transmitted experimentally and in some cases where attempts have been made, *per os* administration of spores has failed to produce infections. Without carefully controlled experimental infections the full effects of these parasites on their hosts cannot be assessed. Future investigation of the factors involved in transmission would be rewarding.

Stunkard and Lux (1965) failed to infect *Pleuronectes americanus* with spores of *Glugea stephani* (Hagenmuller, 1899) and proposed than an invertebrate animal acting as an intermediate or paratenic host, may be involved in the life cycle. Summerfelt and Warner (1970) cited failures of previous authors to infect *Notemigonus crysoleucas* with *Pleistophora ovariae* (Summerfelt, 1964) by administration of spores *per os* and suggested that aging of spores may be important; transovarial transmission might occur in this ovarian parasite.

Per os transmission of microsporidia to fish, ambhibia and mammals has been achieved. Examples are *Glugea anomala* (Moniez, 1887) to sticklebacks, *Pleistophora myotrophica* (Canning, *et al.*, 1964) to toads and *Encephalitozoon cuniculi* Levaditi *et al.*, 1923, to a variety of mammals. Parasites invading through the gut wall must eventually migrate or be carried passively to their preferred sites of infection.   The mechanism of site selection is unknown but it is unlikely that an active searching is involved. Possibly they are carried by blood or lymph from the gut wall to all tissues but develop only in those which provide physiological conditions suitable for their growth and multiplication. Some species are highly site-specific, others, especially those of connective tissue cells, may be found in a variety of organs containing these cells. Some are capable of invading cells of greatly different types: *E. cuniculi* equally infects peritoneal macrophages, brain cells, and kidney tubule cells; other cells, including liver parenchyma, are less commonly infected. The effects of different species may thus be manifested as localized or generalized infections.

Most observations on the effects of microsporidia at the organismal level have been limited to recording externally visible changes and mortality. Observations on behavioural changes in parasitized animals have been made casually on those suffering gross physical deformity and those with nervous symptoms produced by destruction of nervous tissue. No controlled observations have been made on behavioural changes relating to feeding habits, breeding, predation or population dynamics. Such studies would be of great interest, especially in the case of parasitized fish. Examples of gross physical changes in vertebrates are dealt with in this chapter but cellular reactions, which are treated

separately in Chapter seven are only discussed where they have
special relevance to the macroscopic changes in organ structure.

II. EFFECTS OF MICROSPORIDIA ON MAMMALS

Most microsporidian infections in mammals are attributed to
Encephalitozoon cuniculi. Other species *(Nosema connori* Sprague,
1974 in a human infant, a distinct but unnamed species in
Callicebus moloch, and *Thelohania apodemi* Doby *et al.*, 1963,
in *Apodemus sylvaticus)* have not been studied in sufficient detail for the direct effects of the parasites (as opposed to
concomitant debility of the host) to be evaluated.

Many tissues have been reported to contain lesions typical of
encephalitozoonosis (Shadduck and Pakes, 1971). The nervous
system (especially the brain) and kidney tubules are common
sites of infection and lesions have also been found in the liver,
myocardium, adrenal glands, optic nerves, and retina. In the
brain the parasites are often found in large aggregates inside a
cytoplasmic vacuole, host responses such as encapsulation of
parasites and inflammatory reaction being absent. Alternatively,
there are lesions in which parasites are rare or absent, consisting
of a necrotic centre surrounded by a reactional zone of infiltrating
cells. Canning (1967) reported invasion of spore aggregates by
large mononuclear cells that engulfed the spores: the lesions,
with few or no parasites, may have resulted from breakdown of
large aggregates by phagocytes or from an inflammatory reaction
against isolated spores. In the kidney, spores that accumulated
in the tubule cells were liberated into the tubule lumina or
into the surrounding connective tissue by breakdown of the cell
boundaries. Liberation into the connective tissue was followed
by infiltration of mononuclear cells.

No accurate information is available on the relationship between disease and level of infection, six, age or strain of host,
or strain of parasite. The condition of animals infected with
E. cuniculi varies from no visible symptoms, to mild or severe
sickness or death. Infections can be produced *per os* and strong
evidence has been provided for transplacental transmission in
rabbits (Hunt, *et al.*, 1972) and mice (Innes, *et al.*, 1962).
Canning (1971) reported a possible sex difference in susceptibility of LACA mice to *E. cuniculi:* 4 females born to an infected
mother were runts and parasites were observed in two of them
whereas the three males of the litter reached normal size and
were uninfected. The diversity of symptoms in young animals
suggest that infections acquired *in utero* or peri-natally might
be the most severe.

Evidence that *E. cuniculi* often occurs as symptomless infections
in rabbits is provided by the recovery of the organism from
apparently healthy stock animals. By histological examination,
Malherbe and Munday (1958) found that 43 out of 51 healthy adult

laboratory rabbits showed brain or kidney lesions bypical of *E. cuniculi* infections and parasites were demonstrated in the majority of them. Pakes, *et al.*, (1972) found latent infections of *E. cuniculi*, by means of a skin test, in rabbits of both sexes, aged three-twelve months. Chalupský *et al.*, (1973) used an immuno-fluorescent antibody test and found that 35 of 200 normal stock rabbits from laboratory colonies or breeding farms were infected.

Under different conditions *E. cuniculi* can cause a disease in rabbits of varied severity. Wright and Craighead (1922) described an illness used for experiments on poliomyelitis virus in rabbits which they attributed to "Microorganisms," now clearly recognizable as *E. cuniculi*. The symptoms were persistent drowsiness, tremor, and slight or marked motor paralysis. Goodpasture (1924) also found that infected young rabbits appeared drowsy and would sit quietly and not. Cameron and Maitland (1924) observed that elevated temperature, stupor and weakness preceeded paralysis, coma, and death. Pattison, *et al.*, (1971), reporting on an outbreak of encephalitozoonosis in rabbits on a breeding farm, observed that young rabbits showed inco-ordination of limbs and paralysis. Survivors failed to grow at reasonable rate and continued to display nervous symptoms; five doses aborted their fetuses and neonatal mortality in the stock was higher than normal. Some mortality occurred among the rabbits observed in all of these studies. *E. cuniculi* infections of rodents normally produce no symptoms and latent infections are common in laboratory mice (Twort and Twort, 1932; Innes, *et al.*, 1962) and rats (Attwood and Sutton, 1965). Experimental infections, initiated by intraperitoneal inoculation can give rise to abdominal distention (Fig. 1) due to accumulation of peritoneal fluid during the first few weeks. The fluid is later resorbed, the animals return to normal and the mortality is low (Nelson, 1967).

A considerable amount of circumstantial evidence exists to in-dicate that *E. cuniculi* infections in carnivores give rise to severe disease. Plowright (1952), Plowright and Yeoman (1952) and Basson *et al.* (1966) found this parasite in litters of puppies. These authors reported some systemic malaise, such as loss of appetite, fever, vomiting or constipation, but the principal symptoms were of nervous origin. There was weakness and inco-ordination of muscles, convulsions, spasms and change of temper-ment from docile to vicious. The eyes were commonly affected and some puppies became blind. The animals eventually died or were destroyed. A similar illness characterized by severe spasms and and muscular twitching was reported (Van Rensburg and du Plessis, 1971) in littermate Siamese kittens, one of which was infected with *E. cuniculi*. Vavra *et al.* (1971) examined certain carnivores that had become paralyzed and died at the Prague Zoo. The animals included eleven suricats (*Suricata suricatta*), 4 young Arctic foxes (*Alopex lagopus*) and two young clouded leopards (*Neofelis nebulosa*). All were infected with a microsporidian very similar

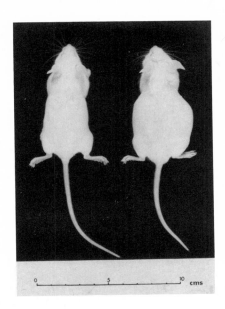

Fig. 1.   Ascitic mouse (right), three weeks after infection with
          the "Nelson strain" of *Encephalitozoon cuniculi* compared
          with normal mouse.

to *E. cuniculi*. Nordstoga (1972) also reported *E. cuniculi* as a
pathogen of blue foxes *(Alopex lagopus)* in Sweden, Finland and
Norway. He studied the pathological changes in 22 blue fox cubs
in Norway, which had died or were killed for pelting when 6 months
old. The cubs had exhibited reduced appetite and growth, thirst,
ataxia, weakness of the posterior muscles and convulsions; some
of the animals wandered in circles. Examination of various
tissues revealed typical *E. cuniculi* lesions in the kidneys and
brain. Chronic arterial lesions, consisting of greatly thickened
and fibrotic transformations of arterial walls, producing in some
cases occlusion of the vessels, were characteristic of the fox
infections. Similar symptoms have not been reported in other
animals. Mohn *et al.* (1974) found severe infections in blue fox
cubs that apparently had been infected transplacentally from
vixen that exhibited no symptoms.
     Most of the microsporidia found in diseased primates have not
yet been positively identified. Some may have been *E. cuniculi*,
others were not. In one fairly well substantiated case of
microsporidiosis in man (Matsubayashi *et al.*, 1959) a nine-year
old Japanese boy suffered a spasmic convulsion and temporary loss
of conciousness, followed by vomiting and headache. The child
made a full recovery after a period of about three weeks. In

another instance, a Ceylonese boy was infected in one eye; the
cornea became opaque and loss of vision occurred (Ashton and
Wirasinha (1973). Spores observed in biopsy material were
larger than those of *E. cuniculi*. Other reported cases of microsporidian infection involved death of the hosts: squirrel monkeys
(*Saimiri sciureus*, Anver *et al.*, 1972 and Brown *et al.*, 1973);
a callicebus monkey (*Callicebus moloch*; Seibold and Fussell
1973); and a human infant (Margileth *et al.*, 1973). To what
extent the microsporidia were involved in causing death of the
hosts was not ascertained.

III. EFFECTS OF MICROSPORIDIA ON BIRDS

The only unquestionable record of microsporidian infection
in birds is that of Kemp and Kluge (1975). They found spores in
renal tubule cells, epithelial cells of the bile duct and intestine, and in hepatocytes of the liver of blue masked lovebirds,
Agapornis personata. Focal necrosis in the liver was the only
sign of inflammatory reaction. The causative agent, identified
as *Encephalitozoon* sp., probably was responsible for the deaths
of 10 out of 14 birds.

IV. EFFECTS OF MICROSPORIDIA ON AMPHIBIANS AND REPTILES

Most of the microsporidian species parasitising amphibians and
reptiles were discovered by histological examinations of tissues;
there was no outward sign of infection. However, *Nosema tritoni*
Weiser, 1960, produced a small whitish cyst on a tadpole of
Triturus vulgaris; Pleistophora danilewskyi (Pfeiffer, 1895) and
P. myotrophica produced elongate white lesions running parallel
with the muscle fibres in their respective reptilian and
amphibian hosts. *P. myotrophica* caused extensive destruction of
voluntary muscles (Fig. 2) in the common toad, *Bufo bufo*,
(Canning *et al.*, 1964) and led to wasting and emaciation in long
standing infections. Invasion by macrophages into the masses of
parasites and subsequent phagocytosis of spores and formation of
sarcoblast nuclei (as a prelude to muscle regeneration) failed
to halt the course of infection. The disease in *B. bufo* ran a
long course and terminated fatally.

V. EFFECTS OF MICROSPORIDIA ON FISH

A. TYPES OF HOST REACTION

In fish, various types of host-parasite relationships occur
that vary in the degree of response by the host.

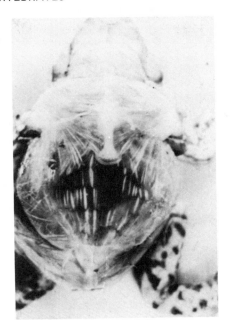

Fig. 2.   Common toad *(Bufo bufo)* showing foci of infection of
Pleistophora myotrophica as white streaks in the abdominal,
pectoral and femoral muscles. X 1.7.

1.   *Infections without cysts*

Some species evoke no response by the host, at least not until
very late in the infectious process. The parasites do not become
sealed at their initial invasion sites and consequently may spread
further in their hosts, either by being conveyed to sites distant
from the original focus or by extending the original lesion in
length and breadth. In the former case there may be numerous
lesions isolated from one another but the effect of each is
restricted to a small swelling in the affected tissue: an example
is *Pleistophora typicalis* Gurley, 1893, in skeletal muscle. If
the parasites spread outwards at the boundary of the original
lesion a large area of tissue may undergo hypertrophy and increased density because of accumulation of spores. Usually only
one or two such sites occur within a single host. The reader is
referred to the report on an infection of *Pleistophora L.
ehrenbaumi* in *Anarrichas minor* by Claussen (1936) for a graphic
example. Macrophage invasion of these lesions is possible because of the absence of limiting membranes but they rarely invade until the later stages of infection and have little effect
in curbing development of the parasites. Although parasites do

not produce the spectacular abnormalities such as caused by
cyst-inducers, they do bring about progressive deterioration of
the tissues.

2. *Infections with cysts*

A common reaction to the invasion of fish by microsporidia is
the laying down by the host of membranes around the parasite to
produce a cyst. The parasites are localized within the host
tissue and are unable to spread. In the mame mammer the cyst wall
prevents macrophage invasion but does not restrict passage of
nutrients to the parasites which are able to develop unhindered
in the enlarging cyst. The origin of the cyst wall components
may be in a single infected cell or in numerous uninfected migratory cells that invade the site of parasitization. The nature of
the different types of tumors caused by microsporidia in fish has
been discussed by Sprague (1969) and is considered by Weissenberg
in Chapter seven.
The idea of a complex consisting of an intracellular parasite
and the hypertrophied host cells acting as a morphological and
physiological entity within normal host tissue was first applied
to a microsporidian relationship with its host by Weissenberg
(1922) and Chatton and Courrier (1923). The latter authors used
the term "complexe xéno-parasitaire" (which had been coined by
Chatton (1920)) for the relationship between *Nosema cotti*
Chatton and Courrier, 1923, and *Cottus bubalis*. The simpler and
more familiar term "senoma" was introduced by Weissenberg
(1949) to replace his original (1922) term "xenon." The xenoma
grows to accomodate the rapidly multiplying parasites while the
original host cell nuclei enlarge or multiply and the cell membranes become thickened to form a cyst to which connective tissue
layers may be added. Some of these cysts are microscopic whereas others reach proportions of several centimeters. Gross
deformities of the fish may result from distention of the affected
organs and compression of neighboring organs. Some of the macroscopic lesions develop as a single cyst e.g., *G. anomala;* others
occurr as closely packed microscopic cysts, each being the site of
a separate invasion by the parasite, e.g., *G. stephani* and
Nosema lophii (Doflein, 1898) Pace, 1908.
Formation of a cyst wall around the parasites and massive invasion of the parasitized area by infiltrating cells has been
studied in *Ichthyosporidium giganteum* (Thélohan, 1895) Swarczewsky,
1914, by Mercier (1921) and in *Ichthyosporidium* sp. Schwartz,
1963, by Sprague (1969). The tumors result from fusion of
neighboring cysts to produce a compound lesion of spectactular
dimensions. After fusion of the cysts to form a large mass of
spores, trabeculae of host tissue appear and, divide the parasitic mass. At first this tissue contains rapidly proliferating
cells and multinucleate giant cells; later, however, there are
only uninucleate cells and the tissue is highly vascularized.

B.   TISSUES AFFECTED

Some microsporidia in fish invade undifferentiated and migratory mesenchyme cells of connective tissue, although this
phenomenon has been determined in only a very few cases by ob-
serving unaltered cells containing early stages of the parasite.
Weissenberg (1968) traced the development of *G. anomala* in this
type of cell.   Parasites of connective tissue might be expected
to have a wide distribution within their hosts and indeed, some
are found in various locations, e.g., *G. anomala* and *G. hertwigi*
Weissenberg, 1911.   Others are organ-restricted such as *G.*
stephani in the gut wall, *P. ehrenbaumi* in the muscles, *N.*
lophii in the nervous system and *Nosema branchiale* Nemeczek,
1911, in the gills of their respective hosts.

1.   Connective tissue

Cysts of *G. anomala* are found in many different sites throughout the body of *Gasterosteus aculeatus, G. pungitius,* and
Gobius minutus.   Weissenberg (1968) put forward the hypothesis
that after hatching of the spores in fish gut, the sporoplasms
penetrated mesenchyme cells in the mid-gut wall and became
distributed from this site by active migration of the cells.
The cell's finally settled when a definite capsule formed at their
surfaces to give rise to the xenoma.   In adult fish the cysts
could be found in the connective tissue of the skin, including
the fins, head, and wall of the branchial chamber; in the cornea;
and in the viscera including gut wall, liver, ovaries, and testes.
In experimentally infected fish larvae, the mid-gut, body cavity,
and ventral skin were commonly infected and xenomas also were
found in the gonads, pancreas, liver, and kidney; on the
peritoneal surface of the stomach and swim-bladder; and in the
muscle layer of the dorsal skin.   Mature cysts attained 3-4 mm in
diameter.   Those in the superficial tissues bulged outward and
caused gross bodily deformity, whereas those in the body cavity
and viscera caused compression of surrounding organs.
The effects of *G. hertwigi* have been studied in smelts *Osmerus*
eperlanus eperlanus of Europe (Weissenberg, 1913) and *Osmerus*
eperlanus mordax of North America (Schrader, 1921; Légault and
Delisle, 1967).   The parasite is most common in the wall of the
intestine but has been reported in other parts of the gut as well
as in the liver, gonads, body cavity, body musculature, and
cornea.   Possibly, like *G. anomala,* it spreads from a primary
site of invasion in the intestine.   Légault and Delisle (1967)
presented a good account of the general appearance of heavily
infected fish.   They studied an outbreak in *O. eperlanus mordax*
in a Canadian lake.   More than 80 percent of specimens examined
that had died of the infection were less than one year old.
Cysts, of which there was an average of 250 per fish, ranged in
size from 0.1 to 8.0 mm in diameter and were found most commonly

in the posterior third of the intestine. The lumen of the gut
was completely occluded and the body wall pushed out in a series
of bulges (Fig. 3). Death was attributed to starvation or
intestinal poisoning. Live specimens with more than 250 small

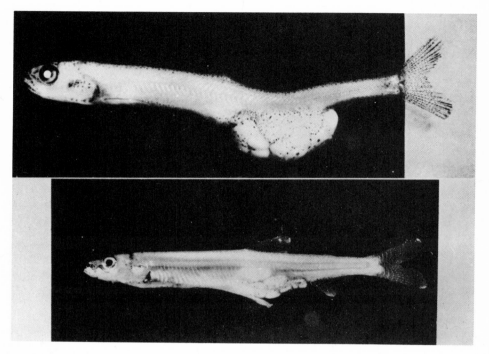

Fig. 3.   Smelt, *Osmerus eperlanus mordax*, showing multiple cysts
           of *Glugea hertwigi* distending the abdominal wall. X 2.5.
           From Légault and Delisle, 1967. Reproduced by permission
           of the National Research Council of Canada from the
           Canadian Journal of Zoology, Volume 45.

cysts were observed to have great difficulty in swimming because
the weight of the cystic agglomeration upset their center of
gravity. They were thus subject to easy predation.
    Sprague and Vernick (1968) found *Apeltes quadracus* infected
with a microsporidian which they named *Glugea weissenbergi*. The
xenomas ranged in size from 1.0 to 6.0 mm and usually were situated beneath the parietal or visceral peritoneum; rarely were
they subdermal. Abdominal distention was not usual because the

cysts normally did not exceed three in number.

The tumors caused by *I. giganteum* in *Crenilabrus melops* and *C. ocellatus* were described by Thélohan (1895). The cysts developed on the mesenteries and merged to form a single mass that distended the abdomen. Mercier (1921) found one *C. melops* measuring only 15 cm long carrying a cyst the size of a chicken's egg. A similar, if not identical parasite, *Ichthyosporidium* sp., was found by Schwartz (1963) in *Leiostomus xanthurus*. The tumors consisted of solid masses of spores, presumably in the body cavity, with four finger-like projections extending back and over the viscera. The abdominal wall was pushed out as a bulge, which could attain a size of 20 mm diameter on fish measuring only 80-110 mm in total length. The bulge usually protruded from an area between the pectoral and pelvic fins (Fig. 4). This species was studied in *L. xanthurus* by Sprague (1969) who found that the site of infection was the subcutaneous connective tissue between the skin and abdominal muscles. He described the bulky lesions, which consisted of masses of parasites and altered host tissue.

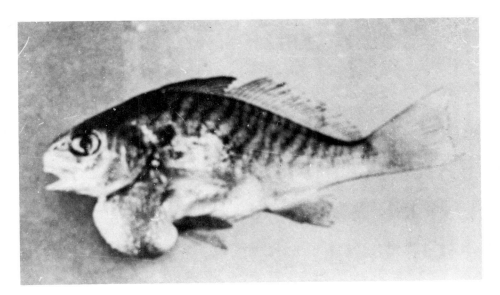

Fig. 4.   Spot, *Leiostomus xanthurus*, with abdominal bulge caused by *Ichthyosporidium giganteum*. X 0.8. From Schwartz, 1963. Reproduced by permission of *Progressive Fish Culterist*, Vol. 25.

Pleistophora cepedianae Putz, *et al.*, 1965, produced large cysts in the body cavity of *Dorosoma cepedianum*. The cyst compressed the viscera against the body wall and sometimes caused a gigantic external bulge measuring up to 1 cm. (Fig. 5). Another species restricted to the body cavity is *Nosema pimephales* Fantham, *et al.* 1941, cysts of which have been found to occlude the abdominal cavity of *Pimephales promelas*.

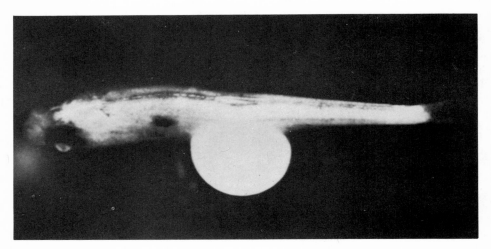

Fig. 5.   Gizzard shad, *Dorosoma cepedianum*, with cyst of
          Pleistophora cepedianae distending the abdominal wall.
          X 3.1.   From Putz, Hoffman, and Dunbar, 1965.   Reproduced
          by permission of the *Journal of Protozoology*, Vol. 12.

2.   *The Gut*

The microsporidian species observed in the gut wall of fish parasitize the connective tissue and extend into the muscular layer; none has been seen in the epithelium. Certain of the connective tissue parasites already discussed attack primarily the gut wall but regularly spread to other tissues. *Glugea stephani* and *Kosema tisae* Lom and Weiser, 1969, are examples of microsporidia that are restricted almost entirely to the gut wall. *G. stephani* invades the gut of *Pleuronectes flesus*, *P. platessa*, *P. limanda*, and *Pseudopleuronectes americanus*. The entire length of the gut from the esophagus to the rectum may be attacked (Fig. 6). In light infections cysts are restricted to the gut wall but in heavy infections other organs are involved. Hagenmuller (1899) found numerous cysts beneath the peritoneum of the liver but none in the parenchyma. Stunkard and Lux (1965) found cysts (0.6-1.0 mm) in the bile duct, liver, mesenteric lymph nodes, and ovaries. Cysts measured 0.6-1.0 mm.

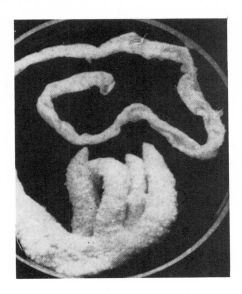

Fig. 6.   Digestive tract of American flounder, *Pseudopleuronectes*
americanus, infected with *Glugea stephani*.   X 0.9.
From Stunkard and Lux, 1965.   Reproduced by permission of
Biological Bulletin,   Vol. 129.

The connective tissue layers may be the primary sites of infection
in the gut but, according to Stunkard and Lux (1965), the whole
thickness of the wall could eventually be supplanted by layers of
cysts, although the epithelium was sloughed rather than invaded.
They found the lumina of the intestine and pyloric caeca reduced or occluded.   The intestine acquired a chalky-white,
pebbled appearance and the wall became thickened and rigid.
Johnstone (1901) studied infections, probably occasioned by
G. stephani, in *P. platessa* whose gut surface was studded with
round white cysts; the internal surface was longitudinally folded
and also covered with cysts.   The wall was 3-4 mm thick.   A con-
trasting type of infection was produced by *N. tisae* in the sub-
mucosa of *Silurus glanis*.   The cysts, measuring up to 0.6 mm in
diameter, were discovered only by microscopic examination (Lom
and Weiser, 1969).

3.   *Gills*

Nosema branchiale causes swellings on the gill filaments of
Gadus aeglefinus.   The disease was first seen by Nemeczek (1911)
and a full description of the pathological effects was given by
Kabata (1959).   The foci of infection were oval swellings

(0.5-1.2 mm long) on the gill filaments; as many as 60 swellings were observed on the filaments of a single gill arch. The parasites were always present in the fibrous connective tissue septum at the center of the filaments. Proliferation of the parasites broke down the fibrous tissue, causing hypertrophy of the filament and displacement of the skeletal rod and blood vessels. Kabata (1959) did not observe a zone of reactional tissue round the parasitic mass. He observed healthy connective tissue separating the parasitized area from the blood vessels, skelatal rod, and respiratory epithelium. Because the respiratory epithelium was entirely unaffected, he concluded that this particular species had no serious effect on the fish. However, more recent studies by J. Lom (personal communication) revealed a typical xenoma: there was hypertrophied cell embedded in a thick layer of irregularly hypertrophied epithelial cells of the gill filament. The wall of the parasitized cell was 1.5 μm thick and stained intensely at its periphery. The vegetative stages of the parasite lined the cyst and the center was occupied by spores as well as one or two agglomerations of degenerate hypertrophied host cell nuclei.

Pleistophora salmonae (Putz, *et al.*1965), in *Salmo gairdneri*, caused similar, smaller swellings restricted to the connective tissue of the gill lamellae. The tips of infected lamellae were badly clubbed. The individual foci which were without a limiting membrane, were quite small (only 200 μm in diameter), and rested in the connective tissue directly overlain by respiratory epithelium (Fig. 7). These investigators (1965) believed that this parasite was identical to the *Plistophora* sp. seen by Wales

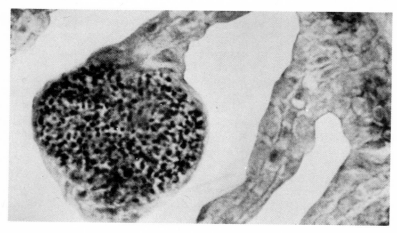

Fig. 7.   Sections of gill lamella of *Salmo gairdneri*, infected with *Pleistophora salmonae*. X 960. From Putz, Hoffman, and Dunbar, 1965. Reproduced by permission of the *Journal of Protozoology*, Vol. 12.

and Wolf (1955) on the gills of *S. gairdneri, Oncorhynchus nerka* and *Cottus* sp. in fish hatcheries. Wales and Wolf (1955) found that cysts containing spores, in contrast to earlier stages, were rare, indicating that the fish probably died early in the infection. Heavily infected gill filaments exhibited rather extensive epithelial proliferation; in domesticated trout, the extent of anaemic gills was correlated with the abundance of parasites. Interestingly, in the absence of a limiting membrane these infections occurred as discrete masses in the localized site rather than as diffuse infiltarations in the connective tissue of the gill arch or elsewhere in the body. More detailed studies may reveal xenoma formation as in *N. branchiale*.

4. *Nervous system*

N. lopii is a common parasite in the nervous system of *Lophius piscatorius*. It produces clusters of spherical cysts that cause conspicuous tumors on the nerve ganglia. The tumors were large and were easily recognized by Doflein (1898) and Weissenberg (1911) in *L. piscatorius* and by Jakowska (1964) in *L. americanus*. Cysts of insignificant size were observed by Jakowska (1965) in sections of the medulla oblongata of *L. gastrophysus* and in the retrorenal region of two *L. piscatorius*. In one specimen of the latter fish the cysts were located in the nerve cell processes of the spinal nerves. No information is available on whether these cysts affected the behavior of the fish.

5. *Skeletal muscle*

An interesting feature of microsporidian infections of fish skeletal musculature is that the foci of infection are rerely delimited by a host cyst. Such infections are similar to those caused by *P. myotrophica* and *P. danilewskyi* in the muscles of amphibians and reptiles. *Glugea shiplei* Drew, 1910, in *Trisopterus luscus (Gadus luscus)* may be an exception. Drew (1910) described opaque white cysts of *G. shiplei*, up to 5 x 3 mm, surrounded by a thin transparent membrane.

Some species cause only slight lesions in their hosts: *P. typicalis* develops in small, nearly spherical cavities in the muscles of *Taurulus bubalis (Cottus bubalis), Myoxocephulus scorpius (Cottus scorpius), Blennius pholis,* and *Pungitius pungitius (Gasterosteus pungitius)* (Thelohan 1895). These spore-filled cavities caused some deformation of the muscle fibres but did not alter their structure or destroy the cross striations (Fig. 8). Other species cause extensive damage in the muscle leading to large tumors that may result in deformity of the body and the affected tissue often appears opaque and white.

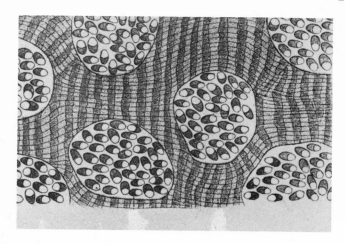

Fig. 8.   Muscle of *Myxocephalus scorpius* infected with
          Pleistophora typicalis. From Thélohan 1895. Reproduced
          by permission of the *Bulletin scientifique de la France
          et de la Belgique* from Vol. 26.

     The course of destruction of the muscle tissue and the host's
reaction have been described in detail in some cases: Early
infection of *Glugea destruens* could be recognized in *Callionymus
lyra* as white flecks in the muscles (Thelohan, 1892).   At this
stage the parasites were surrounded by fibrils which were somewhat
compressed but not otherwise altered.   Later a colorless glassy
refractile substance replaced the muscle fibres adjacent to the
parasites and eventually extended throughout the bundle.   The
hyaline substance was invaded by leucocytes and was replaced by
connective tissue.   *Pleistophora macrozoarcidis* (Nigrelli, 1946)
produced large tumor-like masses in the musculature of
Macrozoarces americanus, especially in the deep muscle near the
vertebral column (Nigrelli 1946).   Areas affected extended for
8 cm or more and caused large bulges on the body.   The parasites
at first occupied the center of the bundle of fibres and caused
the outer layers to become hyaline.   Ultimately, the whole
bundle was destroyed.   Macroscopically, the individual lesions
appeared as whitish streaks along the long axis of the muscle.
Phagocytic activity in the lesions was evident and the host
occasionally reacted by forming connective tissue in the areas
destroyed by the microsporidians.   The parasites were not, however,
localized within cysts and could pass from one focus of infection
to set up another neighobring lesion.   A similar type of infection
was produced by *P. ehrenbaumi.*   According to Duflew-Reichenow
(1953) this parasite was described in *Anarichas lupus* and its
pathological effects were studied more extensively by Claussen

(1936) in *Anarichas minor*. In a specimen of *A. minor* measuring
70 cm long there was a swelling in the dorsal musculature extending
13 cm along the long axis. The swelling measured 5 cm across the
middle and tapered towards the ends. The affected area exhibited
the characteristic milky-white coloration of microsporidian infections but several dark areas were present in the centre of the
lesions.

Claussen (1935) reported that the muscle bundles could be
affected along the whole length but only at a late stage throughout
the width: the center of the bundle was packed with spores whereas the periphery was normal. The fibers at the center of the
bundle were attacked first so that a core of pansporoblasts was
produced surrounded by normal muscle fibers still showing striations. Muscles thus infected represented the milky white areas
of the lesion. Eventually, the infection spread peripherally
so that the layer of normal muscle round the pansporoblasts became narrower and all traces had been destroyed; the spores lay
free in the perimysium. These infected muscles represented the
black-grey areas in the lesion. Early in the infection no host
reaction was detectable. The pansporoblasts were in direct contact with normal muscle fibers and unaltered muscle fibrils were
even present between the pansporoblasts. After total destruction
of the muscle bundles a network of collagen fibers and macrophage-
type cells infiltrated between the spore masses bringing about the
degeneration process which produced grey-black areas.

Pleistophora hyphessobryconis (Schäperclaus, 1941) has been reported frequently as a pathogen of *Hyphessobrycon innesi* and of
other tropical fish. Schäperclaus (1941) accounted in part for
the lack of success sometimes encountered in the rearing of
neon tetra *(H. innesi)* when he found that white flecks in the
abdominal musculature, which disrupted the bright colored bands
along the sides of the body resulting from destruction of muscle
fibers by spherical cysts, each containing numerous spores of this
microsporidian. The organism has been found also in *Hyphessobrycon
gracilis* by Schaperclaus, 1941, in *Brachydanio rerio* and
Hemigrammus ocellifer by Reichenbach-Klinke (1952) and in
Hemigrammus erythrozonus (reported by Thieme, 1956). The unmistak-
able signs of infection were the appearance of white patches on
the body and loss of attractive colors as well as deformity of
the body and abnormal swimming movements. The muscle bundles were
packed with pansporoblasts causing enlargement of the muscle
bundles to several times the normal diameter, interference with
blood circulation and subsequent destruction of parts of the fins
(Reichenbach-Klinke, 1952).

A good description of the course of infection is given by Thieme
(1956). The loss of color begins almost imperceptibly with a few
whitish flecks on the body, which spread until the shining band
of color is interrupted and eventually the whole fish assumes a
greyish, milky-white color. The infection of the musculature

sometimes causes a lateral distortion of the vertebral column with
bending of the body. Fish swim with the tail lower in the water
and towards the end are found almost in a vertical position. There
is loss of weight and difficulty with breathing. Behavioral
differences were noted: continual jerky swimming throughout the
night instead of assuming the characteristic resting position; and
a tendency for infected fish to swim alone instead of in the swarm.

Authors are not entirely in agreement regarding the tissues
other than muscle which may be affected. Schaperclaus (1941)
believed that the ovaries were heavily infected and suggested
that spores sticking to the eggs caused infection in very young
fish. This was quoted also by Geisler (1947). In contrast
Thieme (1956) never found the reproductive system infected. The
testes of infected males were often degenerate, though parasites
were not actually present in them and no infection was ever
detected in the ovaries of females even in those which were
otherwise heavily infected. He found that the skin was a common
site of infection and caused the destruction of the cells and
their pigment which resulted in the loss of color. Reichenbach-
Klinke (1952) and Thieme (1956), found the kidney infected, the
latter reporting that it was more or less destroyed and that
spores were passed through the urinary tract.

Prevalence may be as high as 50 percent (Geisler, 1947) though
Nigrelli (1953) found none in the Neon Tetra of the New York
aquarium. Mortality is high, especially among young fish
(Schaperclaus, 1941).

6. *Reproductive system*

Several microsporidia are parasites of the reproductive organs
of sish. *Pleistophora sciaeniae* was reported from the connective
tissue of the ovary, pressing between the follicles in *Sciaena*
australis (Johnston and Barcnoff, 1919). Other species are
parasites of the follicles themselves. The infected tissues are
reported to be opaque and whitish in color. Thus, the eggs of
Coregonus exiguus bondella infected with *Thelohania ovicola*
contrasted with normal eggs by their milky white appearance
(Auerbach, 1910). *Pleistophora oolytica* in the ovaries of
Leuciscus cephalus and *Esox lucius*, conveyed a white color to the
whole ovary (Weiser, 1949). Sections revealed that 10 and 15
percent of the ovarian follicles were infected in *L. cephalus*
and *E. lucius* respectively. Heavily infected follicles consisted
of closely-packed pansporoblasts superficially resembling the
normal atretic follicles.

Pflugfelder (1952) recognized that the residual bodies found
in the ovaries of several species of exotic fish were defense
reactions against the presence of a microsporidian parasite,
Glugea pseudotumefasciens Pflugfelder, 1952. The reaction was
mainly directed against rod-like stages which preceded spore

formation and involved the deposition of migratory cells in concentric layers around a central detritus of parasites and degenerate host cells. Two or more foci of infection could be encapsulated together leading to bumor-like growths which could be pushed passively out of the ovaries. The parasites often occupied the peripheral parts of the body including the liver, kidneys, spleen, pseudobranchiae, nervous system and retina. Exophthalmia was a common symptom and infection of the nervous system often resulted in interference with equilibrium, deformities of the vertebral column, and death.

P. ovariae has been carefully studied by Summerfelt and Warner (1970) with respect to its effects on the host fish *Notemigonus crysoleucas*. Only females were infected and the major sites were the ovaries although slight infection occurred in the liver, kidney, spleen, and vascular system. Infected ovaries were mottled with white, translucent, or opaque spots and streaks in the ovigerous lamellae. The oocytes developing in the lamellae were replaced by a spore-filled stroma and the white spots were formed by coalescence of several parasitized oocytes into a large amorphous mass. No cyst walls were present. These investigators found no mortality in the golden shiner minnows that were cultured for bait on farms in the United States. There was, however, a greater number of dead eggs in spawning mats of heavily infected fish than of normal fish.

Xenoma formation was reported to (Chatton and Courrier, 1923) to occur in the testes of *Cottus bubalis*. Cysts of *N. cotti* which measured up to 700 μm were easily visible as chalky-white spherical bodies, distinct against the dark, pigmented background of the testes. Each cyst lay free in a fluid-filled space and its surface was covered entirely by a brush border. The outer layers, which were probably derived from infiltrating mesenchymal cells, became modified by nuclear and cytoplasmic fusion and produced an absorptive surface that developed the brush border.

C. MORTALITY OF FISH CAUSED BY MICROSPORIDIA

Information on mortality of host fish occasioned by microsporidian infections is restricted to observations on only a few species. There is no doubt, however, that many microsporidian species can cause death of their hosts. Haley (1953) found 23 percent of the smelt population of the Great Bay region of New Hampshire infected with *Glugea hertwigii* and suggested that the disease may have contributed to the decline in smelts in that area. Legault and Delisle (1967) also found that large numbers of dead smelt in Lake Clay, Canada, mostly "Yong-of-the-year", were infected with *G. hertwigii*. The mean number of cysts per fish was 250. In contrast, fish of the same age group in Lake Heney, was not infected. The factors affecting the severity of infections in the different lakes were not established but deaths

were found to be related to mechanical and physiological damage
to the intestine and other organs rather than to the absolute
number of cysts present. The results of these Canadian workers
supported those of Schrader (1921) who, on finding adult smelt
rarely parasitized with *G. hertwigii*, proposed that the majority
of immature infected fish had died. A similar conclusion was
drawn by Stunkard and Lux (1965) who found the greatest incidence
of *G. stephani* in small flounders. Incidence figures suggested
that fish infected in their first year did not survive into
their second year.

In other incidents *P. salmonae* was the cause of two epizootics
in hatchery rainbow trout, involving almost complete loss of the
stocks (Wales and Wolf 1955). Raabe (1936) reported mortality
of red mullet *(Mullus barbatus)*, continued in aquaria. The fish
showed no external sign of infection but their livers were
hemorrhogic and were peppered with small white spots containing
a microsporidium thought to be *Nosema ovoideum* (Thelohan, 1895)
presumably, the confining conditions may have enhanced the
infection and contributed to the mortality.

CONCLUDING REMARKS

Infections of microsporidia in vertebrates may be diffuse or
localized in cysts. Cysts may compress or obstruct neighboring
tissues or (especially in fish) disturb the balance of the host.
Diffuse infections cause progressive distruction of tissues but
small foci may be partly or wholly destroyed by host cell infiltration.

Microsporidia reveal their full potential as pathogens when
the hosts are reared under intensive conditions. Their economic
importance has already been revealed in the breeding of rabbits
(Pattison, Clegg, and Duncan 1971), blue foxes (Mohn *et al.*, 1974)
and golden shiner minnows (Summerfelt and Warner 1970). As
intensive rearing methods assume greater importance, for example
in fish farming, the search for methods of control by prophylactic
or chemotherapeutic measures may become a necessity.

REFERENCES

Anver, M. R., King, N. W., and Hunt, R. D. (1972). Congenital
encephalitozoonosis in a squirrel monkey. *Vet. Pathol.* 9,
475-480.
Ashton, N., and Wirasinha, P. A. (1973). Encephalitozoonosis
(nosematosis) of the cornea. *Brit. J. Ophthal.*, 57, 669-674.
Attwood, H. D., and Sutton, R. D. (1965). *Encephalitozoon*
granulomata in rats. *J. Pathol. Bacteriol.* 89, 735-738.
Auerbach, M. (1910). Die Cnidosporidien. Eine monographische
Studie. Leipzig. 261 pp.

Basson, P. A., McCully, R. M., and Warnes, W. E. J. (1966). Nosematosis: report of a canine case in the republic of South Africa. *J.S. Afr. Vet. Med. Assoc.* <u>37</u>, 3-9.

Brown, R. J., Hinkle, D. K., Trevethan, W. P., Kupper, J. L., and McKee, A. E. (1973). Nosematosis in a squirrel monkey *(Saimiri sciureus)*. *J. Med. Primatol.* <u>2</u>, 114-123.

Cameron, G. C., and Maitland, H. B. (1924). A description of parasites in spontaneous encephalitis of rabbits. *J. Pathol. Bacteriol.* <u>27</u>, 329-333.

Canning, E. U. (1967). Vertebrates as hosts to microsporidia with special reference to rats infected with *Nosema cuniculi*. *J. Helminthel.* Suppl. 2 *(Protozool.)* <u>2</u>, 197-205.

Canning, E. U. (1971). Transmission of Microsporida, Proc. 4th Int. Coll. Insect Pathol. College Park Maryland, 415-424.

Canning, E. U., Elkan, E., and Trigg, P. I. (1964). *Plistophora myotrophica spec. nov.* causing high mortality in the common toad *Bufo bufo* L. with notes on the maintenance of *Bufo* and *Xenopus* in the laboratory. *J. Protozool.* <u>11</u>, 157-166.

Chalupský, J., Vávra, J., and Bedrnik, P. (1973). Detection of antibodies to *Encephalitozoon cuniculi* in rabbits by the indirect immunofluorescent antibody test. *Folia Parasitol.* (Prague) <u>20</u>, 281-284.

Chatton, E. (1920). Sur un complexe xéno-parasitaire morphologique et physiologique, *Nereisheimeria catenata* chez *Fritillaria pellucida*. *C. R. Acad. Sci.* Paris, <u>171</u>, 55-57.

Chatton, E., and Courrier, R. (1923). Formation d'un complexe xéno-parasitaire géant avec bordure en brosse, sous l'influence d'une microsporidie, dans le testicule de *Cottus bubalis* *C. R. Soc. Biol. Paris* <u>89</u>, 579-583.

Claussen, L. (1936). Mikrosporidieninfektion beim gesleckten Seewolf. *Deutsche. Tierarzt. Wochensch.* <u>44</u>, 307-310.

Delisle, C. (1969). Bimonthly progress of a non-lethal infection by *Glugea hertwigii* in young-of-the-year smelt, *Osmerus eperlanus mordax*. *Can. J. Zool.* <u>47</u>, 871-876.

Doflein, F. (1898). Studien zur Naturgeschichte der Protozoen III. Ueber Myxosporidien. *Zool. Jahrb. Anat.* <u>11</u>, 281-350.

Drew, H. G. (1910). Some notes on parasitic and other diseases of fish. *Parasitology* <u>3</u>, 54-62.

Fantham, H. B., Porter, A., and Richardson, L. R. (1941). Some microsporidia found in certain fishes and insects in eastern Canada. *Parasitology,* <u>33</u>, 186-208.

Geisler, R. (1947). Neon tetra-ten years, *Hyphessobrycon innesi* *The Aquarium, Philadelphia.* <u>16</u>, 254-256.

Goodpasture, E. W. (1924). Spontaneous encephalitis in rabbits. *J. Infect. Dis.* <u>34</u>, 428-432.

Hagenmuller, M. (1 99). Sur une nouvelle Myxosporidie, *Nosema stephani,* parasite du *Flesus passer* Moreau. *C. R. Acad. Sci.* *Paris,* <u>129</u>, 836-839.

Haley, A. J. (1953). Microsporidian parasite *Glugea hertwigii* in American smelt from the Great Bay region, New Hampshire. *Trans. Am. Fish. Soc.* <u>83</u>, 84-90.

Hunt, R. D., King, N. W., and Foster, H. L. (1972). Encephalitozoonosis: evidence for vertical transmission. *J. Infect. Dis.* <u>126</u>, 212-214.

Innes, J. R. M., Zeman, W., Frenkel, J. K. and Borner, G. (1962). Occult endemic encephalitozoonosis of central nervous system of mice. (Swiss Bagg-('Grady strain) *J. Neuropathol. Exp. Neurol.* <u>210</u>, 519-533.

Jakowska, S. (1964). Infeccao Microsporidea das celulas nervosas numa populacao de peixas marinhos, *Lophius americanus*. Ann. *Congr. Lat.-Amer. Zool.*, 2nd <u>1</u>, pp. 265-273.

Jakowska, S. (1965). Infection with neurotropic microsporidians in South American *Lophius Proc. Ann. Meeting Amer. Micr. Soc.* 81st pp. 161-162.

Johnston, T. H. and Bancroft, M. J. (1919). Some sporozoan parasites of Queensland freshwater fish. *J. Proc. Roy. Soc. N. S. Wales.* <u>52</u>, 520-528.

Johnstone, J. (1901). Notes on a sporozoan parasite of the plaice *Pleuronectes platessa*. *Proc. Liverpool Biol. Soc.* <u>15</u>, 184-187.

Kabata, Z. (1959). On two little-known microsporidia of marine fishes *Parasitology*, <u>49</u>, 309-315.

Kemp, R. L., and luge, J. P. (1975). *Encephalitozoon* sp in the blue-masked lovebird, *Agapornis personata:* first report of microsporidian infection in birds. *J. Protozool.* <u>22</u>, 489-491.

Légault, R-O, and Delisle, C. (1967). Acute infection by *Glugea hertwigii* Weissenberg in young-of-the-year rainbow smelt, *Osmerus eperlanus mordax* (Mitchill) *Can. J. Zool.* <u>45</u>, 1291-1294.

Lom, J., and Weiser, J. (1969). Notes on two microsporidian species from *Silurus glanis* and on the systematic status of the genus *Glugea* Thélohan. *Folia Parasitol.* (Prague) <u>16</u>, 193-200.

Malherbe, H., and Munday, V. (1958). *Encephalitozoon cuniculi* infection of laboratory mice and rabbits in South Africa. *J. South Af. Vet. Med. Assoc.* <u>29</u>, 241-246.

Margileth, A. M., Strano, A. J., Chandra, R., Neafie, R., Blum, M., and McCully, R. M., (1973). Disseminated nosematosis in an immunologically compromised infant. *Arch. Pathol.* <u>95</u>, 145-150.

Matsubayashi, H., Koike, T., Mikata, I., Takei, H., and Hagiwara, S. (1959). A case of Encephalitozoon-like body infection in man. *Arch. Pathol.*, <u>67</u>, 181-187.

Mercier, L. (1921). *Glugea gigantea* Thélohan, réactions des tissus de l'hôte a l'infection. *C. R. Soc. Biol. Paris* <u>84</u>, 261-264.

Mohn, S. F., Nordstoga, K., Krogsrud, J., and Helgebostad, A. (1974). Transplacental transmission of *Nosema cuniculi* in the blue fox *(Alopex lagopus)*. *Acta. path. Microbiol. Scand.* Section B <u>82</u>, 299-300.

Nelson, J. B. (1967). Experimental transmission of a murine
    microsporidian in Swiss mice. *J. Bacteriol.* 94, 1340-1345.
Nemeczek, A. (1911). Beiträge zur Kenntnis der Myxo-und
    Microsporidien der Fische. *Arch. Protistenkd.*, 22, 143-169.
Nigrelli, R. F. (1946). Studies on the marine resources of
    Southern New England V. Parasites and diseases of the
    ocean pout, *Macrozoarces americanus. Bull. Bingham
    Oceanogr. Collection* 9, 187-221.
Nigrelli, R. F. (1953). Two diseases of the neon tetra,
    Hyphessobrycon innesi. Aquarium J. San Francisco 24, 203-
    208.
Nordstoga, K. (1972). Nosematosis in blue foxes. *Nord. Vet.
    Med.* 24, 21-24.
Pakes, S. P., Shadduck, J. A., and Olsen, R. (1972). A diagnostic
    skin test for encephalitozoonosis (nosematosis) in rabbits.
    Lab. Anim. Sci. 22, 870-887.
Pattison, M., Clegg, F. G., and Duncan, A. L. (1971). An outbreak
    of encephalomyelitis in broiler rabbits caused by *Nosema
    cuniculi. Vet. Rec.* 88, 404-405.
Pflugfelder, O. (1952). Die sog. Restkörper der Cyprinodontidae
    und Cyprinidae als Abwehrreaktionen gegen Mikrosporidienbefall.
    Z. Parasitenk. 15, 321-334.
Plowright, W. (1952). An encephalitis-nephritis syndrome in the
    dog probably due to congenital *Encephalitozoon* infection.
    J. Comp. Pathol. 62, 83-92.
Plowright, W., and Yeoman, G. (1952). Probable *Encephalitozoon*
    infection of the dog. *Vet. Rec.* 64, 381-383.
Putz, R. E., Hoffman, G. L., and Dunbar, C. E. (1965). Two new
    species of *Plistophora* (Microsporidea) from North American
    fish with a synopsis of Microsporidea of freshwater and
    euryhaline fishes. *J. Protozool.* 12, 228-236.
Raabe, H. (1936). Etudes de microorganismes parasites des
    poissons de mer I. *Nosema ovoideum* Thél. dans le foie dex
    rougets. *Bull Oceanogr. (Monaco).*, 696, 1-11.
Reichenbach-Klinke, H. (1952). Neue Beobachtungen uber den
    Erreger der Neon-Fischkrankheit *Plistophora hyphessobryconis*
    Schäperclaus (Sporozoa, Microsporidia). *Aquarien u.
    Terrarien Zeitschrift* 5, 320-322.
Schaperclaus, W. (1941). Eine neue Microsporidienkrankheit beim
    Neonfisch und seinen Verwandten. *Wochenschrift. für
    Aquarien-u. Terrarrienkunde.* 39/40, 381-384.
Schrader, F. (1921). A microsporidian occurring in the smelt.
    J. Parasitol. 7, 151-153.
Schwartz, F. J. (1963). A new *Ichthyosporidium* parasite of the
    spot *(Leiostomus xanthurus):* a possible answer to recent
    oyster mortalities. *Prog. Fish-Cult.* 25, 181-184.
Seibold, H. R., and Fussell, E. N. (1973). Intestinal micro-
    sporidiosis in *Callicebus moloch. Lab. Anim. Sci.* 23,
    115-118.

Shadduck, J. A. and Pakes, S. P. (1971). Encephalitozoonosis (Nosematosis) and toxoplasmosis. *Am. J. Pathol.*, 64, 657-671.

Sprague, V. (1969). Microsporida and tumours, with particular reference to the lesion associated with *Ichthyosporidium* sp. Schwartz 1963. *Nat. Cancer Inst. Monogr.* 31, 237-249.

Sprague, V., and Vernick, S. (1968). Light and electron-microscope study of a new species of *Glugea* (Microsporida, Nosematidae) in the 4-spined stickleback, *Apeltes quadracus*. *J. Protozool.* 15, 547-571.

Stunkard, H. W., and Lux, F. E. (1965). A microsporidian infection of the digestive tract of the winter flounder, *Pseudopleuronectes americanus*. *Biol. Bull.*, 129 371-387.

Summerfelt, R. C. and Warner, M. C. (1970). Incidence and intensity of infection of *Plistophora ovariae*, a microsporidian parasite of the golden shiner, *Notemigonus crysoleucas*. Special Publication No. 5. *Am. Fish Soc. Washington D. C.*, pp. 142-160.

Thélohan, P. (1892). Observations sur les Myxosporidies et essai de classification de ces organismes. *Bull. Soc. Philom.* 4, 165-178.

Thélohan, P. (1895). Recherches sur les Myxosporidies. *Bull. Sci. France Belg.* 26, 100-394.

Thieme, H. (1956). Erkennung und Wesen der Neonkrankheit *Aquarium u. Terrarium.* 3, 172-175.

Twort, J. M. and Twort, C. C. (1932). Disease in relation to carcinogenic agents among 60,000 experimental mice. *J. Pathol. Bacteriol.*, 35, 219-242.

Van Rensburg, I. B. J. and Du Plessis, J. L. (1971). Nosematosis in a cat: a case report. *J. South Afr. Vet. Med. Assoc.*, 42, 327-331.

Vávra, J., Blazek, K., Lávicka, N., Koczkova, I., Kalafa, S., and Stehlík, M. (1971). Nosematosis in carnivores. *J. Parasitol.* 57, 923-924.

Wales, J. and Wolf, H. (1955). Three protozoan diseases of trout in California. *Calif. Fish & Game.* 41, 183-187.

Weiser, J. (1949). Studies on some parasites of fishes. *Parasitology.* 49, 164-166.

Weissenberg, R. (1911). Beiträge zur Kenntnis von *Glugea lophii* Doflein II. Ueber den Bau der Cysten und die Beziehungen zeischen Parasit und Wirtsgewebe. *Sitz. Ber. Berlin Gesell. Naturf. Freunde.* 149-157.

Weissenberg, R. (1913). Beiträge zur Kenntnis des Zeugungskeises der Mikrosporidien *Glugea anomala* Moniez und *hertwigii* Weissenberg. *Arch. Mikr. Anat.* 82, 81-163.

Weissenberg, R. (1922). Mikrosporidien, Myxosporidien und Chlamydozoen als Zellparasiten von Fischer. *Verhandl. Deutsch. Zool. Gesellsch.* 27, 41-43.

Weissenberg, R. (1949). Cell growth and cell transformation induced by intracellular parasites. *Anat. Rec.* 103, 101-102.

Weissenberg, R. (1968). Intracellular development of the microsporidian *Glugea anomala* Moniez in hypertrophying migratory cells of the fish *Gasterosteus aculeatus* L. an example of the formation of Xenoma tumors. *J. Protozool.* 15, 44-57.

Wright, J. H. and Craighead, E. M. (1922). Infectious motor paralysis in young rabbits. *J. Exp. Med.* 36, 135-140.

Microsporidia in Invertebrates: Host-Parasite Relations at the Organismal Level

Jaroslav Weiser

INSTITUTE OF ENTOMOLOGY
DEPARTMENT OF INSECT PATHOLOGY
CZECHOSLOVAK ACADEMY OF SCIENCES
PRAHA, CZECHOSLOVAKIA

I. INTRODUCTION

In studies on the relationship of the microsporidia to their
invertebrate hosts, the identification of the individual species
is of primary importance. This exercise, however, is becoming
increasingly difficult in view of the growing number of microsporidia
isolated from new hosts and the limited number of diagnostic factors
for species identification. According to a recent world census,
the number of invertebrate species is estimated to be nearly one
million. My experience in distribution of microsporidia of invertebrate hosts indicates that there may be a microsporidian in every
living invertebrate. If only one per cent were new species, there
would be as many as 10,000 species to distinguish. Obviously, it
would be a monumental task to distinguish this large number.
Therefore, the extreme care is necessary to record all characteristics

II. SPECIES IDENTITY AND HOST SPECIFICITY

Whenever data on the structure of a microsporidian under study
are similar to those obtained for other species, the primary
diagnostic feature is range of infectivity by the parasite and
nature of the infection under various conditions. Important
factors of host specificity are: (1) the host tissues in which the
parasite may or may not be able to develop; (2) route of entry
such as by ingestion, penetration of the body cavity by stinging
or puncturing by parasites, or by vertical transmission; and (3)
the availability of the parasite to the host depending upon an
ecological coincidence of transmission in a common locality,
food source, and specific shelters.

III. GERMINATION OF THE SPORES

The way of entry into the host and its significance are discussed
later. In oral transmission, mature spores are carried into the
host with food and liquid. Little information is available on
conditions of spore germination within the gut as well as the
physicochemical processes involved. Sometimes, the autonomy of
these processes is independent of the germ within the spore.
In some cases extrusion of the polar filament is not induced, even
in spores with viable germs, by a variety of stimuli. In other

cases spores with dead germs are able to extrude their filaments
merely as the result of a change in osmotic pressure (Ohshima, 1973).
The site in the host's gut where spore opens differs among the various
microsporidian species. Generally, the first cysts with developing
stages are found in the middle part of the abdomen. It is not
certain whether germs from open spores migrate from the gut wall
to the body cavity and from there invade the salivary glands, the
Malpighian tubules, and the different parts of the gut, or whether
closed spores migrate from the gut to the Malpighian tubules
through their openings in the end of the midgut, or from the mouth
to the salivary glands. This second mode seems unlikely because
the spores are passive migrants and the flow of secretions from the
glands and tubules is against them. Only microsporidia infecting
the gut wall are able to reach the definite site for development
directly by injection of the germ through the polar filament.
Entry through the cuticle also occurs in certain helminths
and molluscs from the outside because there is no
opening to the intestinal tract. Infection of the tape worm
Moniezia benedeni with microsporidia such as *Nosema bischoffi*
suggest an infection of the larval stages in vector mites before
the tape worm invades the final host (Weiser, 1951). The transmission to single segments of the host body may occur during
their growth from the scolex and by direct passage of extruded
germs into the proglotids in the intestine of infected goats.
Passage through the gut of a vertebrate does not damage the microsporidian spores, as was demonstrated by Günther (1959) with
Pleistophora schubergi passed through the gut of a sparrow.

Some authors (e.g., Debaisieux, 1919) observed empty spores in the
infected tissues of blackflies and discussed a possible autoinfection where spores that originate in a host open in the same
individual host and are the source of a new infection. According
to all we know, the autoinfection is not an ordinary step in the
scheme of development of microsporidia in invertebrate hosts. The
reason, however, is not the incapability of the spores to open in
the balanced medium of the hemolymph. Our experiments with injections of *Nosema plodiae* and *N. heterosporum* into *Galleria
mellonella* produced evidence that the use of a number of mature
spores in one series and the same number of vegetative stages in
another, resulted in the same spore counts in infected caterpillars
after eight days (Weiser, 1975a). Spores stored for 8, 14 and 20
days on dry slides at room temperature and injected into *Galleria*
L$_5$-larvae produced infection. This is adequate evidence that spores
of *N. heterosporum* are able to germinate in the hemolymph of
Galleria when injected.

The tertiary zone of limitation of a possible transmission depends on localization and the timing of the transmission.

IV. HOST RANGE OF MICROSPORIDIA

There are groups of infectious agents, in addition to microsporidia, such as viruses, rickettsiae, fungi, coccidia, and
gregarines that are typical of specific habitats. An example is
the group of pests of stored products (Mattes, 1927, Weiser, 1953c,
Kellen and Lindegren, 1968). Other groups are present in blackflies, mosquitoes, and insects that feed on the leaves of deciduous
trees and conifers. Machay (1957) demonstrated that *Nosema
bombycis* is a common pathogen of more than 20 different Lepidoptera
in the environment surrounding silkworm breeding farms in Hungary.
Usually, those microsporidia that invade many different tissues in
the host body are not very host specific (e.g., *Nosema mesnili,
N. heterosporum, N. plodiae, N. ephestiae*). Kaya (1973) demonstrated nine alternate hosts for *Pleistophora schubergi*. In
Europe there are seven more species reported by different authors
(Weiser, 1961).

In addition to logical coincidences of candidate hosts for
experimental transmissions among invertebrates living on the same
food plant, some unexpected transmissions show many possible
combinations. Undeen and Maddox (1973) transmitted *Nosema algerae*
to flies, Lepidoptera, Hemiptera, Odonata, Orthoptera, and crayfish.

V. ADAPTATIONS TO TRANSMISSIONS

Most spores of microsporidia infecting aquatic hosts are adapted
to specific ways of transport. Whereas they are thinwalled in
terrestrial hosts, most of the aquatic hosts have thickwalled,
and sometimes, corrugated or sculptured spores. They resist
desiccation in temporary habitats of mosquito larvae where water
disappears during the summer. Most variable are spores of freshwater species living in streams. One group has elongated spores
(*Mrázekia, Octosporea*). They are typical of hosts occurring in
mud and sand on the bottom of streams (oligochaets, midges,
crustacea etc.). Crescent- or spiral-shaped spores of *Spiroglugea*
and *Toxoglugea* provide for a wide area of spore distribution as
soon as they are liberated from the oval octosporous pansporoblasts. Their passive spinning motion recalls the motion of some
seeds in the air. Spores of *Caudospora*, a pest of blackflies in
streams, have lateral rims and a caudal appendage, very important
for steering them into extended filtering nets of blackfly larvae.
Long needles on pansporoblasts of *Trichoduboscqia*, curled episporal
hairs on spores of *Pleistophora debaisieuxi*, and the three long
appendages on each spore of *Thelohania octospora* probably serve to
retard movement in water; they become entrapped in algae on the
bottom of streams and are exposed to receptive hosts. Specialized
membranes on the surface of *Weiseria laurenti* spores cause them
to rotate around their posterior end.

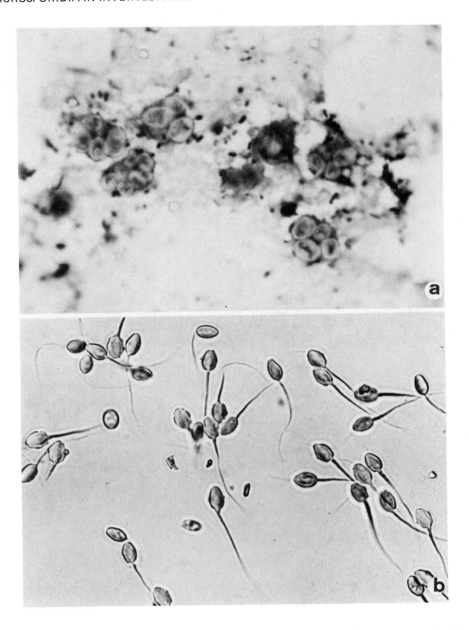

Fig. 1. a, Teratospores of *Thelohania hyphantriae* in the fall
webworm. X 1000; b, *Caudospora simulii*, spores and
sporoblasts with caudal appendage and lateral crests.
X 900.

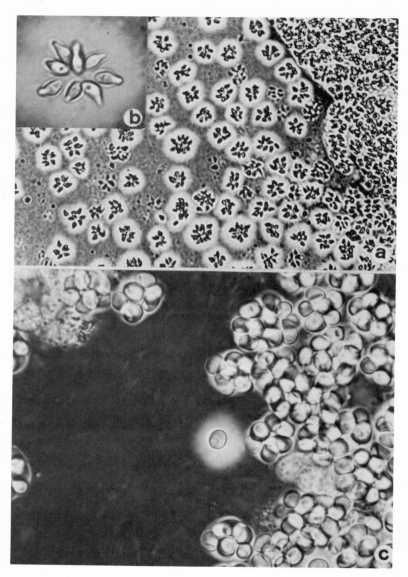

Fig. 2.   a, *Thelohania asterias* with gelatinous capsules, X 800;
b, Single pansporoblast of *T. asterias* with visible
asymetrical spores. X 1000; c, *Thelohania lairdi*, pansporoblasts without apparent mucose flotators and one
free spore with well developed capsule. X 1000.

Another important spore adaptation is the formation of mucous
capsules. They originate from remains of the cytoplasm of plasmodia and are condensed when inside the invertebrate host. They
increase to several times the size of the original spore when
liberated into water. Spores with capsules float for a long
period of time. They have sometimes been described as special
types of planctonic algae, as was the case with *Marssoniella
elegans* which was recently identified by Komárek and Vávra (1968)
as a microsporidian of the genus *Gurleya*. In several cases
(e.g. in *Thelohania lairdi*) the mucus distends the pansporoblast
and breaks the envelope, liberating single spores that float in
water (Weiser, 1964). Mucous floats are invisible in fresh mounts
and can be made visible with India ink. In other microsporidia,
material is concentrated in rigid, non-soluble masses which hold
the spores together in pansporoblasts, e.g. *Telomyxa glugeiformis*.

VI. INFECTIVE DOSE

It is yet not determined whether aggregations of spores in pansporoblasts phylogenetically represents "infective packages" or
minimum infective units for their hosts. Under laboratory conditions, a dose of 40 spores given *per os* produced positive infections with *N. heterosporum* (Weiser, 1975a). Other investigators
were able to demonstrate direct relations between the number of
spores fed to the resulting percentage of infectious such as with
Nosema pyraustae (Lewis and Lynch, 1974) or *N. algerae* (Undeen
and Alger, 1975). This may not be the only way the host interacts
with the parasite. In the above mentioned cases resulting infections were usually not lethal. Kharazi -Pakdel (1968) estimated the LD_{50} of *N. melolonthae* for the European chafer to be
1×10^5 for L_1 and, 5×10^6 for L_2 and L_3 when administered in the
diet. In our own experiments with *N. plodiae, N. heterosporum,
N. mesnili, N. ephestiae,* and *P. schubergi,* we could not identify
the original dose of infective stages on the basis of subsequent
spore counts in the host from the fifth day. In all these cases
the primary development of vegetative stages without sporulation
produced large masses of schizonts, and sporulation occurred at
a time at which all differences in initial spore dosages had
disappeared.

The yield of spores in the infected insect, crustacean, or
mollusc depends on the type of microsporidian and the host. It
may change from 5×10^5 to 1×10^6 in mosquitoes or blackflies,
$5 - 10 \times 10^6$ in beetles (with extreme cases of 2×10^8) to $5 -
10 \times 10^8$ in *Barathra brassicae* (Weiser and Hostounský, 1972)
infected with *N. heterosporum*. In *Antherea pernyi,* the production
of spores in the fat body of the last instar larva was 2×10^9
to 30×10^9. In infected crabs or lobsters the masses of spores
may increase to values of 10×10^{10} and more. In infections of
the fat body for the above mentioned cases, the limiting factor

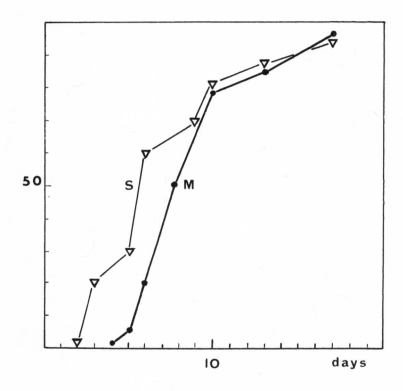

Fig. 3. Mortality curve of *Hyphantria cunea* after administration
of spores of *Thelohania hyphantriae*. S- overdosage and
septicaemia, M- low dose and normal microsporidian infection.

was the volume of the fat body. The final spore count in dead
B. *brassicae* prepupae infected with 9×10^3 to 1×10^5 spores
during the 4th instar was 4 to 5×10^8. This is the number of
spores that nearly fills the available space in the fat body.
Similarly, as many as 1.8×10^8 spores of *Pleistophora schubergi*
were present in the gut of *Feltia segetum* during the final phase
of infection (Nilova, 1967). In our experiments with B. *brassicae*
and *Pleistophora schubergi*, the number of spores in the dissected
gut of the prepupa was 23×10^8, equal to number of spores discarded in the feces during the life of the infected animal.

The final spore count in an infected animal reflects the natural
loss of infective stages during the transmission. Presumably,
infective spores may be transmitted much easier among mosquitoes
and blackflies than among Coleoptera and Lepidoptera. One
important factor, of course, is the stage of instar exposed to
infective spores.

VII. EFFECT OF HOST DEVELOPMENTAL STAGE ON INFECTIVE DOSE

Experimental data derived by different investigators indicate a
sharp increase in the spore dose necessary to infect subsequent
instars. In many instances it was very difficult or even impossible
to infect the latest instars. Milner (1972) indicated that the
difference between LD_{50} of *N. whitei* in *Tribolium castaneum* was
1.8×10^6 spores for L_1 and 1.0×10^{10} spores for L_5 in experiments
in which spores were administered in the food. Analogous results
were obtained upon feeding different instars of *Galleria mellonella*
with spores of *N. heterosporum* or *N. plodiae*. In contrast, injections of high and low spore doses into different instars of the
wax moth larvae resulted in infection. Apparently, infection does
not depend so much on the absolute number of spores introduced into
the host as it does on the gut barrier. Administration of varying
numbers of spores to different instars of a lepidopteran has been
estimated according to the following variables:

	Instars				
	I.	II.	III.	IV.	V.
Length of gut (mm)	2	5	15	20	35
Approximate volume of gut (mm^3)	0.5	1.25	15	80	560
Spore concentration in 1 mm^3 of gut fed 100 spores	200	80	6.6	1.2	0.2
Spore dose necessary to produce equal concentration of 100 spores in 1 mm^3 of gut	100	250	3×10^3	16×10^3	11×10^4

Such calculations are presented to demonstrate the increasing dosage required to produce the same concentration of spores in late instars as in early instars. No correction was made for the polar filament which, at a length of 200 to 400 μm, is able to inject spore germs into the gut wall of minute early in-star larvae but cannot do so very efficiently in late larval instars characterized by a broad gut lumen. These differences may, in part, explain the phenomenon observed by Nordin and Maddox (1974) that closely related hosts occurring in the same locality differ in their susceptibility to parasitation by a certain micro-sporidian. Probably, at the time of distribution of the infective spores, only one of prospective hosts was present in the instar most susceptible to the offered dose.

VIII. MICROSPORIDIAN ADAPTATION

Transmission requires a certain adaptation of the pathogens to a specific cycle of development of the host. Mosquitoes which have died after oviposition on the surface of a breeding place are readily sought by young larvae for food. In several groups of insects, eggs are fixed to the surface of plants by a secretion of special glands or by a mixture of the secretion with feces or, in other cases such as bark beetles, with a mixture of frass. Micro-sporidia are introduced with excretions of infected glands or gut cells. The hatched larvae feed on infected material when they break the egg shells. In this way, infections may be transmitted on single eggs deposited on plants even when there is no trans-mission in the egg, e.g., the sunflower moth, *Homeosoma nebulellum* and its *Nosema* pathogen (Weiser, 1953). Such early infections usually cause high mortality during early larval instars and there is no transfer of the infection into pupae and adults. The in-fection has a "larval" predominance. Healthy adults depose eggs and late larval instars come into contact with the spores from past generation dead larvae. This late infection persists in pupae and adults and has an "adult" predominance. The bimodal alternation of infection occurs mainly in pests of stored products, in animals living in colonies, or in gregarious habits. For example, the maintenance of diseases of blackflies must be ensured mainly in the following way: Spores from dead larvae are transported down-stream and fresh infections can be acquired only with material comming downstream. A steady transfer of infective stages upstream must occur as source of infection. Adults flying to the oviposition-sites must be involved in this transport.

IX. ESTABLISHMENT OF INFECTIONS

The establishment of a microsporidian in its invertebrate host has two different mechanisms. Infections in the gut wall are initiated by injected germs. All further stages develop in infected cells and there is no need for the germs to cross the gut and enter the hemolymph. Destroyed cells burst into the gut and spores leave the host with the feces. Re-entries of germs from spores passing through the gut into other cells of the gut are possible. The therapeutic value of Fumidil B on *Nosema apis* in the honey bee and the action of sufonamides are explained by the action of the drugs on stages in the gut cavity and the reduction of re-entries of germs from the gut.

Infections beyond the gut wall need the transportation of vegetative stages in the hemolymph over the whole body. In some of them a primary development in the oenocytes around the heart and gut is indispensable; in others it seems to be less important. After the first multiplication (which can be the final one in errative infections of *Nosema necatrix* in *Barathra brassicae* or *N. ephestiae* in *Carpocapsa pomonella*), vegetative stages circulate in the hemolymph and are phagocytized by eventual recipient tissues. In their hosts microsporidia have one or several target tissues where they concentrate and develop. The mechanism of this selection is not known. This tissue affinity is often so constant and typical that it can be used as a diagnostic marker. Typical one-tissue-infections are those of the fat body, of the gut, of the Malpighian tubules, or of the muscles. Other microsporidia have affinity to tissues of the same embryonal origin. They use one widely distributed tissue such as the connective tissue which they invade to accomplish proliferation in all adjacent tissues (gonads, muscles, nerve ganglia, etc.). An example is *Nosema bombycis*.

X. SUCCESSION OF INFECTED TISSUES

In other generalized infections one can follow a succession of the infected tissues. In *Nosema plodiae* the oenocytes, salivary glands, and the fat body are infected in succession. In *Nosema stegomyiae*, it is the gut wall, the fat body, salivary glands, Malpighian tubules, hypoderm, neural ganglia, muscles, and ovaries (Weiser, 1961) that are progressively infected. In *Nosema* NFW, in the fall webworm, *Hyphantria cunea*, the sequence is the midgut, the foregut, the hindgut, Malpighian tubules, fat body, gonads, the silk glands, nervous tissue, and the muscle (Nordin and Maddox, 1974). In some infections such as with *Nosema muscularis* and the gypsy moth, the tracheal end cells on the surface of the gut are the first centers of infection (Weiser, 1957).

The extent of damage caused within a given time and the succession of invaded tissues varies with the same microsporidian from host to host. Where it is not possible to use experimental transmission for studies on individual variability, differences in the localization of the infection in different hosts may iniciate descriptions of new species. A remarkable example reported by Weiser and Coluzzi (1972) is *Pleistophora culicis*, which not only

changes the sequence of infected tissues in different secondary
experimental hosts but does not even reinfect the original host
from which the infective spores were isolated. Experimentally
selected new hosts, *Anopheles stephensi*, *A. albimanus*, and
A. gambiae can maintain successive infections originating from
spores of dead larvae of the same species of hosts. In contrast,
Culex pipiens and *Culiseta longiareolata*, (both being the natural
source of the infection), cannot cross-infect each other nor are
they able to acquire the infection when viable spores from any
origin are fed to them. In the original natural locality of
infected mosquitoes there is a thick layer of detritus and dead
bodies of infected larvae on the bottom of the basin that have
accumulated during the year. Continuously hatching new egg rafts
deliver first larvae of different age and different degree of
maturation into contact with spores at the bottom. Consequently,
some of the spores will hatch and infect whereas others pass
through the gut without infecting.

The genus *Parathelohania*, consisting of octosporous microsporidia whose hosts mainly are mosquitoes, produces two different
types of spores, thin-walled and thick-walled, which indicates
differences in their resistance to external climatic conditions
(Hazard and Anthony, 1974).

XI. RELATIONSHIP OF HOST SEX AND MICROSPORIDIAN DEVELOPMENT

All microsporidia attacking terrestrial hosts show no special
association with the sex of the infected animal. In aquatic invertebrates, the situation is different. For laboratory reared
mosquitoes derived from wild eggs, has been established that about
two percent of Florida *Anopheles quadrimaculatus* and *A. crucians*
have a latent infection with *Parathelohania legeri* and *P. obesa*.
The infection was transmitted in the eggs of infected females.
All larvae of the infected stock with visible microsporidian cysts
in the fat body had male gonad-anlagen and died before pupation.
The other larvae with no signs of infection, produced female mosquitoes. Here the microsporidia appeared first during pupation and,
in the case of adult females, in the oenocytes, and the ovaries.
Furthermore, the eggs were infected. The spores from the adult
mosquitoes were thin-walled (Hazard and Weiser, 1968). Both
sexes were equally infected, indicating that there was no induced
shift to one sex or the other. However, the extent of development
and the time required for development was determined by the sex
of the host. Maurand (1973) found in his study that all visibly
infected blackfly larvae were males. In other mosquitoes infected
by microsporidia the differentiation of visibly infected adults
was not so strict because males as well as females emerged from
infected larvae. *Parathelohania legeri* was able to sterilize
infected rearings causing elimination of all males. Other microsporidia heavily reduced the number of males but did not cause
complete kill.

Octosporea effeminans has a sex-determining influence on the offspring of infected *Gammarus duebeni* females where it is localized
in the ovaries (Bulnheim and Vávra, 1968). All infected eggs
developed into females; the infected populations were void of males.
Those males present immigrated from a progeny of noninfected
females. The same phenomenon was observed in another microsporidian
occurring in the same host, *Thelohania herediteria* (Bulnheim, 1971);
however, not all eggs were infected. Sex differentiation of
G. duebeni occurrs some time after hatching and it may depend on
the androgenic gland and its endocrine function. The development
of this gland seems to be inhibited by the microsporidian causing
feminization of the larvae. Thus, the factor ultimately determining
the sex change is the presence of a microsporidian in the body, not
necessarily in the androgenic gland or the ovary.

XII. HORMONAL EXCRETIONS OF MICROSPORIDIA

In some cases, microsporidia have been accused to produce a hormonal
substance that slows down or prevents pupation. Fisher and Sanborn
(1964) found that larvae of *Tribolium castaneum* grew faster, had
supernumerary molts, and pupated rarely, if ever, when injected with
Nosema whitei. Milner (1972), on the other hand, performed similar
experiments but did not find any evidence to support the conclusions
of Fisher and Sanborn. Issi and Maslennikova (1964) recorded a
decrease in susceptibility to diapause, induced normally by
shortening of daylight, in *Apanteles glomeratus* infected with
Nosema mesnili. Replacement of fat and protein reserves in the fat
body of insects with microsporidia cause retardation of the prepupal stage for five to fifteen days, with subsequent death of the
insect or malformation of the pupae. Maurand (1973) identified
three abnormal larval instars produced by larvae of blackflies
with microsporidian infections. Maurand and Bouix (1969) identified
secretions of sulfomucopolysacharides during sporogony of
Thelohania fibrata with substances analogous to juvenile hormones.
In my laboratory in which spores of *N. plodiae, N. heterosporum,*
and T. *ephestiae* were injected into L_4 of the wax moth, doses of
$5 - 8 \times 10^3$ caused retardation of pupation for 10 days whereas
doses over 10×10^3 spores per larva caused dormancy without
pupation and death after two to six weeks. During this time, the
fat body was filled with spores and did not contain any reserve
material for formation of pupal tissues.

XIII. TRANSMISSION OF MICROSPORIDIA BY PARASITES

The transmission of *Thelohania ephestiae* in the flour moth has
been shown to be associated with the parasitic hymenopteran
Habrobracon hebetor (Payne, 1933). Paillot (1918) related the
transmission of *Perezia legeri* with *Apanteles glomeratus*. Blunck
(1952) presented evidence for the transmission of P. *polyvora* in

infected eggs by as many as seven different hymenoterous parasites
of the cabbage butterfly, *Pieris brassicae*, to caterpillars of
this lepidopteran and to caterpillars of *Pieris rapae* and *Aporia
crataegi*. Hostounský (1963) observed that only 50 percent of all
punctures of caterpillars by *Apanteles glomeratus* was for egg
disposition. Issi and Maslennikova (1964) ascertained that the
ovipositor withdraws some hemolymph and fat body cells from
parasitized hosts and subsequently inoculates other hosts. Such
a procedure can initiate infection without actual egg deposition.
Injection of material *via* oviposition puncture produces in
Pieris an infection characterized by spores appearing first in
the hypoderm, the fat body and muscles, and later in the gut wall
or the Malpighian tubules. This selection of infected tissues
corresponds with that described by Paillot (1918) for *Perezia
legeri*. When spores are transmitted in food, the infection con-
centrates in the gut, the Malpighian tubules, the silk glands
and only later does it appear in the muscles and the fat body
corresponding with *P. mesnili*. So, the route of invasion changes
entirely the pattern infection.

XIV. INTERACTION OF MICROSPORIDIA WITH THEIR HOSTS

Interaction of different microsporidia with one host or of
different hosts with one microsporidian involves an assortment
of variations. Sometimes, the infection is acute in one host and
chronic in another. An acute infection results in death of the
host within 10 to 14 days. A chronic infection causes late
mortality before pupation or in the adult stage. A third type,
an inapparent infection, occurs in those cases where spores and
vegetative stages are present but the rate of multiplication is
so low that regeneration replaces all infected cells and there
is no visible alteration of the host. Acute infections do not
produce enough spore material to maintain infection in the population. Consequently, there must be another supply of infective
material from a host with a chronic infection. Extreme cases of
inapparent infections are erratic; they are occasionally introduced infections that are not able to develop effectively in the
host. In most cases, they are characterized by dark tumor-like cysts
such as observed by Henry (1967) in *Nosema acridiophage*. The reaction of many microsporidia to a less suitable host is the formation
of teratospores such as in *Thelohania hyphantriae* (Weiser, 1953a).
Other times, only variation of spore size occurs such as in
Pleistophora culicis (Weiser and Coluzzi, 1972). Some infections
are characterized by increased phagocytosis and formation of
inflamatory responses in the host. Brooks (1971) described such
reactions in *Manduca sexta* infected with *Nosema sphingidis* and

I described another such case for *Ecdyonurus venosus* infected with *Nosema baetis* (Weiser, 1956). The spores were ensheathed in polyphenolic coagula and subsequently destroyed.

A nonreceptive host is infected with the help of a hymenopterous parasite and a hyperparasite (McNeil and Brooks, 1974) or a mixed infection of two microsporidia such as *Thelohania similis* and *Nosema lymantriae* in the brown tail moth (Weiser, 1957). Teratogenesis has been described for *Gurleya sokolovi*, a parasite of the aquatic mite, *Limnochares aquatica* (Issi and Lipa, 1968) in which there was a reduction of maturating sporoblasts from the original eight to four. According to Kellen *et al.* (1966), *Thelohania californica* is not able to sporulate in hybrid mosquitoes *(Culex tarsalis X C. peus)* because the spore wall does not develop completely. In some cases the host is unsuitable for the development of the microsporidian when it migrates to a different environment. *Octosporea effeminans* does not develop in *Gammarus* living in water with 30 percent salinity.

XV. INTERACTION OF MICROSPORIDIA WITH OTHER PATHOGENS

The bacterial flora of the gut determines, in part, whether a given dose of spores will cause a chronic or an acute infection. All results with infective dosages and LD_{50} of insects kept on nonsterile food are valid only for the spore dose as well as the bacterial flora and, thus, have no absolute value. When toxic bacteria such as *Pseudomonas, Serratia* or *Proteus* are present together with microsporidian spores, doses of 5 to 10,000 spores per caterpillar cause primary septicaemias and the caterpilars die within the first five days. In experiments with insects reared on semisterile artificial media, the doses of spores necessary to cause septicemias are much higher (Hostounský, 1973). Multiple perforation of the gut wall with the polar filaments may facillitate entrance by the bacteria. The second group with doses between 1 and 4,000 spores per caterpillar causes toxic stress. Weiser and Veber (1955) demonstrated such a reaction with the browntail moth and *Malacosoma neustrium* infected with *Thelohania hyphantriae* that 30 percent of the larvae remained motionless on leaves for 20 days, did not accept food, and moved only when touched. Eventually, they died. Sometimes, microsporidia that do not infect a host because they are dead or cannot survive in the test insect, cause some abnormal development of the insect (Fig. 4a, b).

Combinations of two different microsporidia do not necessarily cause a more severe noxious effect than an infection with a single organism. The mortality curve for such a combination resembles

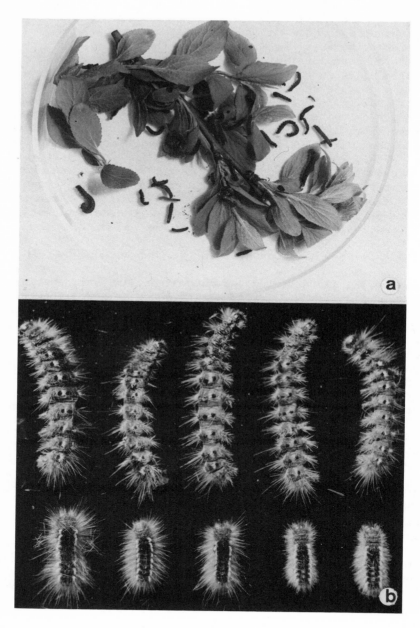

Fig. 4.   a, *Malacosoma neustrium*-caterpillars after infection with
          T. hyphantriae.   Stage of motionless cachexy; b, Normal
          and stressed prepupae of *Euproctis chrysorrhoea* after
          administration of dead *T. hyphantriae* spores.

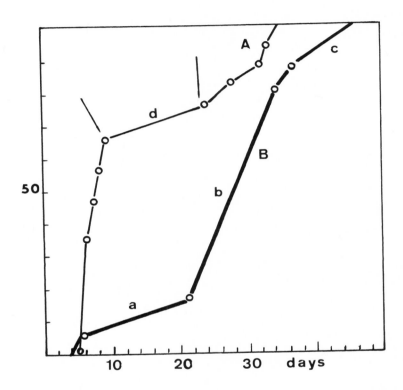

Fig. 5. *Thelohania hyphantriae* in *Euproctis chrysorrhoea*. A,
curve of the infection with the motionless cachexy /d/;
B, normal mortality curve for L_3 with the three distinct
periods of mortality a, b, and c.

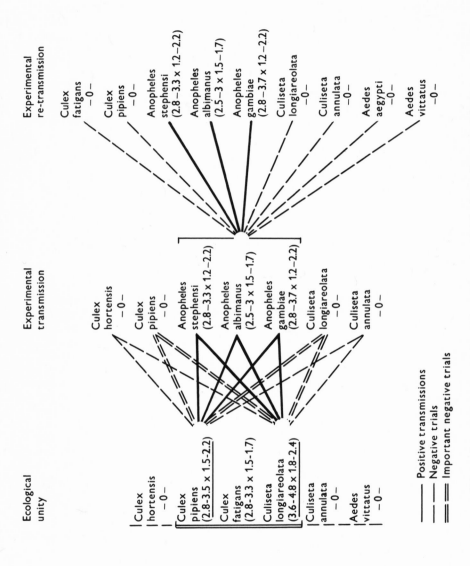

Fig. 6. Experimental transmission of *Pleistophora culicis* to different hosts and the resulting size of spores.

that of the more patogenic microsporidian (Weiser, 1961). Nordin and Maddox (1972) studied interactions of *Nosema* sp., *Pleistophora schubergi hyphantriae*, and a polyhedral virus of the fall webworm caterpillar. The virus alone was more efficient than with the microsporidia or the microsporidia alone. Infections with microsporidia combined with cytoplasmic or pox- viruses did not cause any significant synergism. The same result followed infections with nematodes and microsporidia. The microsporidia *N. otiorrhynchi* supplemented with low doses of insecticides, caused an earlier knock-down and higher mortality (Weiser, 1961).

XVI. CELLULAR AND HUMORAL HOST REACTIONS

Adverse reactions of the host to microsporidia have not been observed at the cellular level. Vegetative stages usually are incorporated into host cells without adverse reactions and parasitophorous vacuoles are formed only during the sporogony as a result of proteolysis occurring around maturating spores (Weiser and Žizka, 1975). Comparative studies on normal, virus- and *Nosema plodiae*-infected waxmoth larvae by polyacrylamide gel electrophoresis of the hemolymph (Weiser and Lysenko, 1972) revealed that some fractions of the hemolymph were changed during the infection. The fractions affected during the infection were different from those affected during virus infection. Peaks of slow-moving high molecular fractions were smaller and migrated to the end of the column. Electrophoretic analysis of hydrophobic and hydrophilic extracts of some microsporidia (Fowler and Reeves, 1974a, b) provided evidence that extracted proteins characterize single species but reveal no significant differences to higher taxa. Spectra of hydrophobic proteins were stable when (1) two different genera of hosts were used for spore propagation, (2) hosts were reared at a variety of temperatures, or (3) proteins were extracted from spores harvested at different stages of sporogenesis. Hydrophilic extracts were unstable in all three instances. The information obtained from these analyses is complex and yet is not clearly understood.

Little data has been collected to characterize any changes in the host insect during a microsporidian infection. Smirnoff (1973) observed a change in the lipid composition of *Archips cerasivoranus* infected with *Nosema cerasivoranae* and *Neodiprion swainei* infected with *Thelohania pristiphorae*. The iodine number characterizing the unsaturated lipids was reduced three-fold in infected insects.

Kučera and Weiser (1973a) found two different types of enzymatic responses to *Nosema plodiae* by *Barathra brassicae*. Specific alanine aminotransferase activity increased on day five of infection whereas alkaline phosphatase and protease activities rose on the 10th day after infection. During the last three larval instars of *Barathra brassicae* infected with *N. plodiae,* the

alanine aminotransferase pattern was 90 percent above that in a
normal larva shortly before the last molt, reaching a maximum at
the end of normal larval development. There was no decrease in
activity similar to that occurring in healthy larvae during the
prepupal stage (Kučera and Weiser, 1973b). The same general
change occurred in the production of alkaline phosphatase
(Kučera and Weiser, 1974); acid phosphatase also was present in
infected larvae. These differences characterize a general
activity of the host metabolism that is different to the normal
decrease in activity before pupation. This fact is in accord
with the general phenomenon mentioned earlier as hormonal activity.
Neither the above studied enzymes nor the recently measured increase of lactate dehydrogenase was in any way related directly
to the parasite itself or to specific processes induced by the
parasitation of fat body cells. There was no specific response of
the infected tissues and the increased enzymatic activity during
the prepupal period merely indicates a general mobilization of the
organism. But this same mobilization was not able to avoid
extreme diapause in L_1 larvae of the browntail moth infected with
Thelohania hyphantriae (Weiser, 1957). The infection was observable
after eight days and remained constant for as long as 180 days
in diapausing caterpillars. Five days after the onset of normal
feeding, mortality was noted and all caterpillars died during the
next 30 days.

XVII. MICROSPORIDIA AS ANTIGENS

It has been demonstrated by an indirect fluorescent antibody test
(Kálalová and Weiser, 1973) that spores of microsporidia are good
antigens producing specific antibodies in the rabbit. A comparison
of 20 different microsporidian materials disclosed that spores of
different species of microsporidia produce species-specific antibodies that give positive reactions with antigens at serum dilutions
up to 32 and 128. Antisera produced after injection of one spore
material gave positive reactions with the same species if spores
were obtained from the original suspension, from fresh infected
tissues of the same host species, or from tissues of different
hosts. Antisera to single species of microsporidia reacted
positively only with the identical species but not with other microsporidia even if they were produced in the same host insect.
Different types of storage did not change the antigenicity of the
spore samples. Material stored for more than 18 years gave the
same reactions as fresh spores. The indirect fluorescent antibody
test did not reflect generic differences.

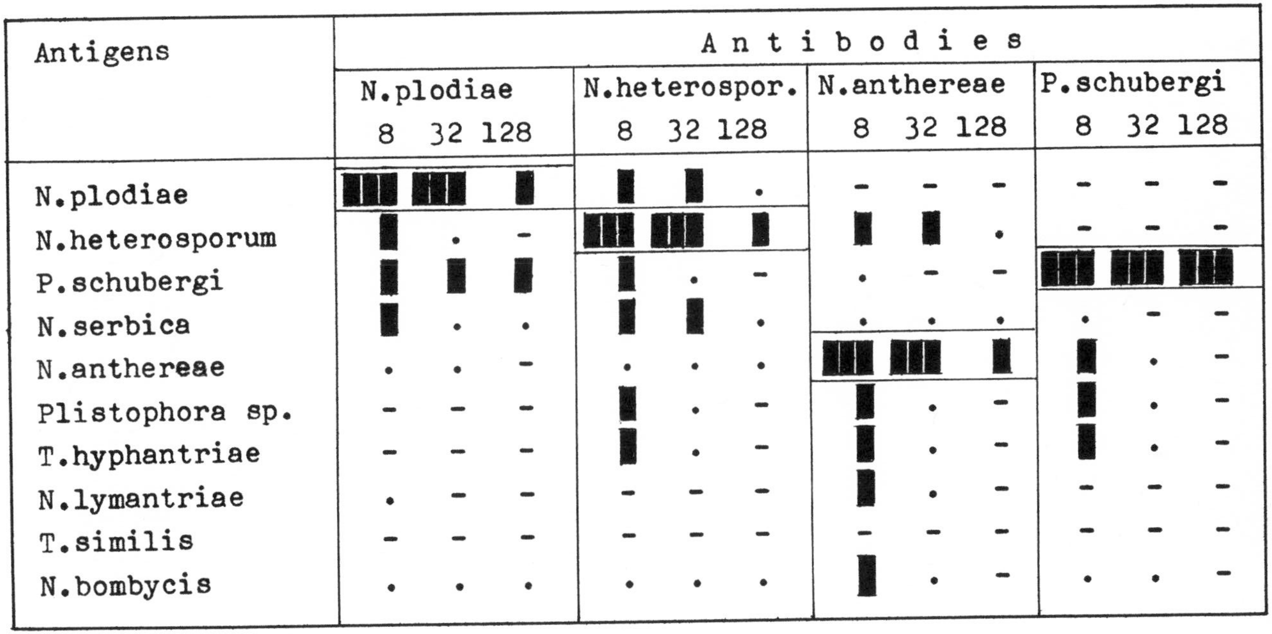

Fig. 7. Reactions of microsporidian spores with antibodies to four microsporidia in indirect fluorescent antibody tests.

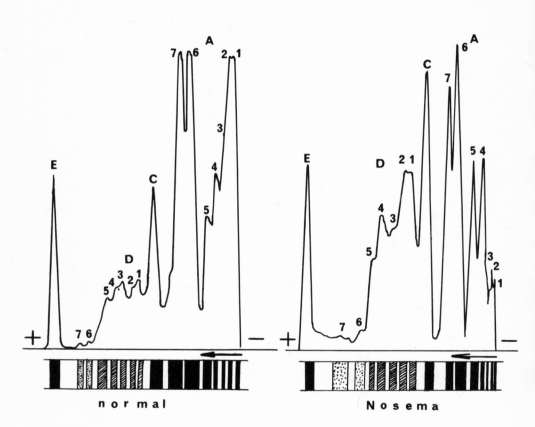

Fig. 8.   Disc electrophoresis of normal and *Nosema plodiae* in-
          fected hemolymph of *Galleria mellonella*.

XVIII. DEVELOPMENTAL CYCLE IN HOSTS

As stated in other chapters, microsporidia are strict intracellular parasites (contrary to the suggestion of Weissenberg,
1970). They use the metabolism of the host cell from which they
receive their nutrition. The rate of development of a microsporidian depends very much on the metabolic activity of the host
cell. They do not develop during the quiescent or diapausing
periods of the host. There are several reports on the duration
of the spore-to-spore cycle in different insects. Generally it
lasts eight days (Weiser, 1961), but for a considerably less time
in fast developing insects. *Octosporea muscaedomesticae*, for
example, needed 80 hours (Kramer, 1965). *Nosema necatrix*
finished the cycle in 200 hours at 21°C after a low dose (Maddox,
1968), but this time was reduced with higher doses and higher
temperature. The shortest generation time was 99 hours at
32°C, the longest was greater than 1000 hours at 15°C. The
generation time for *Nosema mesnili* was 96 to 144 hours depending
on temperature; that for *Pleistophora schubergi* was 188 hours
(Issi and Chervinskaja, 1969). Suitable temperature ranges differ
for the various microsporidians:

Organism	Temperature (degrees C)		
	Optimum	Minimum	Maximum
Nosema mesnili	27	13	34
Pleistophora schubergi	20	17	27
Nosema necatrix	27	15	32
Nosema melolonthae	20	10	25
Thelohania hyphantriae	23	17	35

Spores produced at high temperatures are less viable. Heat
treatment is used for the elimination of microsporidian infections
from eggs and pupae of insects in mass rearings. Heat treatment was
first studied by Karmo and Morgenthaler (1939) on the honey bee and
was used later by Astaurov *et al.* (1952) and Bednjakova and
Verenskaja (1958) on silkworm and oak silkworm, by Allen (1954) on
Macrocentrus ancylivorus, and by many others for mass rearing of
insects. The sterilizing principle is not due simply to destruction
of the microsporidian. More likely it decreases the rate of
development of the microsporidia and kills vegetative stages that
are continuously present in infected tissues. Consequently, the
so-called "vegetative reserve" is not maintained. Temperatures of
40 to 60°C which are used for biosterilization do not harm the
insect host. Probably, they increase the defensive actions of the
host, replacement of infected cells, and development of new
tissues, etc. The method is intriguing but is not a perfect tool
for mass rearings. Some vegetative stages do survive and produce

progeny in treated pupae, adults, or eggs. The only remedy is the older method of Pasteur that involves isolated egg deposition and inspection of each female before use of the eggs. In most infections the eggs are invaded only when large cysts with spores are present in other tissues. An exception may be transovarial transmission of microsporidia in mosquitoes or blackflies mentioned earlier.

The "vegetative reserve" is a typical feature of microsporidian infections. It is a remnant of the primary massive multiplication with masses of schizonts occurring in the infected host. Several divisions of schizonts without continuation to sporogony will completely fill the invaded oenocytes and cells of the hypoderm and offset the original difference in dosage between 40 and 40,000 spores. The primary host cells that absorb the vegetative stages by phagocytosis are not able to destroy the parasite. In contrast, they feed and protect the stages and finally burst. The liberated vegetative stages and spores are distributed within the hemolymph throughout the host body. Whether all these stages are phagocytized by different cells in different tissues or whether they penetrate the host cells by their own activity is yet unknown.

Generally, the relationship of the microsporidian to its host is rather simple. The different stages invade the cells, grow, multiply, and use up the nutritive reserves of the cell. They destroy the cytoplasm and the nucleus autolyzes. Parts of the cells that are filled with spores burst and spill into the gut, Malpighian tubules or into the body cavity. The remains of the cell either regenerate or are replaced by new cells.

XIX. TYPES OF DESTRUCTION AND INFECTION OF HOSTS

One type of infection is diffuse infiltration by vegetative stages that spread throughout the host tissues without any specific accumulation. Single cells burst and liberate some of the spores into the gut. Total numbers of spores in a host can range from 500 to 40,000. Examples are *Nosema carpocapsae*, *N. pyraustae*, *Pleistophora intestinalis*, *Nosema muscularis*, and *N. bischoffi* as well as others (Weiser, 1975).

Another type of infection is an ulcerative process. The microsporidian is confined in foci of cells of large organ where it multiplies intensively. The cells burst and any resulting perforations can be invaded by microorganisms. Although the destruction may be heavy in a limited area, the infection does not spread over the remaining part of the tissue. Usually, this occurs in diseases of the gut, the Malpighian tubules, and the salivary glands, e.g., *Nosema apis* and *Pleistophora schubergi*. Often these infections change into generalized infections causing the infected tissues to become totally disfunctional and to disintegrate, e. g., *Nosema bombycis*, *N. stegomyiae*, *N. algerae*, *Pleistophora culicis*, *P. dixippi*, and others.

One distinct type is a cumulative infection in which the tissues involved become reservoirs of spores. All cells of the fat body are infected and subsequently become filled with spores. As soon as the fat body is filled, further multiplication of the parasite is slowed; the walls of the fat body do not break from the pressure of the parasite. Apparently, all parts of the infected tissue become infected at the same time. Most infections of Lepidoptera localized in the fat body are of this kind. Representative pathogens are *Nosema lymantriae*, *N. plodiae*, *N. heterosporum*, *N. necatrix*, *Pleistophora culicis*, *N. melolonthae*, *Thelohania lairdi*, *T. similis*, *T. mülleri* and many others. The pathogens are released from the tissue of the host only after its death.

Rather rare is the degenerative type of infection. Infection of the tissues is followed by degeneration; destroyed cells are not replaced, spores are rather scarce, and infected animals are somewhat cachectic and dehydrated. *Nosema muscularis* causes this type of infection in *Lymantria dispar*.

XX. THE XENOPARASITIC COMPLEXES

A special category of host-parasite interactions distinctly different from simple infections is the xenoparasitic complex ("complete xenoparasitaire" of Chatton, 1920). It is defined as an entity consisting of the host cell, tissue and parasite living together to form a distinct physiological and morphological unit within the host's body. Weissenberg (1922) applied this concept to the *Glugea*-cyst, for which he introduced the term "xenon" (later changed to "xenoma"). Recently, Maurand (1973) proposed to substitute his term "tissue parasitaire" with the term "xenoma" and used this designation for several infections in invertebrates where the host cells desintegrated and formed a common plasmodium. Studies of the relationship of *Pleistophora debaisieuxi* of *Odagmia ornata* revealed the presence of a typical xenoparasitic complex in insects (Weiser, 1976). The invaded cell in this specific complex presents itself to the maternal body as the parasite. The xenoma is characterized by functional nuclei and by a specific development of invaded cells that are active through complete formation of all the spores. Xenoparasitic complexes with microsporidia are represented by two main types: (1) syncytical xenomas with host cells confluent in one common syncytium, and (2) neoplastic xenomas in which the parasite provokes an increase in the number of host cells inside the lobe of infected tissue.

In syncytial xenomas the infected fat bodies dissolve the cell membranes inside the lobe and the resulting syncytium is progressively invaded by microsporidia. During the last instars of blackflies when the fat body is filled with fat droplets, the disappearance of cell walls is regarded by some investigators as a normal physiological feature. The cell walls of the

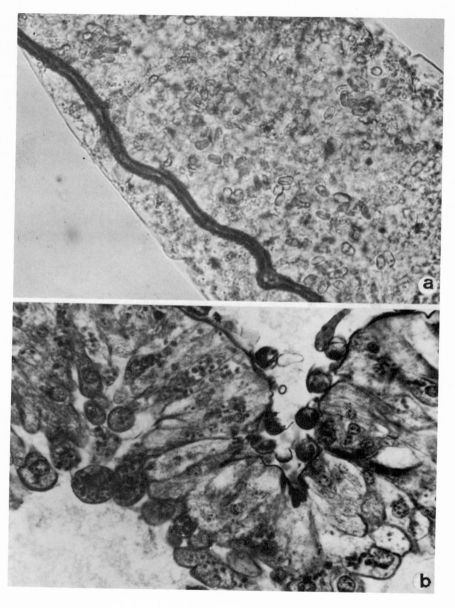

Fig. 9.   a, Diffuse infiltration of *Pleistophora periplanetae* in
the Malpighian tubules of *P. americana*. X 1000; b, Early
infection of the midgut of the honey bee with *Nosema apis*,
diffuse infiltration later changing to ulceration. X
700.

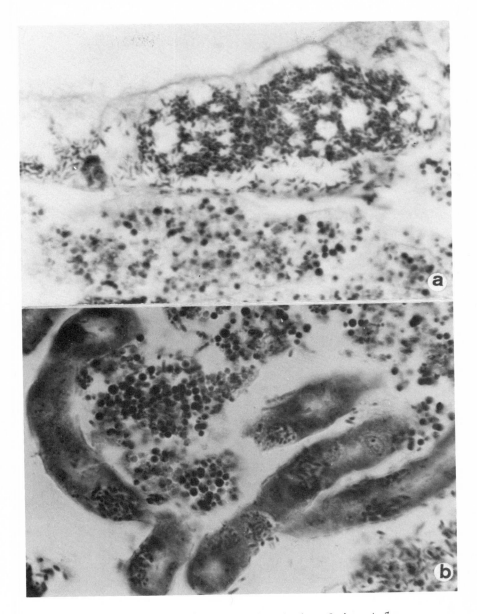

Fig. 10.   a, *Nosema mesnili* in the fat body of *Apanteles
           glomeratus*. The spores concentrate in the internal part
           of the tissue. X 500; b, Ulcerative type of infection,
           Nosema mesnili in the larva of *Apanteles glomeratus* in
           the white cabbage butterfly. Destructions of the walls
           are visible. X 500.

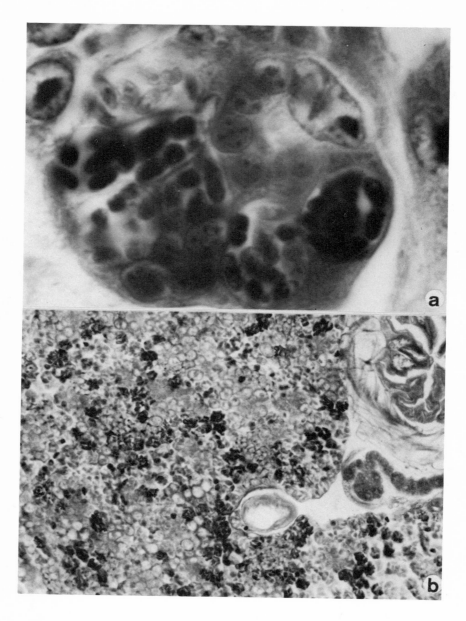

Fig. 11. a, *Pleistophora culicis*. Primary nodule in the gut wall
of *Culiseta longiareolata*. Slight hypertrophy of the
host cell nuclei. X 1000; b, Lobe of the fat body of
Simulium-larva with a cumulative infection with microsporidia *Thelohania bracteata*. X 1000.

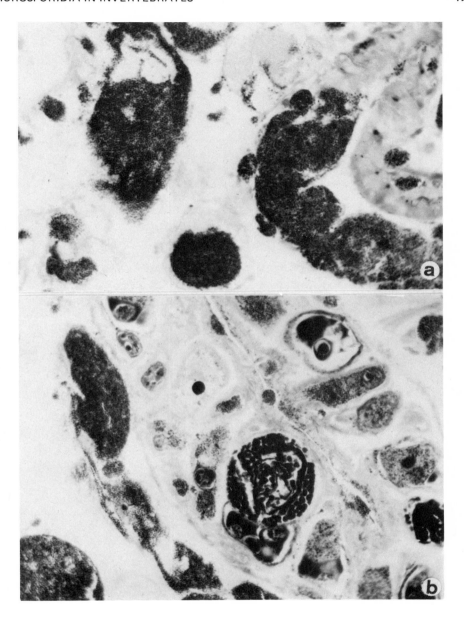

Fig. 12. a, *Nosema stegomyiae* in *Anopheles gambiae*. Infected
        Malpighian tubules and gut changed into black masses of
        spores. X 300; b, The same infection, destructions in
        the ovary. Only one follicle normal, all other
        infected. X 300.

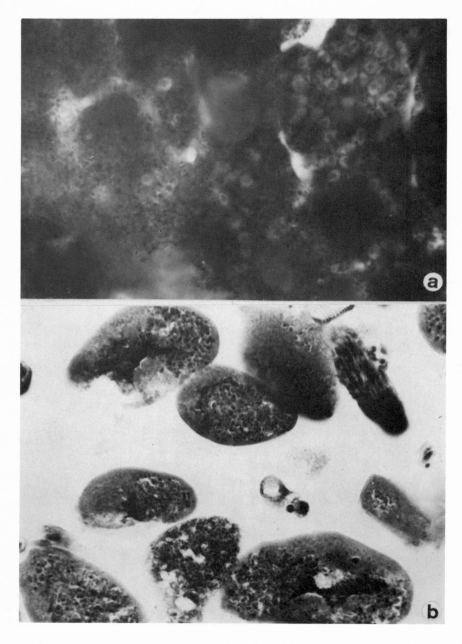

Fig. 13.   a, Spores of *Nosema otiorrhynchi* in the infected egg of
           Otiorrhynchus ligustici. X 700; b, Oenocytes of
           Pieris brassicae with *Nosema mesnili*.   X 500.

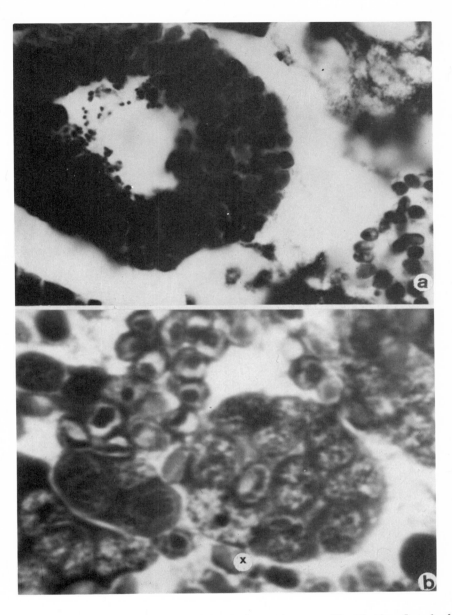

Fig. 14.   a, Hypertrophy of the nucleus in a cell of the fat body
           of the ephemerid infected with *Nosema baetis*. X 1000;
           b, Smear of the fat body of *Odagmia ornata* with
           Pleistophora debaisieusi. Cells are single xenomas/
           senocytes/, 1200 X.

Fig. 15.   a, Young xenocytes, X, of *Pleistophora debaisieuxi*
           in the fat body of *Odagmia ornata*, 12,000 X; b, Final
           stage of the developing pansporoblast of *Pleistophora*
           debaisieuxi.   The xenocyte is vacuolated and with many
           processes on the surface.   The nucleus of the xenocyte
           /X/ is well visible. 15,000 X.

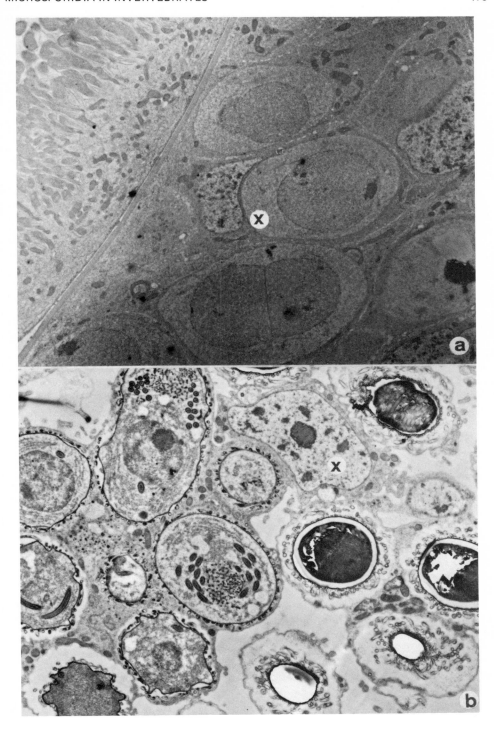

surrounding uninfected lobes of the fat body persist and only the infected lobes form the syncytia. The number of the nuclei in such syncytia does not differ from the number of nuclei in a non-infected lobe. This kind of complex was described by Maurand (1973) for *Pleistophora simulii*.

Syncytia with hypertrophied nuclei are produced in the fat body or in the salivary glands of insects and they also have been observed in gonads of fishes. The nuclei hypertrophy in the area of the developing parasite. Compared to the original number of nuclei, the number of giant nuclei is reduced 10- to 30-fold. The nuclei attain ten times their original size and the polytene chromosomes break down into chromatin blocks. Finally, the nuclei break leaving long chromatin smudges that eventually disappear. Maurand (1973) proported *Thelohania bracteata* to incur this kind of xenoma. Giant nuclei are present also in tissues infected with *Stempellia simulii*, *S. magna*, *Nosema baetis*, *Thelohania chaeto-gastris* and *Pleistophora longifilis*. Nuclear hypertrophy also occurs in host tissues infected with *Gurleya francottei*. In each case, the details of the syncytial organization and the xenoparasitic complex are slightly different.

The transition between a syncytial and neoplastic xenoma is a "*Glugea*-cyst." Its unicellular origin in the infected phagocyte of a fish host, as in insect xenomas, was postulated first by Debaisieux (1919a, 1920) and confirmed experimentally by Weissenberg (1922). Neoplastic xenomas of vertebrates occur in lamellar cysts surrounded by a sinus of the blood stream. The venous sinus supplies the necessary oxygen and nutrition. Characteristic of this xenoma is the conservation of a viable nucleus that divides or fragments into tens or one hundreds nuclei localized beneath the cyst membrane. The fragmented nuclei are normal structured in an area of well organized cytoplasm beneath the cyst wall. Structural organization is less perfect toward the centre of the cyst where the mature spores concentrate. This organization differs from the xenoma in insects. Fragmentation of the nuclei and an subdivision of the adjacent cytoplasmic areas appears to be the result of decreased oxygen supply under the thick cyst wall as well as the reaction to the developing parasite. Insect xenomas can be characterized as a special type of neoplasia directly influenced by the parasite.

Neoplastic xenomas without an enveloping cyst wall are typical in insects. Electron micrographs of *Pleistophora debaisieuxi* in *Odagmia ornata* revealed a system in which sporonts induce division of the infected host cell. Each original host cell divides according to the number of sporonts contained within and a lobe of the fat body harbors three to five times the original number of cells. Each sporont develops into a multisporoblastic pansporoblast inside the host cell and this cell with a typical active nucleus containing granular chromatin, active mitochondria, and a lobate surface remains as such until the spores mature. The

sporoblasts and maturing spores release a proteolytic enzyme
that digests periparasitic vacuoles around each sporoblast and
spore. Eventually, the entire xenoma host cell is dissolved and
the spores are liberated. A chemical stimulus may initiate
primary division of the host cells.

REFERENCES

Allen, H. W. 1954. *Nosema* disease of *Gnorimoschema operculella*
    Zeller and *Macrocentrus ancylivorus* Rohw. *Annals Entomol.*
    Soc. Amer. 47, 407-424.
Astaurov, B. L., Ovanesjan, T. G. and Lobshanidze, V. I. 1952.
    Desinfection of pebrinous eggs of the silkworm by short
    treatment with hot water. *Dokl. VASCHNIL* 3, 44-51.
Bednjakova, T. A. and Verenskaja, V. N. 1958. Sterilizing action
    of high temperatures on infections of the silkworm, *Bombyx*
    mori L., with *Nosema bombycis* Naeg. during the different
    stages of diapause. *Doklady Akad. Nauk SSSR* 122, 737-740.
Blunck, H. 1952. Ueber die in *Pieris brassicae* L., ihren Parasiten
    und Hyperparasiten schmarotzende Mikrosporidien. *Trans. 9th,*
    Int. Congress of Entomol., Amsterdam 1951, pp. 432-438.
Brooks, W. M. 1971. The inflammatory response of the tobacco
    hornworm, *Manduca sexta*, to infection by the microsporidian
    Nosema sphingidis. J. Invertebr. Pathol. 17, 87-93.
Bulnheim, H. P. 1971. Entwicklung, Uebertrangung und Parasit-Wirt
    Beziehungen von *Thelohania herediteria* sp. n.. *Z. Parasitenk.*
    35, 241-262.
Bulnheim, H. P. and Vávra, J. 1968. Infection by the microsporidian
    Octosporea effeminans sp. n., and its sex determining influence
    in the amphipod *Gammarus duebeni. J. Parasitol.* 54, 241-248.
Chatton, E. 1920. Sur un complexe xéno-parasitaire morphologique
    et physiologique, *Neresheimeria catenata* chez *Fritillaria*
    pellucida. C. R. Acad. Scie., France 171, 55-57.
Debaisieux, P. 1919. Microsporidies parasites des larves de
    Simulium: Thelohania varians. La Cellule 30, 47-79.
Debaisieux, P. 1919a. Hypertrophie des cellules animales para-
    sités par des Cnidosporidies. *C. R. Soc. Biol.* 82, 867-869.
Debaisieux, P. 1920. Etudes sur les Microsporidies. IV. *Glugea*
    anomala Moniez. *La Cellule* 30, 217-243.
Fisher, F. M. and Sanborn, R. C. 1964. *Nosema* as a source of
    juvenile hormone in parasitized insects. *Biol. Bull.*
    126, 235-252.
Fowler, J. L. and Reeves, E. L. 1974a. Detection of relationships
    among microsporidian isolates. Hydrophobic extracts. *J.*
    Invertebr. Pathol. 23, 3-12.
Fowler, J. L. and Reeves, E. L. 1974b. Detection of relation-
    ships among microsporidian isolates by electrophoretic
    analysis: Hydrophilic extracts. *J. Invertebr. Pathol.*
    23, 63-69.

Günther, S. 1959. Ueber die Auswirkung auf die Infektiosität
  bei der Passage insektenpathogener Mikrosporidien durch den
  Darm von Vögeln und Insekten. *Nachrichtenbl.f.d.Deutsch.*
  Pflanzenschutzd. 13, 19-21.
Hazard, E. I. and Anthony, W. D. 1974. A redescription of the
  genus *Parathelohania* Codreanu 1966 Microsporidia: Protozoa
  with a reexamination of previously described species of
  Thelohania Henneguy 1892 and descriptions of two new species
  of *Parathelohania* from anopheline mosquitoes. USDA
  Techn. Bull. 1505, 26 pp.
Hazard, E. I. and Weiser, J. 1968. Spores of *Thelohania* in
  adult female *Anopheles:* development and transovarial
  transmission and redescriptions of *T. legeri* Hesse and
  T. obesa Kudo. *J. Protozool.* 15, 817-823.
Henry, J. E. 1967. *Nosema acridophagus* sp.n., a microsporidian
  isolated from grasshoppers. *J. Invertebr. Pathol.* 9,
  331-341.
Hostounský, Z. 1963. *Pieris brassicae,* its continual rearing and
  transmission of its infections with parasites. Ph.D Dissert.,
  Czech.
Hostounský, Z. and Weiser, J. 1972. Production of spores of
  Nosema plodiae Kellen and Lindegren in *Mamestra brassicae*
  L. after different infective dosage. I. *Věst. Čs. spol.*
  zool. 36, 97-100.
Hostounský, Z. and Weiser, J. 1973. Production of spores of
  Nosema plodiae in *Mamestra brassicae* after different dosage,
  II. *Vest. Cs. spol. zool.* 37, 234-237.
Issi, I. V. and Lipa, J. 1968. *Gurleya sokolovi* sp.n., a micro-
  sporidian parasite of the water mite *Limnochares aquatica*
  L. Acarina:Hydrachnellae, and a note on a gregarine infection
  in the same mite. *J. Invertebr. Pathol.* 10, 165-175.
Issi, I. V. and Maslennikova V. A. 1964. The effect of microspori-
  diosis upon the diapause and survival of *Apanteles glomeratus*
  L. and *Pieris brassicae* L. *Entomologiceskoe obozrenie* 43,
  112-117.
Issi, I. V. and Chervinskaja, V. P. 1969. On the influence of
  temperature on the development of *Nosema mesnili* and
  Plistophora schubergi (Microsporidia, Nosematidae). *Zoolog.*
  zhurnal 48, 1140-1146.
Kaya, H. K. 1973. Pathogenicity of *Pleistophora schubergi* to
  larvae of the orange-striped oakworm and other lepidopterous
  insects. *J. Invertebr. Pathol.* 22, 356-358.
Kálalová, S. and Weiser, J. 1973. Identification of microsporidia
  by indirect fluorescent antibody tests. *Abst. V. Int. Conf.*
  Insect Pathol. 5th, Oxford, p. 111.
Karmo, E. and Morgenthaler, O. 1939. The development of *Nosema*
  apis at various temperatures. *Bee World,* 20, 57-58.

Kellen, W. R., Clark, T. B., Lindegren, J. E. and Sanders, R. D. 1966. Development of *Thelohania californica* in two hybrid mosquitoes *Expt. Parasitol.* 18, 251-254.

Kellen, W. R. and Lindegren, J. E. 1968. Biology of *Nosema plodiae* sp. n., a microsporidian pathogen of the Indian meal moth *Plodia interpunctella* Hbn. Lepidoptera: Phycitidae. *J. Invertebr. Pathol.*, 11, 104-111.

Kharazi-Pakdel, A. 1968. Recherches sur la pathogenie de *Nosema melolonthae* Krieg. *Entomophaga*, 13, 289-318.

Komárek, J. and Vávra, J. 1968. In memoriam of *Marssoniella* Lemm. 1900. *Arch. Protistenk.*, 111, 12-17.

Kramer, J. P. 1965. Generation time of the microsporidian *Octosporea muscaedomesticae* Flu in adult *Phormia regina* Meig. (Diptera, Calliphoridae.) *Z. Parasitenk.* 25, 309-313.

Kučera, M. and Weiser, J. 1973a. Alanine aminotransferase, alkaline phosphatase and protease activity in *Mamestra brassicae* during microsporidian infection. *J. Invertebr. Pathol.* 21, 121-122.

Kučera, M. and Weiser, J. 1973b. Alanine aminotransferase in the three last larval instars of *Barathra brassicae* infected by *Nosema plodiae*. *J. Invertebr. Pathol.* 21, 287-292.

Kučera, M. and Weiser, J. 1974. Alkaline phosphatase in the last larval instar of *Barathra brassicae*/Lepidoptera/infected by *Nosema plodia*. *Acta entomol. bohemoslov.* 71, 289-293.

Lewis, L. C. and Lynch, R. E. 1974. Lyophilization, vacuum drying and subsequent storage of *Nosema pyraustae* spores. *J. Invertebr. Pathol.* 24, 149-153.

Machay, M. L. 1957. Occurrence of *Nosema bombycis* Naegeli among wild Lepidoptera. *Folia Entomol. Hungarica* 10, 359-363.

Maddox, J. V. 1968. Generation time of the microsporidian *Nosema necatrix* in the larvae of the armyworm, *Pseudaletia unipuncta*. *J. Invertebr. Pathol.* 11, 90-96.

Mattes, O. 1927. Parasitäre Krankheiten der Mehlmottenlarven und Versuche über ihre Verwendbarkeit als biologischer Bekämpfungsmittel. *Sitzber. Ges. Bedford. d. ges. Naturwiss.*, *Marburg* 62, 381-417.

Maurand, J. 1973. Recherches biologiques sur les microsporidies des larves de simulies. *Dissert.*, 200 pp, Montpellier University.

Maurand, J. and Bouix, G. 1969. Mise en évidence d´un phénomene secretoire dans le cycle de *Thélohania fibrata* Strickland 1913, microsporidie parasite des larves de Simulium. *C. R. Acad. Sci.*, *Paris* 269, 2216-2218.

Milner, R. J. 1972. *Nosema whitei*, a microsporidian pathogen of some species of *Tribolium*. III. Effect on *T. castaneum*. *J. Invertebr. Pathol.* 19, 248-255.

McNeil, J. N. and Brooks, W. M. 1974. Interactions of the hyperparasitoids *Catolaccus aeneoviridis* and *Spilochalcis side* with the microsporidians *Nosema helithidis* and *N. campoletidis*. *Entomophaga* 19, 195-204.

Nilova, G. N. 1967. Number of spores of two microsporidia in the caterpillars of *Feltia segetum*. *Vestnik selchoz. nauki*

Nordin, G. L. and Maddox, J. V. 1972. Effects of simultaneous virus and microsporidian infections on larvae of *Hyphantria cunea*. *J. Invertebr. Pathol.* 20, 66-69.

Nordin, G. L. and Maddox, J. V. 1974. Microsporidia of the fall webworm, *Hyphantria cunea*. I. Identification, distribution, and comparison ὁf *Nosema* sp. with similar *Nosema* spp. from other Lepidoptera. *J. Invertebr. Pathol.* 24, 1-13.

Ohshima, K. 1973. Change of relation between infectivity and filament evagination of debilitated spores of *Nosema bombycis*. *Annot. Zoolog. Japon.* 46, 188-198.

Paillot, A. 1918. *Pérezia legeri* nov. sp. microsporidie nouvelle, parasite des chenilles de *Pieris brassicae*. *C. R. Soc. Biol.* 81, 187-189.

Payne, N. M. 1933. A parasitic hymenopteron as a vector of an insect disease. *Entomol. News* 44, 22.

Smirnoff, W. A. 1973. Biochemical exploration in insect pathology. *Current Topics in Compar. Pathobiol.* 2, 89-106.

Undeen, A. H. and Alger, N. E. 1975. The effect of the microsporidian, *Nosema algerae*, on *Anopheles stephensi*. *J. Invertebr. Pathol.* 25, 19-24.

Undeen, A. H. and Maddox, J. V. 1973. The infection of nonmosquito hosts by injection with spores of the microsporidian *Nosema algerae*. *J. Invertebr. Pathol.* 22, 258-265.

Weiser, J. 1951. A contribution to the knowledge of the microsporidia of parasitic helminths. *Věst. čs. spol. zool.* 15, 252-264.

Weiser, J. 1953a. Parasiten der Raupen der Sonnenblumenmotte, *Homesoma nebulellum* Hbn. mit besonderer Rücksicht zur Art *Mattesia povolnyi* sp. n. *Folia zool. et entomol.* 15, 252-264.

Weiser, J. 1953b. To the knowledge of the parasites of the fall webworm, *Hyphantria cunea*. Vest. cs. spol. zool. 16, 228.

Weiser, J. 1953c. Schizogregarines of the flour pests. I. Věst. čs. spol. zool. 16, 199-212.

Weiser, J. 1957. Mikrosporidien des Schwammspinners und der Goldafter. *Zschr. Angrew. Entomol.* 40, 509-527.

Weiser, J. 1956. Studien über Mikrosporidien in Süsswasserinsekten. *Čsl. parasitologie* 3, 193-202.

Weiser, J. 1961. Die Mikrosporidien als Parasiten der Insekten. Beihefte zur Angewandten Entomologie, 149 pp, P. P. Parey, Hamburg.

Weiser, J. 1965. Zwei Mikrosporidien aus Köcherfliegen Larven. *Zool. Anzeiger* 175, 229-234.

Weiser, J. 1973. Transmission of microsporidia *via* injection. *Proc. Int. Conf. Insect Pathol. 4th, Oxford,* p. 13.

Weiser, J. 1976. The *Pleistophora debaisieuxi* xenoma. *Z. Parasitenk.* 48, 263-270.

Weiser, J. 1976. Responses of insects to injections of
    microsporidia. *Věst. Čs. spol. zool.* In press.
Weiser, J. and Coluzzi, M. 1972. *Plistophora culisetae* in
    different mosquito hosts. *Folia parasitol.* <u>19</u>, 197-202.
Weiser, J. and Lysenko, O. 1972. Protein changes in the hemolymph
    of *Galleria mellonella* infected with virus and protozoan
    pathogens. *Acta entomol. bohemoslov.* <u>69</u>, 97-100.
Weiser, J. and Veber, J. 1955. Ueber die Möglichkeiten des
    biologischen Kampfes gegen *Hyphantria cunea.* *Čsl. parasitol.*
    <u>2</u>, 191-199.
Weiser, J. and Žizka, Z. 1976. Stages in the sporogony of
    Plistophora debaisieuxi Jirovec. *Acta Protozoologica,*
    In press.
Weissenberg, R. 1922. Mikrosporidien, Myxosporidien und Chlamydo-
    zoen als Zellparasiten von Fischen. *Verh. Deutsch. Zool.*
    Ges. <u>27</u>, 41-43.
Weissenberg, R. 1970. Some remarks upon the taxonomy of the
    genera *Glugea* and *Nosema* (Protozoa, Microsporidia). *J.*
    Parasitol. 56/4, Sec. II, Part I., 363-4, Abstr. 668.

Microsporidian Interactions With Host Cells

RICHARD WEISSENBERG[1]

---

[1]Deceased. The text of Professor Weissenberg's manuscript for this volume had just been completed when he died. The editors found it necessary to condense the contents of the paper but they have been very careful to preserve the meaning. A brief biographical sketch is included at the end of this chapter.

I. INTRODUCTION

In the life cycle of microsporidia, the two essential periods of
development, schizogony and sporogony, take their course, generally,
within the host cells. Intrusion into the nucleus does not occur[2].
Within the cytoplasm, microsporidia multiply as schizonts and
later undergo sporogony. During the life cycle, they may infiltrate the cytoplasm as sprouting schizonts or extend within it as
compact colonies; the cytoplasm itself may become reduced and
finally replaced almost completely by the spores of the parasite.
This latter situation is especially true in arthropods. Thus,
damage is frequently done to the host cell and often death occurs
as a result of the invasion.

There is extreme variation in the cytopathology of microsporidian
diseases. It is of great significance whether the invasion of the
host cell progresses through the entire cytoplasm or remains
localized within the cell. Further, there are essential variations
in the reaction of the host cell to the invasion. A very conspicuous effect of the cell infection can be a stimulation of the
host cell by the schizonts to initially undergo hypertrophic
growth.

Certain morphological features such as structure, shape, and
spore size have been used as a practical basis for classification
of microsporidia. Similarity of these features, however, by no
means indicates strict similarity of all biologic characteristics
of the species compared such as the type of life cycle or development in the host cell, etc. Because biological characteristics
are known for only a small number of microsporidia biological
parameters have not yet been used extensively to arrange microsporidia into taxonomic groups. However, there are essential
differences in the kinds of cell parasitism and the effect of
invasion on the host cell to define at least three biologic types.
The first type includes the majority of microsporidian species,
in which the multiplying schizonts, under favorable conditions,
may spread without limitation through the entire cytoplasm of
the invaded cell. This type of cell parasitism can damage and
finally destroy host cells producing severe illness of the host.
This relationship of the microsporidia to invaded cells generally
is characterized as hostile.

The second type of invasion is rare and has been observed only in
the infection of ganglion cells of the angler fish *Lophius* by
Nosema lophii. The development of the colony of the parasite in
this case remains restricted to the region of the cell from which
the axon extends. The host cells undergo a marked hypertrophy
and the unoccupied portion of the ganglion cells, which contains

---

[2]A recent study revealed the presence of *Nosema bombycis* in the
host cell nucleus (Takizawa, H., E. Vivier, and A. Petitprez.
C. R. Acad. Sci. Paris, 277, 1769-1771, 1973).

the cell nucleus, becomes considerably enlarged. It loses its
function within the nervous system, and specific cell organelles
responsible for differentiation such as Nissl granules and
neurofibrils can no longer be observed in it. Generally however,
the structure of the cytoplasm and nucleus appear undamaged and
they may continue hypertrophic growth for an extended time.
Whereas the hypertrophied cytoplasm of the occupied cell portion
becomes distended by growth of the colony and takes on the
appearance of a thin covering layer around the colony, the
unoccupied cell portion does not become utilized by the parasite.
In old lesions, the unoccupied portions of the host cells
disappear; after regressive changes, only masses of spores are
usually still present. More detail of the cytopathology of this
peculiar microsporidian are discussed in section III.
     The third type of host cell invasion is exemplified by the cyto-
pathology of the fish parasite *Glugea anomala*. Cell invasion in
this case likewise remains localized but the unoccupied portion of
the host cell and the developing microsporidian colony form a symbiotic complex that resembles a biological unit (Weissenberg, 1922a,
1922b, 1968). Again, details will be discussed section III.
     In addition to changes of the invaded cells, very often
changes also occur in the neighboring cells and tissues such as
mesenchyme or connective tissue. Thus, a connective tissue
capsule carrying blood vessels may often be formed around the
hypertrophying invaded cells. At later stages, it frequently
may be observed that several cells of the connective tissue
capsule develop into phagocytes, penetrate the cytoplasm of the
hypertrophic invaded host cell and, by engulging groups of spores,
may finally destroy much of the degenerating host cell.

II. REPLACEMENT OF HOST CELL CYTOPLASM BY MICROSPORIDIA

     Progressive infiltration of the cytoplasm of invaded host cells
by multiplying schizonts can finally lead to an almost complete
replacement of the cytoplasm by the accumulating microsporidian
spores. This phenomenon is especially true in cells of arthropods.
The mechanism(s) responsible for shrinking of the cytoplasm has
not yet been determined. Competition may exist between the cell
parasites and the normal constituents of the cytoplasm for
nutrients within the cell. If the schizonts are able to obtain
an advantage in this kind of competition, such an event may be
sufficient to induce atrophic changes in the cytoplasm. It has
been conjectured that the schizonts of microsporidia, produce
proteolytic enzymes which catalyze the dissolution of the host
cell cytoplasm (Stempell, 1909). It seems unlikely to me that
multiplying schizonts which utilize nutrients absorbed by the
host cell from intercellular fluids should need additional
nourishment from dissolved cytoplasm as an extra source of

nourishment. However, during spore maturation, it is possible
that extracellular proteolytic enzymes are excreted. A number of
observations of destruction of cytoplasmic structures have been
evaluated in favor of lysis by a proteolytic enzyme. In addition
to the lysis of cytoplasm in the host cells of *Nosema bombycis*
proported by Stempell, reference is made to the studies of
Petri (1965, 1966) on rat sarcoma cells invaded by *Nosema cuniculi*.

III. TYPES AND EXAMPLES OF CELLULAR INVASION AND PARASITISM

It is characteristic of the first type of cellular invasion
described in the Introduction to this chapter that under favorable conditions colony formation in the host cell cytoplasm may
proceed without limitation throughout the whole cytoplasmic
region of the host cell. Listed below are some examples that
demonstrate variety in the cytopathology of this kind of invasion.

A. *NOSEMA APIS ZANDER, 1909*

This microsporidian frequently produces an infection of a
number of epithelial cells in the midgut of adult honey bees. It
is chiefly the midgut portion ("ventriculus") where the parasite
invades cells of the epithelium. Within the cytoplasm of an
invaded epithelial cell, the schizogony progresses and the
production of spores follows. Finally, the infected cell may
appear as a rounded sac in which the cytoplasm is replaced by
numerous spores. A specific reaction of the invaded host cells
to the infection by the sporoplasms and to the multiplication of
the schizonts has not been observed. Especially, the host
cells do not undergo a hypertrophic growth.

B. *NOSEMA BOMBYCIS NÄGELI, 1857*

The infection produced by *Nosema bombycis* in caterpillars of
the silk-moth *Bombyx mori*, the so-called silkworms, represents
a severe microsporidian disease. It affects first the midgut
but sporoplasms of spores germinating in the lumen of the midgut
can also pass the barrier of the intestinal wall and reach the
blood through hemocoelic spaces, such germs are transported to
various distant organs and can establish colonies in cells of
these organs. Just as is true for the cell parasitism of
Nosema apis, also in the cytopathology of *N. bombycis* disease,
hypertrophy of the invaded cells does not occur. In contrast,
infiltration of a larger part of the host cell by schizonts leads
to dissolution of cytoplasmic remmants whereas the outer cell
membrane and the cell nucleus remain intact for some time.

Among the various parts of organs and tissues that can become
invaded by sporoplasms floating in the hemocoel are egg cells
within ovaries. According to Stempell (1909), the developed
schizonts are assembled in the central region of the egg, a
location where they will not impede the formation of the
embryonic organs, during the time of embryo formation. In later
stages of the embryo, schizonts enter newly formed embryonic
cells, especially of the gut, and there multiply. Thus, in
young hatched silkworms, sometimes the entire epithelium of the
midgut may be found infiltrated by schizonts and spores.

C. *THELOHANIA TIPULAE* WEISSENBERG, 1926

A third example among the multitude of microsporidian infections of the first type is invasion of fat body cells of
insect larvae. Usually, cells of the fat body react to invasion
by undergoing a pronounced hypertrophy. Fig. 1 shows a section
through an uninfected portion of the fat body of a larva of the
dipteran *Tipula lateralis*. Fig. 2 depicts several cells filled
with groups of spores of *Thelohania tipulae* Weissenberg, 1926.
Comparison of the two drawings reveals considerable cell
hypertrophy due to invasion. This is especially evident for the
nuclei, the diameters of which have increased about four times.
Also, the cells have become much larger. The average diameter
of an uninfected uninucleate cell is 22 µm. Infected cells
increased to sizes of 90 x 80 µm. The cytoplasm of the uninvaded
cells in Fig. 1 contains a number of vacuoles that had been
filled with stored fat droplets. A considerable number of
groups of spores are chief components of the cell bodies of
invaded cells (Fig. 2). Only the outer cell membranes are still
present in the invaded cells. The inner layers of the cytoplasm
together with their fat vacuoles disappear completely. The cell
nuclei, which never become invaded, undergo very conspicuous
hypertrophy (Fig. 2). The cytoplasm of the cells is now filled
with numerous spore-groups. In some regions of the cell, they
are very densely arranged. In other areas they are more sparsely
distributed. The complete lack of cytoplasmic remnants around
them indicates dissolution of the cytoplasmic substance, possibly
due to enzymatic action. Due to a lack of information on
Tipula lateralis, it is not known whether hypertrophy of the cells
preceded infiltration of the cytoplasm by multiplying schizonts
or whether the two processes progressed in the cells simultaneously. Nevertheless, it is apparent that the hypertrophy
afforded enough additional cytoplasm for the spreading of
schizonts through the cell. Consequently, the parasite had the
opportunity to develop many more spores in the invaded cell than
would have been possible in a non-hypertrophic host cell. An
invaded cell is presumed alive as long as the structure of the
nuclei does not show regressive changes. Upon the disappearance

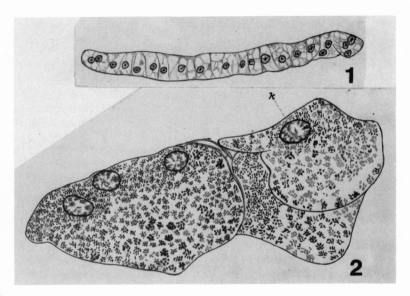

Fig. 1.   Section of a normal larval fat body of *Tipula lateralis*.
          Formalin, Delafield's hematoxylin. X 310.   After
          Weissenberg (1926).

Fig. 2.   Section of diseased fat body of *T. lateralis*.   Cells have
          become hypertrophic due to invasion by *Thelohania tipulae*.
          Delafield's hamatoxylin and safranin. X 310.   After
          Weissenberg (1926).

of fat droplets, however, the host cell has lost its storage
unction.

The second type of cell parasitism in whith the invasion of the
host cell remains restricted to a portion of this cell has
hitherto been observed only in the live cycle of a single microsporidian species, *Nosema lophii*. Very early stages of the cell
infection are still unknown. However, the portion of the life
of this species is of great biological and morphological interest.

D. *NOSEMA LOPHII*

Nosema lophii frequently invades ganglion cells of the
peripheral nervous system of the marine fish *Lophius piscatorius,
L. budegassa,* and *L. americanus* as well as nerve cells of
the central nervous system [namely, in the medulla oblongata
(Mrázek, 1899) and in the spinal cord (Weissenberg, 1909)]. The
cytopathology of *N. lophii* is characterized by considerable
hypertrophy of the invaded ganglion cell or nerve cell. Invasion
of several cells leads to the development of colonies (1-2 mm in
diameter) of the microsporidian that can be seen as whitish nodules
on the ganglia. Usually, they are arranged in grape-like clusters
often reaching the size of a pea. In old lesions, after replacement of most of the nervous tissue by layers and strands of
connective tissue, tumors the size of a cherry may result. Many
of the ganglion cells in the spinal ganglia as well as in ganglia
of cerebral nerves are multipolar, elongated cells with a thicker
basal portion containing the nucleus. The bulbous part of the
ganglion cell is the proximal portion. The axon extends from the
attenuated distal portion. The microsporidian colonies develop
only in the distal portion of the host cell. Under stimulus from
the parasite, the infected cell undergoes considerable hypertrophy.
The cytoplasm as well as the nucleus and its components undergo
hypertrophy. Possibly, the cells become invaded at relatively
early stages when their proximal portions having the largest
transversal diameters of about 40-60 µm. Upon propagation of the
schizonts, the host cell becomes stimulated to enter hypertrophic
growth. During the course of such growth the proximal portion of
the cell may attain a width of about 850 µm. Oval microsporidian
colonies in the distal cell portion have grown to diameters of
more than 1,500 µm by this time. A section through a ganglion
of the nervous vagus, shown in Fig. 3, is from one of the earliest
known cases of the disease (Weissenberg, 1911b). Among numerous
normal ganglion cells, which at low magnification appear as small
bodies (g), five hypertrophous cells in the center of the field are
very conspicuous. In two of them (h_1 and h_2) not only the proximal
portion but also the distal portion containing the microsporidian
colony is observed. Numerous spores, appearing as black spots,
are formed in the oval colonies. The growth of the colony considerably distends the distal portion of the ganglion cell so that

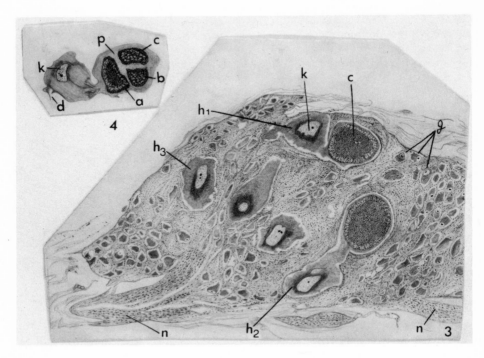

Fig. 3. Section of chief extracranial ganglion of the vagus
nerve of *Lophius piscatorius* (25 cm long) showing
relatively early infection by *Nosema lophii*. g, normal
ganglion cells; n, bundles of nerve fibers; h_1, h_2, h_3,
infected hypertrophic ganglion cells. Proximal and distal
portions of cells h_1 and h_2 are distended by a colony, c,
of *N. lophii*. Formalin, Dalafield's hematoxylin and
safranin. X 50. After Weissenberg (1911b).

Fig. 4. Longitudinal section of a spinal ganglion cell of *L.
piscatorius* (23 cm long) at a stage of infection earlier
than shown in Fig. 3. The bulge of the distal cell portion
shows three small colonies of *N. lophii* a, b, and c in the
hypertrophic cytoplasm, p. k, cell nucleus in the proximal
portion; d, entrance of cell processes, interpreted as
dentrites. Flemming's fluid, iron-hematoxylin after
Heidenhain. X 50. After Weissenberg (1911b).

this part of the cell appears as a bulge. This phenomenon is better seen in Fig. 4 which at the same magnification illustrates the earliest stage of material studied. Instead of single oval colonies with a diameter of about 350 μm in the section of the vagus ganglion, a group of three smaller colonies occur in the spinal ganglion cell. As components of the originally attenuated distal portion of the cell, they distend this particular area. Around the colonies, the hypertrophied cytoplasm (p) is distinct.

A much more advanced stage of a *Nosema* tumor in a spinal ganglion of *Lophius* is portrayed in Fig. 5. In a central cell, the oval colony (A) has reached a length of 1300 μm. Its distended cytoplasmic cover consisting of hypertrophied cytoplasm of the distal portion of the cell is clearly recognizable. The hypertrophied proximal portion of the cell, cut longitudinally, has a triangular shape. The basis of the triangle, compared with the corresponding structure of the preparation of Fig. 4, has increased in length about three-fold. Two noninfected ganglion cells (g_1 and g_2) are shown on each side of the neighboring double colony (B) to allow immediate comparison of the size differences. Colony A in Fig. 5 represents the peak of the growth period. Several colonies in the section of the tumor show regressive changes, such as reduction of the cytoplasmic cover of the colonies (D and E) or fragmentation in the certical zone of colonies beginning at the layer of the double colony (B). Details of the regressive changes have been described (Weissenberg, 1911b).

Hypertrophic growth of nerve cells invaded by microsporidian cell parasites is not the only type of response observed in *Lophius*. Certain uninvaded nerve cells growth unusually large due to hereditary factors. In such cases, cell enlargement is not as extreme as in corresponding cells infected by a microsporidian parasite. Holmgren (1899) has shown that the size of spinal ganglion cells of *Lophius piscatorius* increases with the growth of the *Lophius* specimen.

Heidenhain's iron hematoxylin staining reveals that the colonies of the *Lophius* parasite contain two kinds of components (Figs. 3, 4, and 5). First, there is a granulated mass of intensively stained particles that consists chiefly of spores and a few sporoblasts. The darkly stained structures are chiefly accumulated in the central region of the colonies. Their smooth surface also forms a thin superficial layer of the colonies. This thin marginal layer is separated from the central granulated mass by a stripe of very lightly stained structures. High magnification (Fig. 6A and B) shows that these latter structures consist of multiplying schizonts. In the *Lophius* parasite they are very delicate cytoplasmic structures with a diameter of about 1.5 – 2 μm. They have a tiny nucleus and are surrounded by a layer of glossy capsule. Multiplication of the schizonts is indicated by several factors. Often, two structures of similar appearance

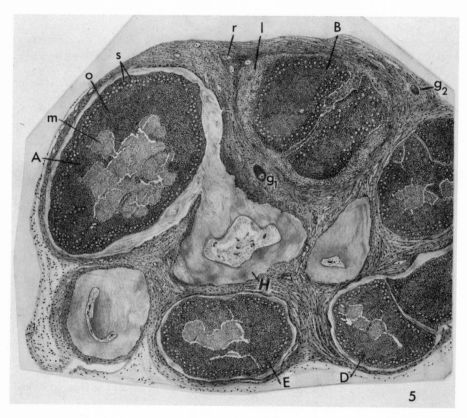

Fig. 5.   Section of a spinal ganglion of *L. piscatorius* specimen
(22 cm long) showing three large hypertrophic ganglion
cells and a group of five colonies of *N. lophii* advanced
in growth.   A, The distal portion of central ganglion cell
distended by a colony; H, base of the triangular section
through the proximal portion of the central ganglion cell;
o, mass of oval spores; m, accumulation of cylindrical
spores; s, areas containing schizonts; g_1 and g_2, uninfected ganglion cells on the sides of a colony, B.
Fixation and staining as in Fig. 4.   X 50.   After
Weissenberg (1911b).

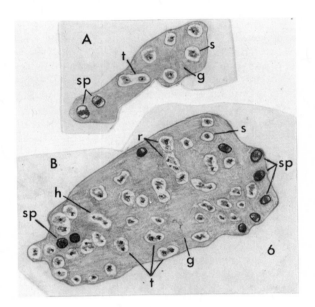

Fig. 6. Highly magnified (X 1500) schizogony portions (A and B) of a *N. lophii* colony in a spinal ganglion cell shown in Fig. 4. t, divided schizonts; h, division stage in which the nuclei of the daughter schizonts are connected by a delicate bridge; r, chain of schizonts; g, homogenous ground substance; sp, oval spores. In portion A, the cytoplasm of the schizonts was more distinctly marked than in portion B. After Weissenberg (1911b).

are located not far from one another (see structure   t in Fig. 6B).
In some groups the nuclei are connected by a stained filament (h
in Fig. 6B). Also chain arrangements have been observed (r).

The fate of the hypertrophied proximal portion of the
ganglion cell has not yet been investigated in detail. In the
nodes of old *N. lophii* tumors, strands of connective tissue
fibers are present as well as masses of spores from former
colonies; no remnants of the proximal portions of the ganglion
cells occur. How the ganglion cells perish is still unknown
althouth it appears that the stage of the central ganglion cell
with the large cytoplasmic bridge between the proximal and distal
portions of the cell (Fig. 5) is followed by a stage in which
the connection of the two portions is reduced and finally lost.
Advanced stages of the disease have been observed in *Lophius
americanus* in which the large bridge between the two portions of
the ganglion cell was replaced by very thin connections
(S. Jakowska, personal communication). This replacement may be
interpreted as a preliminary step to separation of the two portions.
Intermediate colonies that have lost their cytoplasmic cover
but have not been attacked by phagocytes probably continue their
growth within the host cell as long as they contain multiplying
schizonts. This condition typifies all the colonies of the
tumor shown in Fig. 5.

The occurrence of nodules containing microsporidian spores
on ganglia of *Lophius* was first described by Thélohan (1895).
Only three years later, Doflein (1898) described the disease
in greater detail and presented an instructive diagram of the
distribution of nodule groups on spinal and cerebral nerves. He
named the parasite *Glugea lophii*. However, Doflein did not recognize the relation of microsporidian colonies to hypertrophied ganglion cells and contended that smaller ganglion cells as well as
connective tissue become invaded by the microsporidian. Supposedly,
upon disintegration of the small infected cells, groups of spores
formed that ultimately would create colonies. In contrast Mrázek
did not observe invasion of connective tissue, but discovered that
the colonies are closely associated with ganglion cells that
become hypertrophied. The alleged early stages of the infection
of connective tissue cells were characterized by Mrázek as
phagocytes that engulfed spores of partially disintegrated colonies.

In 1909 and 1910, I had the opportunity to study this interesting disease of *Lophius* at the Zoological Station of Naples.
My investigations (1911a and b) essentially confirmed the observations of Mrázek published in his classic paper (1899). There
is only one major point in which I differ from Mrázek's interpretation. According to Mrázek, the microsporidian colony is
typically located within the neurite (axon) of the ganglion cell
after its exit from the cell. In my opinion, the microsporidian
colony grows not far from the exit of the axon, but still within
the ganglion cell itself and distends the attenuated distal
region of the cell to form a bulge (Weissenberg, 1911b). In

addition to this confirmation of Mrázek's results, my four
publications on the microsporidial disease of *Lophius* in the
period of 1909-1911 contained a study of the distribution of the
microsporidal colonies in the nervous system (1909) and detailed
investigations of the schizonts (1911b) and of regressive changes
in the colonies (1911a, b). No generation of sporont cells was
observed between schizonts and sporoblasts. The belief that
schizonts are directly transformed into sporoblasts led me
(1911c) to change the name of the parasite *Glugea lophii* to
Nosema lophii. Later, I learned that Pace (1908) had also made
a brief study of the *Lophius* parasite and had independently
transferred it to the genus *Nosema*.

Probably the microsporidium reaches the *Lophius* host as a
parasite of a prey fish. The spores of *Nosema lophii* then
germinate in the lumen of the gut of *Lophius*. Furthermore,
the sporoplasms presumably enter the intestinal wall as aneuro-
trophic germs and become attached to neurofibrils in the
epithelial layer of the gut or in the intestinal connective
tissue or muscular layer. If the neurofibrils become assembled
into a nerve fiber, which connects the gut wall with a ganglion
of the vagus nerve or with a ganglion of the autonomic trunk
as a neurite, the possibility exists that the microsporidian
germ may migrate along such a neurite in the direction of the
central nervous system and finally reach the distal portion of
its ganglion cell were a colony of schizonts and sporoblasts
become established. Such an hypothesis is supported by the early
observations of Mrazek (1899) who sometimes found microsporidian
colonies on the neurites at a considerable distance from the
ganglion cells. In my own view, that location of colonies is ex-
ceptional; I believe that the colony normally develops in the
distal portion of the ganglion cell where the axoplasma of the
neurite has continued into the neuroplasma of the ganglion cell.

A systematic investigation of the development of the microsporidian parasite of *L. americanus*, which would allow a comparison
with the observations on the two European species, has not yet
been performed. There are, however, preliminary studies by
Jakowska and Nigrelli (1959) in which the authors have reported
a distribution of the microsporidian colonies in ganglia of
cerebral and spinal nerves and on the medulla oblongata of
L. americanus. This finding corresponds very well to the results
obtained with the European species. However, Jakowska and Nigrelli
(1959) did not observe colonies developing within the cytoplasm
of hypertrophied ganglion and nerve cells. It seems very probable
that the *L. americanus* specimen that Jakowska and Nigrelli studied,
like the two European species previously studied, had already
completed an earlier developmental stage in which the hypertrophic
growth of invaded nerve cells and the intracytoplasmic position
of the developing colonies would be conspicuous. Jakowska (1964)

also believed that microsporidian colonies develop in the cytoplasm of hypertrophied ganglion cells of the North American
anglerfish. I have personnally studied some of Jakowska's
preparations. Some of special interest were sections through the
medulla oblongata region of a young *Lophius* measuring 13 cm in
length. Jakowska had interpreted intracytoplasmic structures
in ganglion cells of such young material as microsporidian
colonies in which spores were not developed. However, I
observed that intracytoplasmic sprouts from blood capillaries
of the surrounding connective tissue were responsible for some
diagnostic errors, especially because it is not easy to fix
schizonts in *Lophius* lesions. Mrázek (1899) found that connective
tissues and blood vessels in *Lophius* may form intracytoplasmic
insertions in normal ganglion cells. Thus, because transformation of these intracytoplasmic structures into colonies has
not been demonstrated, they can not be interpreted definitely as
groups of schizonts preceding the formation of spores.

A common feature of the first type of invasion discussed
earlier is that the parasites do not remain restricted to the
cytoplasmic region of the host cell that is initially invaded.
In contrast, they tend to invade neighboring regions of the host
cell cytoplasm and finally may infiltrate the entire cytoplasm
of the host cell with sprouts of multiplying schizonts. *Nosema
lophii*, which represents the second type of invasion, remains restricted to the distal portion of the host cell cytoplasm. The
proximal portion does not become infiltrated although it undergoes hypertrophic growth. Figs. 3-5 distinctly reveal areas of
multiplying schizonts that appear as islands within the medium
zone of the surrounding spore mass in the colonies. The proximal
hypertrophied cytoplasmic area is not invaded at all[3].

---

[3]In the original manuscript Dr. Weissenberg was of the opinion
that these unique features of the host-parasite relations justify
the creation of a new genus and a new family for *Nosema lophii*.
Therefore, he proposed *Spraguea* g. n. with *S. lophii* as type
species, and *Spraguidae* f. n. He said these taxa would "Be
characterized by (1) the formation of colonies of the microsporidian parasite only at the cytoplasmic zone of the host cell
where the invasion had originally started and (2) by the location
of groups of multiplying schizonts only at a median layer of the
colony." The editors agree in thinking Weissenberg attributed too
much value to these characters but they do not agree on whether
any value at all should be attributed to them at this time. The
matter is presented in the form of a footnote as a compromise
between the opinions of the editors on the one hand and their
obligation to the author on the other hand.

In the third type of microsporidian infection, the entire cytoplasm of the host cell becomes invaded. Host cell and parasite work together as a single unit to build a complex structure which, in highly developed cases, reaches macroscopic dimensions with a long life span. In the case of *Thelohania tipulae*, an example of host cell hypertrophy of a larval fat body cell of an insect was described. Most of the host cell cytoplasm is replaced by a rather large colony of the intracellular parasite. Regressive changes in the host cytoplasm leading to the loss of stored cell products is prominent. However, in the third type of invasion, the hypertrophied host cell displays some progressive changes. The most conspicuous of these changes is exemplified in cells infected by *Glugea anomala* and *G. hertwigii*.

E.   GLUGEA ANOMALA *(MONIEZ, 1887) GURLEY, 1893*

When *G. anomala* or *G. hertwigii* invade a receptive host, the host cell nucleus undergoes amitotic multiplication. Consequently, many hundreds of its descendants become distributed in the cortical cytoplasm of the host cell; most of the sprouting schizonts multiplies in the intermediate and central region of the host cell. There is, however, no sharp demarcation of the cytoplasmic layers and their contents. Another progressive change of the host cell is the production of a conspicuous cuticular cell capsule. The encapsulated complex of host cell and parasite colony appears as a cyst. Subsequently, the capsule becomes surrounded by connective tissue layers abundantly laden with blood vessels. The capsule structure is homogeneous and allows passage of nutrients from the intercellular fluids and blood to the microsporidian colony as well as the passage of metabolic products to the outside. The capsule delimits the complex structure from the surrounding tissue.

G. *anomala* parasitizes the three spined stickleback *Gasterosteus aculeatus*. Invaded cells become hypertrophied and often reach a diameter of 3-4 mm. Observations of early stages of the infection indicate that the invaded host cell is at first a uninucleate migratory cell in the mesenchyme of young fishes. The microsporidium is probably entrapped by phagocytosis. Figure 7 shows an early stage of the microsporidium surrounded by an eccentrically located vacuole (v). The vacuole is embraced by a crescent-shaped nucleus that has formed the bulge of a lobe. In Fig. 8 the host cell nucleus is trilobed and the parasite has developed into an oval schizont equipped with a large nucleus displaying a large karyosome in a clear zone. The invaded cells of Figs. 7 and 8 have a diameter of about 7 μm.

In the two focal planes of Fig. 9 cell enlargement is distinct. The oval cell attains a diameter of 12 μm (Fig. 9A). Also, amitotic multiplication of the host cell nucleus has

Fig. 7.   Early stage of the invasion of a mesenchyme cell of a
          young three-spined stickleback (*Gasterosteus aculeatus*)
          by an amoebula of *Glugea anomala* on the 12th day of
          infection. The parasite lies in a vacuole, v. The
          vacuole is embraced by the crescent-shaped host cell
          nucleus that has formed a lobe, l. Acidified alcohol,
          Delafield's hematoxylin. X 2600. After Weissenberg (1968).

Fig. 8.   A more advanced stage of cell invasion. The nucleus of
          the schizont has developed a large karyosome. The host
          cell nucleus is trilobated. Fixation, staining, and
          magnification as in Fig. 7. After Weissenberg (1968).

Fig. 9.   Infected mesenchyme cell is shown in two focal planes,
          A and B. The vacuole, v, in the upper plane, A, contains
          one schizont. In the lower plane, B, a plurinucleate
          plasmodium is contained in the vacuole. The host cell
          nucleus has produced a number of peripherally located
          nuclei by a series of amitotic divisions; the arrow points
          to a deep indentation of one of them. Acidified alcohol,
          Delafield's hematoxylin. X 2,250. After Weissenberg
          (1968).

Fig. 10. Oval host cell on the 18th day of infection (sieze is 52 X
          45 μm). The marginal section shows numerous hypertrophied
          division products of the host cell nucleus that have con-
          tinued to multiply amitotically (see formation of lobes,
          l, and sprouts, s). The progressive schizogony has formed
          plurinucleated cylinders of schizonts, of which four are
          cut lognitudinally; others are sectioned transversaly, r.
          A cuticular capsule occurs as a thin membrane, m, around
          the host cell. Flemming's fluid, Heidenhain's iron-
          hematoxylin. X 1,550. After Weissenberg (1968).

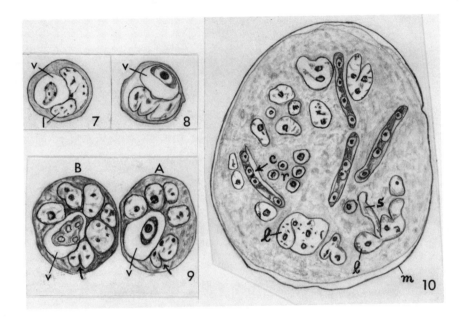

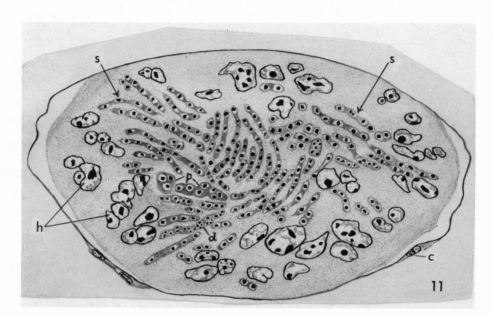

Fig. 11.   Longitudinal section of ovoid host cell (135 x 90 μm) on
           the 22nd day of infection. The cytoplasmic region is
           filled with sprouting polynucleated schizont-cylinders,
           s. The cortical cytoplasmic zone contains a large number
           of large vesicular nuclei, h, derived by amitotic
           divisions of the host cell nucleus. At p there is a
           thicker schizont-plasmodium surrounded by a vacuole in
           preparation for subdivision into sporonts ("Vakuolenzellen"
           d, double-layered schizont-cylinder; c, fibroblast attached
           to cuticular capsule. Fixation and staining as in Fig.
           10. X 870. After Weissenberg (1968).

progress in the cortical cell zone. The vacuole (v) contains
stages of schizogony, namely a plasmodium in the lower focal
plane (Fig. 9B). In the next stage (Fig. 10) the oval host
cell in the marginal section measures 45 x 52 μm. The schizonts
have developed into plurinucleate cylinders sprouting into
the hypertrophying cytoplasm. Narrow clear spaces around them
are probably remnants of the former vacuole. The amitotic multiplication of the host cell nuclei has continued in the cortical
zone indicated by formation of lobes and sprouts (s). The cell
capsule appears as a thin membrane (m).

The oval host cell then enlarges to a size of 90 x 135 μm
(Fig. 11). The deeper cytoplasmic zone is infiltrated by a
number of plurinucleate cylinders (s) of schizonts. The cortical
zone contains the large vesicular nuclei (h) descended from the
host cell nucleus. The cell capsule has become thicker.

The beginning of sporogony is marked by the development of
a vacuole around a plasmodium (P, Fig. 11). Such a plasmodium
(compare also U in Fig. 12) will become subdivided into uninucleate
cells through a sequence of multiple divisions. The division products (Fig. 13), which I called "Vakuolenzellen" (Weissenberg, 1913),
are sporonts. Each of them (Figs. 14 and 15) divides into two
sporoblasts that are transformed into spores. Fig. 16 shows a row
of invaded host cells from the wall of the coelomic cavity of a
young stickleback with diameters of more than 200 μm. Numerous
sporogony vacuoles have developed in the middle zone of these
cells and have fused in their central areas, forming a storage
space for the spores. The thick cortical zone contains schizogony
stages and the external areas hold host cell nuclei. A more
advanced stage of a corresponding cell of a smelt invaded by
Glugea hertwigii displays nuclear multiplication by amitosis
during sporogony (Fig. 17). Of special interest are the
connecting bridges (marked by arrows) between daughter nuclei
that have not completely separated. Fig. 18 portrays a terminal
stage of *G. anomala* cyst development in the wall of the coelomic
cavity of a young stickleback. The cyst (c) with a diameter of
more than three mm nearly fills the lumen of the cavity. Most
of the developmental stages of schizogony and sporogony are not
present and the cyst contains a mass of mature spores. The number
of vesicular host cell nuclei, distributed within the distended
cortical zone of the cyst, is much reduced. However, several
of these nuclei (K, Fig. 19) are contained beneath the thick
capsule (cy). Thus, the developmental process ends with the
formation of a cyst containing a large mass of spores. The cyst
is built by active participation of the host cell, which not only
became distended by the multiplying intracellular parasites but
also grew by continuous enlargement of its own cytoplasm. Whereas
distension of the host cell by accumulation of *Nosema lophii*
spores (mentioned earlier) makes difficult the recognition of

Figs. 12-19. Sporogony stages of *G. anomala* or *G. hertwigi* in
              hypertrophied mesenchyme cells of *Gasterosteus
              aculeatus* or *Osmerus eperlanus*.

Fig. 12.   Schizont-cylinder, s, within the marginal region of the
           cytoplasm, pr, of a *G. anomala* cyst (2,000 μm in diameter).
           u, two sporogony-plasmodia cut longitudinally surrounded
           by vacuoles; t, cross-sections of sporogony-plasmodia.
           Flemming's fluid, Heidenhain's iron-hematoxylin method.
           X 2500. After Weissenberg (1913).

Fig. 13.   Group of sporonts ("Vakuolenzellen") that have originated
           from a sporogony-plasmodium. Fixation, staining, and
           magnification as in Fig. 12. After Weissenberg (1913).

Fig. 14.   Group of sporonts ("Vakuolenzellen") dividing into two
           sporoblasts. This stage is of long duration; the nucleus
           has divided into two daughter nuclei, which have moved to
           the poles of the elongated cells and are still connected
           by a distinct filament. The cytoplasm of the elongated
           sporonts has not yet been divided. Fixation, staining
           and magnification as in Fig. 12. After Weissenberg (1913).

Fig. 15.   Progressive division of the sporont cytoplasm. The fila-
           ment which connected the sporoblast-nuclei has disappeared.
           Fixation, staining, and magnification as in Fig. 12.
           After Weissenberg (1913).

Fig. 16.   Sagittal section of mid-gut of a young stickleback (29th
           day of infection). m, mid-gut lumen; dm, dorsal muscles;
           vs, ventral skin; ov, portion of the ovary; C, E, F,
           complex structures consisting of hypertrophied multinuc-
           leate mesenchyme cells of the wall of the coelomic cavity
           that have formed around *G. anomala* colonies and represent
           highly developed "xenomas". The largest xenoma F has a
           diameter of 270 um. The host cell cytoplasm of the xenomas
           contains numerous sporogony-vacuoles, which in the central
           region of the xenomas have formed a storage space for the
           accumulating spores. Fixation in Sanfelice's mixture of
           chromic acid, formalin, and acetic acid; staining with
           Heidenhain's iron-hematoxylin. X 66. Original photo-
           micrograph.

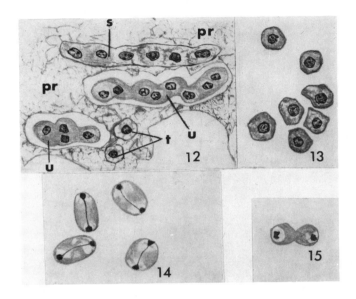

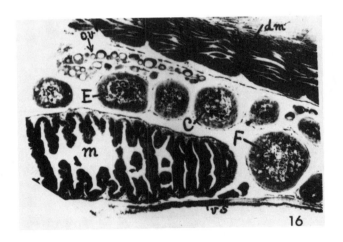

Fig. 17. Amitotic multiplication of the descendants of the host
          cell nucleus in hypertrophied mesenchyme cell of the
          smelt *Osmerus eperlanus* infected by *G. hertwigii*. When
          the buds of the nuclei become moved apart, connecting
          bridges (see arrows) between the daughter nuclei are
          frequently recognizable. Formalin, Delafield's
          hematoxylin. X 550. After Weissenberg (1913).

Fig. 18. Transverse section of a young stickleback affected by a
          large *G. anomala* cyst (3,000 μm in diameter). The cyst
          has developed in the mesenchyme of the wall of the
          coelomic cavity and nearly fills the lumen. c,
          cyst;   d, gut; o, ovary; ch, chorda dorsalis; r,
          spinal cord; m, muscles. X 15. After Weissenberg (1913).

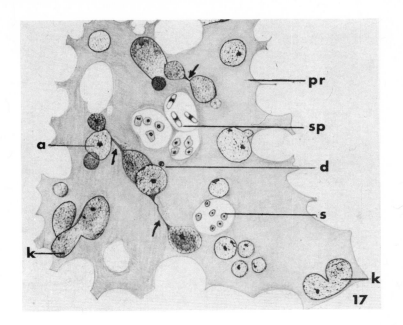

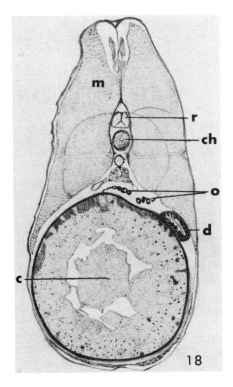

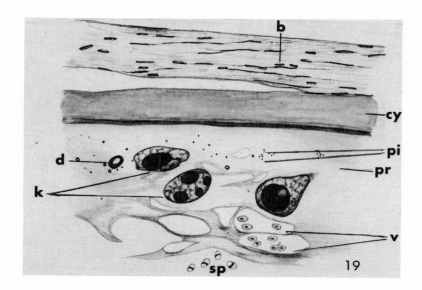

Fig. 19.   Transverse section of part of the ventral cortical zone
           of a large *G. anomala* cyst (see Fig. 18). b,
           connective tissue; cy, cuticular capsule of the hyper-
           trophied host cell; pr, host cell cytoplasm; k,
           remnants of the sprouts of the host cell nucleus; sp,
           microsporidian spores. Formalin, Delafield's
           hematoxylin. X 570. After Weissenberg (1913), but
           (see especially K) with partial change of interpretation
           based on the results of Weissenberg (1921): pr, became
           recognized as cytoplasm of the host cell; k, was recog-
           nized as remnants of sprouts of the host cell nucleus.

gradual hypertrophic growth of the cytoplasm in advanced stages, there are two progressive changes in *G. anomala* parasitism that disclose active participation of the host cell in cyst formation. These are the remarkable amitotic multiplication of the host cell nucleus and the production of the conspicuous cell capsule.

IV. THE GLUGEA ANOMALA CYST

A. EARLY INTERPRETATIONS

At the beginning of the twentieth century, *Glugea anomala* cysts were interpreted by several investigators as parasitic protozoa of gigantic size. Stempell (1904) concluded that the mature *G. anomala* cyst represents a single large protozoon of macroscopic size with numerous nuclei in its cytoplasm as well as developing and mature spores. Pérez (1905) agreed with Stempell after studying a microsporidium that forms cysts in the barnacle *Balanus amaryllis*. Awerinzew and Fermor (1911) and Pérez (1905) believed that the host cell nuclei represent large "vegetative nuclei" of the supposed multi-nucleate protozoon.

Several other investigators such as Schröder (1909), Schuberg (1910), and Mrázek (1910) observed that host cells invaded by small microsporidia can be stimulated to undergo a remarkable hypertrophy; their enlarged nuclei may then be found between microsporidian developmental stages. These investigators become very skeptical of Stempell's interpretation regarding large vesicular nuclei in *Glugea* cysts as vegetative nuclei of a gigantic protozoon. Rather, they presumed that hypertrophic growth of host cells and enlargement of host cell nuclei is also involved in the development of *G. anomala*.

I investigated the schizogony and sporogony of the microsporidian in detail in growing cysts (Weissenberg, 1911a) but could not confirm the development of sporogony stages from nuclei claimed to be the vegetative nuclei of a large protozoon. However, I did discover a *Glugea* cyst on a fin of a young stickleback with a diameter of about 80 μm that displayed schizont-cylinders in such excellent condition that I considered the small cyst to be an early normal stage of the microsporidium. Vesicular nuclei were not seen in the cyst but iron hematoxylin stain revealed a number of small intensively stained compact bodies scattered throughout the cytoplasm as well as the schizont-cylinders. I interpreted the compact bodies as "primary nuclei" and then believed that they were the common root from which both the vesicular nuclei and additional schizonts arose. Therefore, I concluded that this was evidence favoring Stempell's interpretation of *G. anomala* as a large protozoon. However, I knew that definitive clarification of the problem awaited discovery of earlier developmental stages of the cysts.

B. FINAL INTERPRETATIONS

To obtain early developing stages of *G. anomala*, I infected young sticklebacks by feeding them some young *cyclops* that had ingest-

ed *Glugea* spores (Weissenberg, 1913). After several weeks, there
appeared *Glugea* cysts with a diameter of about 300 μm. Two of
the fishes were sacrificed on the seventh and ninth days of infection. Sections through the seven day and nine day infected fish
showed numerous migratory cells in the mesenchyme of the midgut
and in the coelomic cavity. Some of the cells were small uninucleate; others were larger plurinucleate forms. Vacuoles in the
host cell cytoplasm contained either a small single celled protozoon or binucleate stages. A number of these forms resembled
schizogony stages of *G. anomala* that I had observed earlier in
growing cysts (Weissenberg, 1913). Obviously, the migratory
cells in the mesenchyme has engulfed early stages of *G. anomala*
by phagocytosis. Hypertrophic growth of the migratory cell had
begun and was accompanied by amitotic multiplication of the host
cell nucleus. Thus, the *G. anomala* cyst is a complex of two
components: (1) the host consisting of a hypertrophied,
multinucleate fish cell, and (2) the parasite composed of an
enclosed microsporidian colony.

C. COMPARATIVE ANALYSIS: DESIGNATION OF "XENOMA"

The *G. anomala* cyst, characterized by amitotic multiplication
of the host cell nucleus, represents the most complex formation of
a hypertrophic host cell and an enclosed colony of intracellular
microsporidian parasites. Furthermore, it represents a rare
variation of hypertrophic cell growth occasioned by parasitic
invasion. Hypertrophic growth is a rather common response to
parasitic invasion, but usually, the enlarged nucleus remains undivided. Amitotic nuclear division has been observed only in a
few species of one family of microsporidia besides *Glugea anomala*
and *G. hertwigii*. Mrázek described this family of organisms as
Myxocystidae (1897, 1910), later classified by Léger and Hesse
as Mrazekidae (1916). Some members of this family are parasites
of oligochaete worms; some species invade lymphocytes as well as
spermatocytes of the worms. Fig. 20 shows a hypertrophied
lymphocyte of *Limnodrilus* invaded by *Mrazekia caudata* wherein
amitotic multiplication of the host cell nucleus occurs.

Interestingly, Mrázek (1910) also observed hypertrophic invaded cells in the seminal sacks and coelom of the worm
Lumbriculus which contain a single gigantic nucleus surrounded
by numerous microsporidian cells. He also studied initiation of
amiotic division of the hypertrophied cell nucleus in invaded
lymphocytes of *Limnodrillus*. As Fig. 21 demonstrates, the budding
of the hypertrophied nucleus of the lymphocyte on the left side
shows similarity to amitotic division products of the host cell
nucleus observed in infections by *G. hertwigii* (see Fig. 17);
especially noteworthy are the nuclear bridges that persist and
connect some of the division products.

Jírovec (1930) has observed hypertrophic growth without
nuclear division of cells of the perch *Acerina cernus* invaded by
Glugea acerinae. He discovered numerous hypertrophied cells
of gut connective tissue filled with spores. The largest cysts
mainly in the tunica propria were about 200–350 μm in diameter.
The youngest cysts averaged 20–30 μm in diameter and contained a
centrally located undivided host cell nucleus. Jírovec observed
some schizont-cylinders and isolated schizonts in addition to
sporogony stages and spores. Probably schizogony was limited
in *G. acerinae* relative to that in *G. anomala* (Fig. 11). The
larger *G. acerinae* cysts contained mostly masses of mature spores.
The cyst capsules attained a thickness of about 0.2–0.5 μm.

The main difference in *G. acerinae* and *G. anomala* cysts is
the fate of the host cell nucleus. As demonstrated above,
sprouting of schizonts in *G. anomala* is accompanied by conspicuous
amitotic multiplication of the host cell nucleus that becomes
divided into a number of nuclear buds; the buds then swell and
become vesicular nuclear forms. The division products continue
amitotic division so that the cortical region of the host cell
cytoplasm is filled with hundreds of amitotic division products.
In the first period of sporogony the division products of the host
cell nucleus are well developed; later, they are reduced in
number, apparently by degeneration. In *G. acerinae*, no division
of the host cell nucleus was observed by Jírovec (1930) nor any
abnormality in the structure of the nucleus. In cells that had
accumulated spores, the nucleus was beginning to degenerate.
Eventually, the spores broke the nucleus filling its lumen.

Based on the *G. anomala* cyst complex, I proposed a name for
such an association derived from the Greek work xenon or xenoma
(Weissenberg, 1922a,b).[4] Because xenon was already used for a
chemical element, I later changed the name to xenom or xenoma
(Weissenberg, 1949). The latter designation, xenoma, has a certain similarity to tumor. If the word tumor is used for local
enlargement of living matter in an organism, one of the most
important kinds is a neoplasm that results from rapid cellular
proliferation. However in the case of a xenoma, localized enlargement of tissue is the result of cellular hypertrophy stimulated by intracellular parasites. Certainly, it is advantageous
to the invaded organism to have parasite colonies localized within hypertrophied cells rather than to have the infection spread
to other parts of this tissue. The advantage to the parasite is
that it can develop within a protecting and hospitable host cell
under excellent nutritional conditions. In this regard, the xenoma
is a symbiotic complex because the association is beneficial to
the parasite, which can accumulate macroscopic colonies, and to

---

[4]The fact that a parasite and its host cell are intimately
related, structurally and physiologically, was already recognized by Chatton (1920) and by Chatton and Courrier (1923) who
used the name "complexe xeno-parasitaire" for such an association.

Fig. 20.   Hypertrophied lymphocyte of the oligochaete annelid
            worm, *Limnodrilus*, invaded by *Mrazekia caudata*. The
            large nuclei are amitotic division products of the
            host cell nucleus. The small cells in the cytoplasm
            of the lymphocyte are schizonts of the cell parasite.
            After Mrázek (1910).

Fig. 21.   Early stage of amitotic sprouting of the nucleus of a
            lymphocyte of *Limnodrilus* infected by a microsporidian.
            The nuclear buds on the left side of the nucleus are
            still connected with one another or with the chief
            portion of the nucleus by nuclear filaments. The small
            cells in the cytoplasm of the lymphocyte are stages of
            the microsporidium (schizonts and spores). After Mrázek
            (1910).

Fig. 22.   Part of a transverse section through the midgut of a
            larva of *Tipula gigantea*. d, nucleus of a cylindrical
            epithelial cell; z, cone-shaped epithelial cell; e,
            transversal sections of elastic fibers above circular
            muscle fibers; g, ground substance of the tunica
            elastico-muscularis; l, transversal sections of longi-
            tudinal muscle fibers; a, b, c, cysts of *Nosema
            binucleatum*. Sublimate-alcohol after Schaudinn,
            hematoxylin, and safranin. X 367. After Weissenberg
            (1926).

Fig. 23.   Early stage of a *N. binucleatum* cyst. A, sketch of fresh
            preparation. X 1750; B, preparation fixed with sublimate-
            alcohol and stained with hematoxylin. After Weissenberg
            (1926).

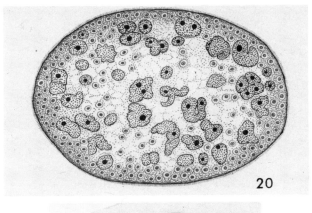

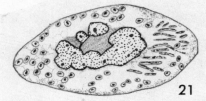

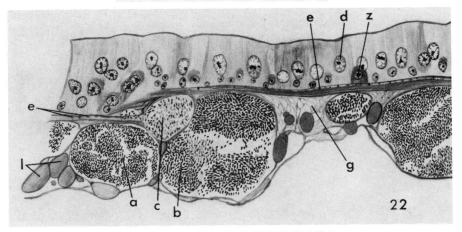

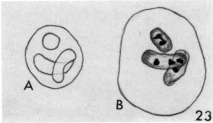

the host cell because it is stimulated to form large amounts of cytoplasm. In highly developed cases, this cytoplasmic build-up is accompanied by production of numerous nuclei derived from the original host cell nucleus and these formative processes are associated with a long cell life.

V. VARIATIONS OF METAZOAN HOST CELL INVASIONS

Not all microsporidia stimulate their host cells to hypertrophic growth. Sometimes, the host cell is destroyed by the multiplying microsporidia as in the case of *Nosema bombycis* or occasionally there is little cytopathological effect by the cellular parasites, e.g., *N. apis*. One unique infection is that caused by the nerve cell parasite, *Nosema lophii*. Considerable hypertrophy of the host cell is induced by the microsporidium but colony formation is restricted to the distal portion of the cell; proximal cell portion is not utilized at all by the parasite.

The highest degree of host cell-microsporidian association is reached when the symbiotic complex is of long duration, for which the designation "xenoma" is appropriate. Of course, there are simple or rudimentary xenomas and highly developed complexes. An example of a rudimentary form is the *Glugea acerinae* xenoma of connective tissue cells in the perch *Acerina cernua*. Here the host cell nucleus remains undivided and degenerates at an early stage. A highly developed xenoma is caused by *C. anomala* and *G. hertwigii* in which the host cell nucleus produces several hundred descendants by a series of amitotic division. The *G. hertwigii* xenomas sometimes develop in great numbers in the tissues. The *G. anomala* xenomas usually develop in small numbers of mesenchyme cells throughout various organs of the three-spined stickleback *Gasterosteus aculeatus*. But, these xenomas frequently become gigantic, reaching 3-4 mm in diameter. Cell hypertrophy usually occurs only in invaded cells but there are a few exceptions. For example, Schuberg (1910) observed in the epithelium of the seminferous tubules of *Barbus fluviatilis*, infected by *Plistophora longifilis*, hypertrophy of nucleus and cytoplasm not only of invaded cells but also of some neighboring uninvaded ones.

VI. MICROSPORIDIA AS PARASITES OF PROTOZOA

Among the protozoa, a few myxosporidians and gregarines are recognized as hosts of microsporidia. The microsporidium *Nosema marionis* is a frequent parasite of the myxosporidium *Ceratomyxa coris*. However, even in cases of heavy infection of the myxosporidium by the microsporidium, there is no apparent harm to the host. For example, spore formation of *Ceratomyxa* is not disturbed by its microsporidian parasite (Stempell, 1919). If *Nosema notabilis* parasitizes the myxosporidium *Sphaerospora polymorpha*

only slightly, spore formation of the host proceeds normally.
If, however, the infection is heavy, the host nuclei undergo
hypertrophy and degeneration and spore formation does not occur
(Kudo 1939, 1944). Therefore, *N. notabilis* may be considered a
true pathogen of a myxosporidium.

The invasion of *Cephaloidophora* (syn. *Frenzelina) conformis*
by *Nosema frenzelinae* [Léger and Duboscq (1909a, 1909b, 1909c)]
is an example of microsporidian infection of gregarines. It is
of great interest that the microsporidian infection has a pathogenic effect on the developmental processes of the gregarines.
Within the cysts of the infected paired gregarines the development of gametes is not completed normally. As result of cell
degeneration, conjugation of male and female gametes becomes
prevented, which is considered by Léger and Duboscq as a parasitic
castration. The schizonts of the microsporidia develop into
spores within the cysts and completely fill the gregarines.

VII. MICROSPORIDIAN INVASION OF GLANDULAR CELLS OF DIPTERA

The salivary glands of Diptera larvae are sometimes invaded
by microsporidia. Roberts *et al.* (1967), Diaz *et al.* (1969),
Jurand *et al.* (1967), Pavan *et al.* (1969) have described microsporidian invasion of several members of Sciaridae and its
effects on the polytene chromosomes. Characteristically, the
size of the polytene chromosomes increases under the
stimulus of cell invaders. The width of the polytene chromosomes increases as does the amount of deoxyribonucleic
acid. Furthermore, synthesis of ribonucleic acid is enhanced.
Interestingly, during pupation of *Sciara ocellaris* some other
Sciaridae many of the infected cells do not become destroyed.
Consequently, infected salivary gland cells have been isolated
from adult flies (Jurand *et al.*, 1967; Pavan *et al.*, 1969;
Pavan *et al.*, 1971. There were no signs of degeneration observed in the isolated cells. Pavan *et al.* (1971) advocated that
such cells of Sciaridae have become a separate entity something
like a unicellular tumor. These investigators considered that the
host cytoplasmic organelles may have been functionally replaced,
in part, by corresponding organelles of the parasite.

VIII. DEVELOPMENT OF NOSEMA BINUCLEATUM CYSTS IN TIPULA GIGANTEA LARVAL MIDGUT CELLS

A peculiar development of cysts of *Nosema binucleatum* frequently occurs in the midgut wall of *Tipula gigantea* larvae
(Weissenberg, 1926b). The histological aspects of the midgut are
depicted in Fig. 22. The epithelial layer is surrounded by the
tunica elasticomuscularis. Beneath a network of elastic fibrils
(e), the tunica consists of a homogenous ground substance (g) into
which fibers of muscle cells are inserted. An inner layer of

rather thin circular muscle fibers (r) is followed by an outer
layer of thicker muscle fibers arranged in longitudinal direction.
As Fig. 22 demonstrates, it is the layer of the longitudinal
muscle fibers where, in an infected larva, cysts of *N. binucleatum*
(a,b,c) develop. Frequently, such cysts reach diameters of about
120 μm. Depending on the climatic season stages of sporogony
and schizogony vary. In the fall, for example, earlier development stages of an average diameter of 15 μm (Figs. 23 A and B).
Such cysts are rare in specimens collected during the spring. The
smallest cysts observed contain only a few schizonts sprouting in
a vacuole space, which in fresh conditions (Fig. 23A) is filled
with fluid. There is no remnant of a host cell nucleus in such
vesicles. Apparently, the cysts do not originate in host cells.
How the sporoplasms of ingested spores reach the ground substance
of the gut wall is in question. Possibly, they do so by moving
between the longitudinal muscle fibers and vacuoles then form
around them. In such a manner they are delimited from the ground
substance by the vacuolar membranes. In addition to the sprouting
of the parasites within the small cysts, such vesicular structures,
filled with fluid, may become distended as the result of diffusion
of nutrients through their cyst membrane until the cysts become
full-sized (about 120 μm in diameter).

Generally schizogony of microsporidia takes its course within
the cytoplasm of a host cell. Development of cysts of *N.
binucleatum* may represent an exception.

REFERENCES

Awerinzew, S., and Fermor, K. (1911). Studien über parasitische
    Protozoen. Zur Frage über die Sporenbuildung bei *Glugea
    anomala. Arch. Proteistenk.* <u>23</u>, 1-6.
Chatton, E. (1920). Un complexe xéno-parasitaire morphologique
    et physiologique *Neresheimeria paradoxa* chez *Fritillaria
    pellucida. C. R. Acad. Sci. (Paris)* <u>171</u>, 55-57.
Chatton, E., and Courrier, R. (1923). Formation d'un complexe
    xénoparasitaire géant avec bordure en brosse, sous l'in-
    fluence d'une microsporidie, dans le testicule de *Cottus
    bubalis. C. R. Soc. Biol. (Paris)* <u>89</u>, 579-583.
Diaz, M., and Pavan, C. (1965). Changes in chromosomes induced
    by microorganism infection. *Proc. Nat. Acad. Sci. (Wash.)*
    <u>54</u>, 1321-1327.
Diaz, M., Pavan, C., and Basile, R. (1969). Effects of a virus
    and a microsporidian infections in chromosomes of various
    tissues of *Phynchosciara angelae* Nonato and Pavan. *Rev.
    Bras. Biol.* <u>29</u>, 191-206.
Doflein, F. (1898). Studien zur Naturgeschichte der Protozoen.
    III. Ueber Myxosporidien. *Zool. Yahrb. Anat.* <u>11</u>, 281-350.
Jakowska, S. (1964). Infeccao microsporidea das celulas
    nervosas numa populacao de peixes marinhos, *Lophius americanus.
    Annals 2nd Congr. Lat. Amer. de Zool.*, Sao Paulo, 1962. pp.
    265-273.

Jakowska, S., and Nigrelli, R. F. (1959). Nosematiasis in the American Anglerfish. *J. Protozool. 6 (Suppl.)*, 7.

Jírovec, O. (1930). Über eine neue Microsporidienart *(Glugea acerinae* n.sp.) aus *Acerina cernua. Arch. Protistenk.* 72, 198-213.

Jurand, A., Simoes, L.C.G., and Pavan, C. (1967). Changes in the ultrastructure of salivary gland cytoplasm in *Sciara ocellaris* (Comstock, 1882) due to microsporidian infection. *J. Insect Physiol.* 13, 795-803.

Kudo, R. (1939). Observations on *Nosema notabilis* n. sp. parasitic in a myxosporidian. *Anat. Rec.* 75, 153.

Kudo, R. (1944). Morphology and development of *Nosema notabilis* Kudo, parasitic in *Sphaerospora polymorpha*, a parasite of *Opsanus tau* and *O. beta. Illinois biol. Monogr.* 20, 1-83.

Léger, L., and Duboscq, O. (1909a). Sur une microsporidie parasite d'une gregarine. *C. R. Acad. Sci. (Paris)* 138, 733-734.

Léger, L., and Duboscq, O. (1909b). Microsporidie parasite de *Frenzelina. In:* Etudes sur la sexulité chez les grégarines. *Arch. Protistenk.* 17, 117-119.

Léger, L. and Duboscq, O. (1909c). *Perezia landesteriae* n.g., sp., microsporidie parasite de *Lankesteria ascidiae* Ray-Lank *Arch. Zool. exp.* 41, (5), v. 1, Notes et revue No. 3, 89-94.

Léger, L., and Hesse, E. (1916). *Mrazekia* genre nouveau de Microsporidies a spores tubuleuses. *C. R. Soc. Biol.(Paris)* 79, 345-348.

Mrázek, A. (1897). Uber eine neue Sporozoenform aus *Limnodrilus. S.-B. Kon. bohm. Ges. Wiss. Prag,* math.-nat. Kl. Pt. 1, Art. 8, 1-5.

Mrázek, A. (1899). Sporozoenstudien II. *Glugea lophii* Doflein. *S.-B. Kon. bohm. Ges. Wiss. Prag,* math.-nat. Kl. 34, 1-8.

Mrázek, A. (1910). Sporozoenstudien. Zur Auffassung der Myxocystiden. *Arch. Protistenk.* 18, 245-259.

Pace, D. (1908). Parasiten und Pseudoparasiten der Nervenzelle. Vorlaufige Mitteilung uber vergleichende Parasitologie des Nervensystems. *Z. Hyg. Infekt.-Kr.* 60, 62-74.

Pavan, C., Biesele, J., Riess, R. W., and Wertz, A. V. (1971). Changes in the ultrastructure of *Rhynchosciara* cells infected by Microsporidia. *In:* Studies in Genetics VI. *Univ. Texas Publ.* 7103, 241-267.

Pavan, C., Perondini, A.L.P., and Picard, T. (1969). Changes in chromosomes and in development of cells in *Sciara ocellaris* induced by microsporidian infections. *Chromosome* (Berl.) 28, 328-345.

Pérez, Ch. (1905). Sur une *Glugea* nouvelle parasite de *Balanus amaryllis. C. R. Soc. Biol.* (Paris) 58, 150-151.

Petri, M. (1965). A cytolytic parasite in the cells of transplantable, malignant tumours. *Nature* (Lond.) 205: 302.

Petri, M. (1966). The occurrence of *Nosema cuniculi (Encephalito-zoon cuniculi)* in the cells of transplantable malignant tumours and its effect upon tumour and host. *Acta Path. Microbiol. Scand.* 66, 13-30.

Roberts, P. A., Kimball, R. F., and Pavan, C. (1967). Response of *Rhynchosciara* chromosomes to microsporidian infection. *Exp. Cell Res.* 47, 408-422.

Schröder, O. (1909). *Thelohania chaetogastris,* eine neue in *Chaetogaster diaphanus* Gruith schmarotzende Microsporidienart. *Arch. Protistenk.* 14, 119-133.

Schuberg, A. (1910). Uber Microsporidien aus dem Hoden der Barbe und durch sie verursachte Hypertrophie der Kerne. *Arb. Gesundh.-Amte* (Berl.) 33, 401-434.

Stempell, W. (1904). Uber *Nosema anomalum. Arch. Protistenk.* 4, 1-42.

Stempell, W. (1909). Ueber *Nosema bombycis* Nägeli. *Arch. Protistenk.* 16, 281-358.

Stempell, W. (1919). Unterschungen über *Leptotheca coris* sp. und das in dieser schmarotzende *Nosema marionis* Thélohan. *Arch. Protistenk.* 40, 113-157.

Thélohan, P. (1895). Recherches sur les Myxosporidies. *Bull. Sci. France et Belg.* 26, 100-394.

Weissenberg, R. (1909). Beiträge zur Kenntnis von *Glugea lophii* Doflein. 1. Ueber den Sitz und die Verbreitung der Mikro-sporidiencysten am Nervensystem von *Lophius piscatorius* und *budegassa. S.-B. Ges. Naturf. Fr.* Berlin No. 9, 557-565.

Weissenberg, R. (1911a). Ueber einige Mikrosporidien aus Fischen. *(Nosema lophii* Doflein, *Glugea anomala* Moniez, *Glugea hertwigii* nov. spec.) *S.-B. Ges. Naturf. Fr.* Berlin No. 8, 344-351.

Weissenberg, R. (1911b). Ueber Microsporidien aus dem Nerven-system von Fischen *(Glugea lophii* Doflein) und die Hypertrophie der befallenen Ganglienzellen. *Arch. Mikr. Anat.* 78, 383-421.

Weissenberg, R. (1913). Beiträge zur Kenntnis des Zeugungskreises der Microsporidien *Glugea anomala* Moniez und *hertwigii* Weissenberg. *Arch. Mikr. Anat. 82 (Abt. 2),* 81-163.

Weissenberg, R. (1921). Zur Wirtsgewebsableitung des Plasma-körpers der *Glugea anomala*-Cysten. *Arch. Protistenk.* 42, 400-421.

Weissenberg, R. (1922a). Fremddienliche Reaktionen beim intra-zellulären Parasitismus, ein Beitrag zur Kenntnis gallen-ähnlicher Bildungen im Tierkörper. *Verh. dtsch. zool. Ges.* pp. 96-98.

Weissenberg, R. (1922b). Mikrosporidien, Myxosporidien und Chlamydozoen als Zellparasiten von Fischen. *Verh. dtsch. zool. Ges.,* pp. 41-43.

Weissenberg, R. (1926). Microsporidien aus Tipulidenlarven.
(Nosema binucleatum n. sp., *Thelohania tipulae* n. sp.).
Arch. Protistenk. 54, 431–467.
Weissenberg, R. (1949). Cell growth and cell transformation
induced by intracellular parasites *Anat. Rec.* 103, 517–518.
Weissenberg, R. (1968). Intracellular development of the microsporidan *Glugea anomala* Moniez in hypertrophying migrating
cells of the fish *Gasterosteus aculeatus* L., an example of
the formation of "Xenoma" tumors. *J. Protozool.* 15,
44–57.

BIOGRAPHICAL SKETCH

JULIUS RICHARD WEISSENBERG

1882-1974

Professor Weissenberg was born on 18 March 1882 in Breslau,
Germany. After completing studies at the Universities of
Freiburg and Berlin he became the assistant of Oscar Hertwig,
Director of the Anatomical-Biological Institute of the University
of Berlin. In 1907 he received the Doctor of Medicine from the
University of Berlin and in 1913 became Assistant Professor of
Histology and Embryology at the Institute. He served as military
physician in the German Army from 1915–1918. In 1923 Dr.
Weissenberg became Associate Professor at the Institute and
continued to teach embryology until 1933 when he lost his position
because of Nazi regulations against professors of non-arian
descent. In 1937 he came to the United States where he held
positions in the following institutions: Washington University
School of Medicine, St. Louis (1937); Wistar Institute of
Anatomy (1937-1940); Middlesex University Medical School,
Massachusetts (1940-1945); Middlesex University School of
Veterinary Medicine (1945-1948); Woman's Medical College of
Pennsylvania in Philadelphia (1948-1957). Meantime, (1944)
Professor Weissenberg became a U.S. citizen. He retired in 1957
but remained active in scientific work.
Most of Professor Weissenberg's teaching activities and many
of his publications were medically oriented. However, his main
research interest was intracellular parasitism and a majority of
his publications dealt with this subject. More particularly, he
worked periodically for well over a half of century on some
organisms associated with xenoma formation in fish, the virus
Lymphocystis and different Microsporidia.

Microsporidia and Mammalian Tumors

MICHAEL PETRI

THE UNIVERSITY INSTITUTE OF
  PATHOLOGICAL ANATOMY
COPENHAGEN, DENMARK

I. INTRODUCTION

In the majority of affected species mammalian microsporidiosis
is a mild disease and often it is not a disease at all, being
"latent" without symptoms or signs. Different stimuli may activate
the infection and in the literature a number of such cases has been
documented, primarily among laboratory animals (Petri, 1969;
Shadduck & Pakes, 1971). One notable exception is encephalitozoonosis of blue fox (Nordstoga, 1972) in which the disease carries
an extremely high mortality due to lesions very much similar to
polyarteritis nodosa in humans. Outbreaks have occurred also in
Denmark and in a number of cases studied by the author (Petri,
1975) the lesions were multiple and severe. The significance of
encephalitozoon infection in laboratory animals, therefore, is
not primarily one of a pathogenic organism but one of interference
with experimental results. The parasite is actually less pathogenic
to the animals than to the experiment. The stress imposed upon a
laboratory animal by an experiment may activate a silent infection,
the signs of which will blend with those of the experiment.

In animals with spontaneous encephalitozoonosis the parasites are
found mainly in the brain and kidney but when introduced into the
peritoneal cavity they multiply zealously, causing in many cases
the formation of a large quantity of ascites. Though obviously
a fertile soil for *Encephalitozoon sp.* peritoneal involvement in
spontaneous disease has not been reported. This is important as
the association between *Encephalitozoon cuniculi* and tumors occurs
mainly in ascites tumors, i.e. fluid tumors composed of cells
growing in the peritoneal cavity.

II. EXPERIMENTAL TUMORS

Although "tumor" literally means "swelling," the term is restricted to neoplastic growth that involves the formation of new
and abnormal masses of tissue. For descriptions of the biology
and pathology of tumors (neoplasms) the reader is referred to
standard textbooks of pathology (Capelle & Anderson, 1971;
Anderson, 1971, Payling Wright, 1960). The experimental study of
cancer is based on tumors in laboratory animals of three types:
spontaneous, induced, or transplanted. By employing animals of
inbred strains that are genetically identical, tumor tissue can
be transplanted for many generations without the interference of
transplantation immunity due to tissue incompatibility. Transplanted tumors that have been established from spontaneous or
induced primary tumors of different types are major tools in cancer
research. They are valuable and extensively used because they are
malignant, fast growing tumor models composed of uniform cell
populations with a highly reproducible performance (see Stewart
et al., 1959). Some can be converted into ascites tumors, a few
of which have been maintained by continuous transfers for many

years, e.g., the Yoshida rat ascites sarcoma (see Petri, 1969).
Although spontaneous ascitic tumors do not occur in nature, the
transplanted laboratory forms are convenient cancer models. In
the present context it is important to realize that, being fluid,
they contain no stromal cells and that they consist of an almost
pure culture of malignant cells.

III. THE YOSHIDA ASCITES SARCOMA AND ENCEPHALITOZOON CUNICULI

This tumor is one of the traditional ascites tumors, its origin
dating to 1943 (Yoshida, 1949). It has been carried in continuous
transfers in different strains of rats since then in many laboratories. The strain used in this author's laboratory still is
morphologically identical to the original tumor; the cells in the
ascitic fluid resemble monocytes, though they have malignant
features such as cellular and nuclear pleomorphism, mitosis, and
large nucleoli. When the ascitic tumor is transplanted into the
subcutaneous tissue or interstitial connective tissue in other
parts of the body, a solid tumor is formed that can in return be
converted into the fluid form by transplantation into the peritoneal
cavity (see Petri, 1969). The cells multiply vigorously and after
4 to 5 days several milliliters of fluid can be obtained with a
pure population of tumor cells (approximately 100,000 cells per
μl).
I have observed parasitation of the ascitic tumor cells by
E. *cuniculi* (Petri 1965, 1966). The first sign was slight
irregularities in the otherwise reproducible behavior of the tumor.
However, in spite of only minor impairment of its performance and
maintenance of malignancy, the parasites were found in large
numbers in many of the tumor cells. Although total growth was
less vigorous than in the uninfected tumor, the majority of infected cells maintained the capacity for division and cells were
found in all stages of mitosis. When observed by phase-contrast
microscopy or in fixed and stained smears, the majority of parasites
were mature spores found in vacuoles whereas developmental stages
were seen either in the periphery of vacuoles or in other parts of
the cytoplasm. Occasional spores were found in the extracellular
fluid, some in the process of being released by degenerated cells.
I also have observed that the germ and filament are released out
of the infected cell and extrusion presumably does not occur into
other parts of the same cell. Furthermore, the length of the filament,
which is extruded in a straight line, clearly exceeds that of most
tumor cells. When a drop of ascites is spread under a cover-glass
ånd observed directly by phase-contrast a small number of free
germs (sporoplasms) can be observed in the extracellular fluid.
Observations of the ascitic fluid or tissue cultures infected
with E. *cuniculi* under ideal circumstances would be important in
determining the entry of the sporoplasm into a new cell. There
can be little doubt that the life cycle from sporoplasm to spore

is intracellular and that the sporoplasm must be introduced into
the cell by some mechanism.

The association between *E. cuniculi* and the Yoshida ascites
sarcoma is remarkably stable; by regular weekly transfers this
tumor has been kept in my laboratory for a number of years with
only minor fluctuations. By subcutaneous transplantations, however,
the parasitized tumor does not grow into a solid tumor; a major
part of the transplanted cells do not contain parasites. Perhaps
the life cycle does not occur only within one cell; other cells
may be intermediate. Though speculative, this hypothesis is
supported by the fact that many nonparasitized cells contain
vacuoles that are morphologically similar to parasitic vacuoles.

The mortality of animals with the infected ascites sarcoma is
somewhat lower than those with the noninfected tumor. Survivors
are immune to further tumor transplantation and in some rats a
state of mutual adaption between tumor and host is produced with
persistence of malignant cells for prolonged periods. After an
interval of one to two years some survivors may develop intraperitoneal rhabdomyosarcomas, i.e. malignant tumors derived from
skeletal muscle (Petri, 1968). The pathogenesis of this bizarre
phenomenon has not been established, but longtime experiments
with newborn rats given cell-free tumor extracts have so far been
negative (Petri, unpublished data) and an oncogenic virus has
therefore not been found.

The mortality caused by the infected sarcoma is due to growth
of the tumor. Rats resistant to tumor growth tolerate large
amounts of infected sarcoma (Petri, 1969). Although infected as
well as noninfected sarcoma cells, because of their malignant
potential, invade adjacent structures in the peritoneal cavity,
only few parasites are found in the host cells. Undoubtedly,
the life cycle of *E. cuniculi* takes place in the tumor, the
tumor being the actual host. The animal-tumor-parasite association is a kind of hyperparasitism.

IV. OTHER TUMORS

(1) Ehrlich ascites carcinoma in mice was infected in one mouse
with *E. sp.* and the infected tumor was carried on in noninfected
mice. Though only occasional cells became parasitized during the
course of the experiment, the survival time was significantly
prolonged compared with a control group (Petri, 1969).

(2) Arison *et al.* (1966) noted a microsporidian infection in the
Ehrlich carcinoma. The parasite was observed to retard the
growth of several other experimental tumors, solid as well as
ascites forms, whereas the Ehrlich tumor cells disappeared from
the fluid. The prolonged survival time in mice bearing 3, 4, 7,
9-dibenzpyren-induced solid fibrosarcomas is an interesting
observation, but this phenomenon may be a nonspecific effect.

(3) Infection with *E. cuniculi* in an ascitic plasmacytoma in the golden hamster was found to be due to *E. cuniculi* (Meiser *et al.*, 1971). Organisms were not found in solid tumors.

(4) Structures seen in a human pancreatic carcinoma were claimed to be microsporidia (Marcus *et al.*, 1973). The evidence, however, in my opinion is not convincing because the structures seen in the published figures are more heteromorphous than typical spores and do not possess polar vacuoles. Although ascites with typical nosema spores were in fact produced in mice by intraperitoneal injection of the tumor, this situation may have been due to activation of latent nosematosis in the test animal.

DISCUSSION

The multiplication of *E. sp.* and of other microsporidia require special conditions because it is dependent on the extrusion of a sporoplasm. Although the nature of these conditions cannot be stated with certainty, a few generalizations may be made. To establish itself, the parasite must find a suitable type of cell that is able to supply its metabolic requirements and from there it must be able to propagate other cells. It is reasonable to assume that conditions allowing free extrusion of the sporoplasm and its intrusion into new cells will be favorable. Ascites tumors seem to offer these conditions because the cells multiply rapidly, have a high metabolic activity, and free-floating un-infected cells are readily available at any time. By extrusion the germ may take one of two paths: extrusion occurs directly into a neighboring cell or, after extrusion into a fluid inter-cellular compartment, the germ becomes attached to the surface of a cell and from there either enters the cell actively or is phagocytosed into an intracellular vacuole. The first pathway has been described in detail by Weidner (1972) with spores of *Nosema michaelis*. He used an experimental system with a fluid medium in which the sporoplasms were extruded directly into various types of invertebrate and vertebrate cells, including ascites tumor cells. Spores of *E. sp.* however, do not multiply in solid tumors although the tumor cells lie in close contact. The second route which is readily acceptable for ascitic tumors has not been observed directly but it may have general application for other tissues. Perhaps both mechanisms are used depending upon species and type of tissue.

The two mechanisms apparently have one feature in common: the need for a fluid space or interspace. The pathological features of encephalitozoonosis may lend some support to this idea. In this disease, the parasites are found mainly in certain locations that are close to a fluid compartment such as epithelial cells of the distal part of the nephron and in endothelial cells. In diseased blue foxes, the parasite has an affinity for endothelial cells and vessel walls (Petri, 1975). In nerve cells the spores may even extrude into the cytoplasm of the same host cell due to its large size; however, Brightman and Reese (1969) have presented evidence that clearly demonstrated the existence of a fluid inter-space between nerve cells. Obviously, the fluid space offers a minimum of mechanical resistance. This may explain why the spores do not propagate in solid tumors whose cells are surrounded by connective tissue.

Microsporidiosis of tumors probably is a nonspecific phenomenon created by the favorable environment offered to the parasites by fast growing ascites tumors. No evidence is yet available to directly link the causation or progression of spontaneous malignant tumors in mammals to microsporidia. Microscopic monitoring for microsporidia (Petri, 1969) should be carried out regularly on all transplanted ascites tumors.

The association between microsporidia, primarily *E. cuniculi*, and malignant tumors is significant in cancer research mainly because of its influence upon experiments with transplanted ascites tumors. The high incidence of latent encephalitozoonosis in many laboratory animals and the subtlety of its interference with experimental data has been amply documented.

REFERENCES

Anderson, W.A.D. (1971). "Pathology", Vol. I-II, sixth edition. C. V. Mosby, St. Louis.

Arison, R. N., Cassaro, J. A., & Pruss, M. P. (1966). Studies on a murine ascites producing agent and its effect upon tumor development. *Cancer Res.* 26: 1915-1920.

Brightman, M. W., and Reese, T. S. (1969). Junctions between intimately apposed cell membranes in the vertebrate brain. *J. Cell. Biol.* 40: 648-677.

Capelle, D. F. and Anderson, J. R. (1971). "Muir's Textbook of Pathology", ninth edition. Edward Arnold, London.

Marcus, P. B., van der Walt, J. J. & Burger, P. J. (1973). Human tumour microsporidiosis. *Arch. Pathol.* 95: 341-343.

Meiser, J., Kinzel, V. & Jirovec, O. (1971). Nosematosis as an accompanying infection of plasmacytoma ascites in Syrian golden hamsters. *Pathol. Microbiol.* 37: 249-260.

Nordstoga, K. (1972). Nosematosis in blue foxes. *Nord. Vet. - Med.* 24: 21-24.

Payling Wright, G. (1960). "An introduction to Pathology", third edition. Longmans, London.

Petri, M. (1965). A cytolytic parasite in the cells of trans-plantable, malignant tumours. *Nature* (London) 205: 302.

Petri, M. (1966). The occurrence of *Nosema cuniculi (Encephalitozoon cuniculi)* in the cells of transplantable malignant tumours and its effect upon tumour and host. *Acta Pathol. Microbiol. Scand.* 73: 1.12.

Petri, M. (1969). Studies on *Nosema cuniculi*. *Acta Pathol. Microbiol. Scand.*, suppl. 204.

Petri, M. (1975). Unpublished observations.

Shadduck, J. A. & Pakes, S. P. (1971). Encephalitozoonosis (nosematosis) and toxoplasmosis. *Am. J. Pathol.* 63: 657-671.

Stewart, H. L., Snell, K. C., Dunham, L. J. and Schlyen, S. M. (1959). "Transplantable and transmissible tumors of animals". Atlas of Tumor Pathology, Section XII, Fascicle 40. Armed Forces Institute of Pathology, Washington 25, D. C.

Yoshida, T. (1949). The Yoshida sarcoma, an ascites tumour. *Gann.* 40: 1-18.

Epizootiology and Microbial Control

Y. TANADA

DIVISION ENTOMOLOGY & PARASITOLOGY
UNIVERSITY OF CALIFORNIA
BERKELEY, CALIFORNIA

I. INTRODUCTION

The microsporidia are among the most common pathogens found infecting insects under natural field conditions. This is increasingly evident as greater numbers of insect pathologists become acquainted with these obligatory minute pathogens. Their numbers and those of susceptible insect hosts have increased significantly during the past decade, especially where extensive studies with specific groups of insects, e.g., mosquitoes, have been conducted in search of promising pathogens for use in microbial control.

The interest in microsporidia has resulted in numerous reviews, mainly in the area of epizootiology and microbial control (Steinhaus, 1949, 1954, 1957; Weiser, 1956, 1961a, 1963, 1966, 1970; Dutky, 1959; Tanada, 1959, 1963, 1967; Franz, 1961a,b; Cameron, 1963; Hall, 1963; Lipa, 1963; Kramer, 1968a; Heimpel, 1969; McLaughlin, 1971, 1973). The more specific reviews, e.g., those dealing with pathogen-host interrelationships and with aquatic insects, will be considered later. The reviews reveal that even though increasing numbers of microsporidia are being recorded from insects, the number of studies on epizootiology and field application is rather limited.

The present chapter treats epizootiology and microbial control separately, but these fields are closely interrelated and many principles in epizootiology will also apply to microbial control, particularly in the case of long-term or "permanent" control. In other words, microbial control can be considered as the applied branch of epizootiology where man plays a role in introducing and enhancing the pathogen for the control of insect pests. In the case of epidemiology of vertebrate diseases, man attempts to manipulate the environmental and host conditions, and often even the pathogen, to reduce or eliminate the outbreaks of disease in human and domestic animal populations. In a few cases, such as the use of virus against rabbits in Australia, man may apply pathogens in the microbial control of a vertebrate pest.

II. EPIZOOTIOLOGY

The principles and factors of epizootiology of infectious diseases of insects have been discussed by several workers (Steinhaus, 1949, 1954; Franz, 1961a; Tanada, 1963, 1964). These principles should also apply to the microsporidian diseases, but there is a serious lack of field studies to support this assumption. Most studies have been conducted in the laboratory, and there is some question whether results from such studies also apply to field situations.

The primary factors that are involved in the cause, initiation, and development of epizootics are the pathogen population, the host population, and an efficient means of transmission. All of these factors are affected by the abiotic and biotic environments. I shall first discuss the properties of the pathogen population that are most significant in epizootics. These are (i) virulence and infectivity, (ii) capacity to survive or persist, and (iii) capacity to disperse.

A. VIRULENCE AND INFECTIVITY

There are apparently no records of the natural occurrence of
microsporidian strains which vary in their virulence. It is likely
that such strains exist, but the difficulty is in being able to
detect them with reliable methods, e.g., bioassay, serology, chromatography, transmission and scanning electron microscopy, etc.
Fowler and Reeves (1974a,b) extracted hydrophilic and hydrophobic
proteins from microsporidian spores and subjected them to polyacrylamide gel electrophoresis. They detected differences and concluded
that this method could be used in identifying microsporidians.

In the laboratory, there are four methods that have been applied
to increase the virulence of a pathogen: (i) passage through susceptible hosts, (ii) dissociation in culture into more virulent
and less virulent strains, (iii) introduction of the microorganism
together with substances that may aid in increasing its invasive
powers, and (iv) mutualistic association with other microorganisms
that may render it more capable of invading tissues than it would
be otherwise (Steinhaus, 1949). There are only a few studies reporting the use of these methods in microsporidia.

Nosema sp. (probably Nosema algerae), after passage through 20
generations of Anopheles quadrimaculatus, has greatly increased in
virulence for this mosquito (Hazard and Lofgren. 1971). Most microsporidians have been passed through several insect species without
any apparent alteration in their virulence and infectivity to their
former host. Thus, Smirnoff (1968) successfully adapted Thelohania
pristiphora, a microsporidian of the larch sawfly, Pristiphora erich-
sonii, to the tent caterpillars, Malacosoma disstria and M. americanum, which were more easily reared than the larch sawfly. The
microsporidian remained virulent for the larch sawfly even after six
passages in the Malacosoma spp. Smirnoff (1968) recommended the
use of M. disstria because in M. americanum, the microsporidian appeared to predispose the larvae to a nuclear-polyhedrosis-virus
infection. Subsequently, Smirnoff (1974) adapted T. pristiphora to
other species of sawflies. On the other hand, the successive passages in alternate hosts may result in a loss in virulence of the
microsporidian for the original host (Hall, 1954; Weiser, 1969).
Hall (1954) mass produced Nosema infesta in the potato tuberworm,
Gnorimoschema operculella, an insect much more amenable to mass
production than the target insect, the sod webworm, Crambus bonifatellus. After successive passages through the potato tuberworm,
the yield of spores began to drop and the microsporidian became less
virulent towards the tuberworm. In the above examples, strains of
microsporidians probably were dissociated by the passage through
alternate hosts.

When two or more microsporidians infect an individual larva, the
infection may not be more virulent than the infection by only one
of the microsporidian species (Weiser, 1956, 1961a, 1963), but in
others, the infection may increase in virulence. In still others,

a microsporidian species may enable other host-specific microsporidia to infect another host. Thus, *Nosema lymantriae*, which normally infects only *Lymantria monacha*, can infect *Euproctis chrysorrhoea* when combined with *Thelohania similis*, which is pathogenic for these two insects (Weiser, 1957a). Apparently, *T. similis* conditions the host, *E. chrysorrhoea*, in some unknown manner to enable *N. lymantriae* to infect this host. A similar situation may occur in the Indian meal moth, *Plodia interpunctella*, in which *Thelohania nana* has only been observed in a dual infection with *Nosema heterosporum* (Kellen and Lindegren, 1969). In *Culex tarsalis*, *Nosema lunateum* has been observed also only in dual infection with *Thelohania californica* (Kellen *et al.*, 1967).

The virulence and pathogenicity of a microsporidian may depend on the infective dose, the host larval instar, and the organ or tissue infected by the microsporidian (Weiser, 1963). In general, the higher the dosage, the more acute is the infectious process and the shorter the period of lethal infection. The younger larvae are generally not only more susceptible but succumb faster from a microsporidian infection than the older larvae, which in some species may even be refractory to infection. Microsporidians which infect the gut and musculature and those which are systemic produce acute infections. Those which confine the infection mainly to the fat body cause chronic infection, with a long period of lethal infection or even be nonlethal. From his epizootiological study with several insect pests and their microsporidians, Lipa (1963) concluded that the pathogenicity of the microsporidian infection might be related to the manner of invasion into the host. Peroral invasion was more pathogenic, transovarial transmission less pathogenic, and transmission by the hymenopterous vector was intermediate between these two. Weiser (1963) has concluded ". . . acute infections are quite infrequent in epizootics, where they are lost with the death of the hosts. The most common of all are chronic, adapted infections, which are able to maintain a stable distribution in a given population." In an acute infection, the host insect dies so rapidly that the replication of the pathogen is limited, whereas in a prolonged infection, there is an abundant production of spores (Weiser, 1963; Kramer, 1968a; McLaughlin, 1971; Maddox, 1973).

B. PERSISTENCE

The microsporidian spores can survive in the external environment. However, for more than 95% of the known microsporidian species, there is no information on the extent to which their spores can withstand the vicissitudes of nature (Kramer, 1970). Most studies on spore longevity have been conducted in the laboratory (Weiser, 1956, 1961a, 1963; Kramer, 1970; Maddox, 1973). From the available evidence, Kramer (1970) has suggested that (*i*) differences in the ability to survive vary from species to species, (*ii*) spores of

some species are bound in feces or in dried cadavers and may remain
viable for one or more years under room conditions, (*iii*) the longevity of naked dried spores under room conditions generally does
not exceed 3 to 4 months and may range from about 2 weeks to over
1 year, and (*iv*) naked spores in a cold clean aqueous medium may
survive for 7 to 10 years. Thus the spores are favored generally
by moist conditions and low temperatures and by being protected in
feces or cadavers. The spores of *Nosema algerae* are killed when
dried for 5 minutes (Alger and Undeen, 1970). In the soil, the
microsporidian may survive for at least 12 months (Weiser, 1956,
1961a). When the larvae of *Colias eurytheme* and *Trichoplusia ni*
were fed alfalfa leaves contaminated with the soil from an alfalfa
field, they became infected with a microsporidian, *Nosema* sp. (Tanada and Omi, 1974).

In many microsporidians, especially those which are transmitted
transovarially by the host, the persistence in the biotic environment, which may consist of the primary and secondary hosts, parasites, predators, scavengers, and other carriers, may be more important than the persistence of the spores in the physical environment. According to Kellen *et al*. (1965), this is especially the
case with certain *Thelohania* spp. of univoltine mosquitoes. The
microsporidians survive in the hibernating mosquito during the long
period when no larval stage is available for infection. Kellen *et
al*. (1965) believe that the microsporidian spores are not capable
of surviving outside of the host during this period. Weiser (1961a)
reports that the larvae of *Euproctis chrysorrhoea* infected with
Thelohania hyphantriae just prior to hibernation may retain in a
latent form the infection from October to April. When the larvae
commence feeding, the microsporidian develops and causes high mortality to the larvae. This microsporidian persists in the hibernating larvae of *Nygmia phaeorrhoea* Weiser and Veber, 1957).

The persistence of microsporidian often cannot be dissociated with
its dispersal and transmission. Taking this into account, Maddox
(1973) concluded in his thorough review: "Theoretically, the ideal
characteristics for ultimate persistence of a microsporidian would
include: spores which are very resistant to environmental conditions; a wide host range; a low infectious threshold; a tolerance
to high spore dosages; transmission transovarially and by parasites,
as well as oral transmission; a short generation time; spores passed
in the feces of hosts for long periods of time; many spores produced
in the course of infection; and a great latitude in the thermal limits of development."

C. DISPERSAL

Physical factors, such as wind, rain, stream, river, etc., may
disperse microsporidian spores. However, there is very little, if
any, information concerning the effect of these factors, primarily

because of the lack of studies involving the persistence of spores in the physical environment. Certain microsporidian spores have appendages or are covered with a gelatinous capsule that enables them to float in water and thereby be carried with water movements (Weiser, 1963). The effect of wind and rain on the dispersal of microsporidian spores has not been investigated. If the spores persist in the soil or on the plant parts, such factors may play a part in dispersal.

The primary method of dispersal is closely associated with the persistence of the microsporidian in the biotic habitat. In some cases, the infected hosts transmit the microsporidian within or on the surface of the egg whose larva becomes infected. The movements of the infected hosts disperse the microsporidians, which are deposited in the environment in regurgitations, fecal deposits, and in the disintegrating bodies after death. Some microsporidians infect several different species, including parasites, which are found in the same biotope. All of these insect species serve not only in the persistence but also in the dispersal of the microsporidian. The principal host of *Thelohania hyphantriae* is the fall webworm, *Hyphantria cunea*, but this microsporidian also infects *Malacosoma neustria*, *Euproctis chrysorrhoea*, and *Hyponomeuta malinellus*, which also spread the microsporidian (Weiser and Veber, 1955). *H. cunea* migrated from America to Europe and after 5 years became infected by *Pleistophora schubergi*, a microsporidian infecting *E. chrysorrhoea* and *M. neustria* (Weiser, 1961a). The hymenopterous parasites of *Pieris brassicae* (Blunck, 1954; Hostounský, 1970), *Pieris rapae* (Tanada, 1955), *Heliothis zea*, and *H. virescens* (Brooks and Cranford, 1972) are also susceptible to the microsporidians which infect their host insects. Other examples of alternate hosts of microsporidians are given in several other sections of this chapter.

When the microsporidian infects the midgut epithelium and malpighian tubes, the feces of the infected hosts are highly contagious (Weiser, 1956; Günther, 1956; Tanabe, 1971; Maddox, 1973). The larvae of *Choristoneura fumiferana* infected with *Nosema fumiferanae* discharge viable spores not only in the feces but also in their regurgitated fluids (Wilson, 1973). Maddox (1973) points out that the type of tissues infected largely determines how effectively the microsporidian is dispersed throughout the host populations. Relatively little dispersal occurs when the infection is restricted to the fat body, whereas infection in the digestive tract results in widespread distribution. The generation time (spore to spore development) and the absolute numbers of spores also influence dispersal.

Nonsusceptible insects and vertebrate animals may serve as carriers and disseminators of microsporidians. *Thelohania hyphantriae* is distributed vertically on the trees by ants and beetles, and laterally among the trees by adults of *Hyphantria cunea* (Weiser, 1963). The spores of *T. hyphantriae* retain their virulence after being excreted by predators and scavengers, such as *Calosoma sycophanta*, *Xylodrepa quadripunctata*, *Cantharis fusca*, *Formica rufa*, and the mite, *Tyro-*

phagus noxius (Weiser, 1957b). However, in *Nosema curvidentis*, which infects the fat body of the bark beetle, *Pityokteines curvidens*, the spores are not passed through the feces of the beetle but are distributed in the feces of scavengers, such as mites and a staphylinid beetle, which feed on the dead bark beetles (Weiser, 1961b). Since 2.8% of larvae, 68% of feeding adults, and none of the freshly emerged adults and pupae were infected, Weiser (1961b) concluded that the larvae which started their galleries from the original egg pockets rarely came in contact with the spores, but the adult bark beetles feeding in the old gallery before egg deposition might ingest spores deposited by the carriers. Scavengers also play a role in the dispersal of *Nosema plodiae*, a pathogen of the stored product insect, *Plodia interpunctella* (Kellen and Lindegren, 1971). The spores of *Pleistophora schubergi* and *Nosema polyvora* retain their virulence for their insect hosts after passage through the alimentary tract of a bird or that of an earwig (Günther, 1959).

According to Weiser (1956, 1963), the microsporidian-infected insects are favorable hosts for predators and scavengers which may aid in the dispersal of the microsporidians. In some cases, however, such predators may remove the microsporidian-infected hosts from the biotope (Weiser and Veber, 1957).

III. TRANSMISSION

Canning (1970) has reviewed the transmission of microsporidia in insects and vertebrates. The major route of transmission in insects is through the mouth. Transmission may also take place through the egg of the host and by the oviposition of hymenopterous parasites. In the case of transovum transmission, the microsporidian may enter the egg by way of the ovary (transovarial) and other reproductive organs or it may occur on the surface of the egg by being smeared with feces or anal hairs contaminated with spores. The hymenopterous parasites may themselves be susceptible to the microsporidian infecting the host or may be refractory to infection. The microsporidian may gain entrance into the host by the contaminated parasite ovipositor or, when the parasite is infected, by the infected embryo.

Successful transmission through oral ingestion may be dependent on the characteristics of the host alimentary tract, such as pH and enzymes. This aspect will be discussed further in the section, Host Population.

The transovarial transmission of *Nosema bombycis* in the silkworm is the classical example first established by Pasteur. Subsequently, transmission through the egg has been shown to occur commonly in microsporidian-infected insects. This is especially the case when the infection occurs in the ovary and in the alimentary tract. In the mosquitoes, transovarial transmission appears to be the principal, if not the only, means of transmission in certain genera (Kellen

and Lipa, 1960; Kellen *et al.*, 1965, 1966a, 1967; Canning, 1970;
Chapman *et al.*, 1970a; Chapman, 1973, 1974a). The mosquito species
in which peroral transmission has succeeded easily in the laboratory
are *Pleistophora culicis*, *Nosema stegomyiae* or *N. algerae*, and a
Stempellia sp. (Chapman, 1973, 1974a). *Thelohania californica* appeared to perorally infect *Culex tarsalis* when the spores were placed
together with the larvae in water and soil from a pond that was
naturally contaminated with the microsporidian (Kellen and Lipa,
1960). Kellen and Lipa (1960) concluded that the spores had to be
conditioned by wetting and drying before they became infectious when
eaten by the larvae. However, later attempts failed in transmitting
the microsporidian (Kellen and Wills, 1962). According to Chapman
(1974a), the Lake Charles Laboratory staff made many attempts at
peroral transmission with various species of *Thelohania* from about
20 mosquito species but had not been successful.

Peroral transmission of microsporidia to mosquitoes in the field
has been successful in some cases. First-instar mosquito larvae
were placed into screened plastic containers, that were set in the
field for about 1-4 weeks, and then the larvae were reared in the
laboratory. Some of these larvae became infected indicating that
peroral transmission had occurred (Kellen *et al.*, 1966a; Chapman
et al., 1970b).

The extreme difficulty of obtaining peroral transmission with certain microsporidian species indicates that their spores must first
undergo some conditioning before they infect mosquito larvae. The
conditioning may result from physical factors, e.g., desiccation,
minerals, pH, etc., or from biotic factors, e.g., alternate hosts
or products produced by the organisms. Whatever the factors may
be, their knowledge is essential for the use of these promising
pathogens in the control of mosquitoes.

Adult males may transmit the microsporidian to their progeny. The
infected males of the spruce budworm, *Choristoneura fumiferana*,
transmit *Nosema fumiferanae* to some of their offspring (Thomson,
1958). In *Plodia interpunctella*, the males infected with *Nosema
plodiae* transmit the spores to females, which in turn transmit the
microsporidian to the offspring (Kellen and Lindegren, 1971).

The role of insect parasites in the transmission of microsporidians
to the host insects has been thoroughly reviewed by Brooks (1973).
Paillot (1933) was first to suggest that *Apanteles glomeratus* transmitted *Perezia legeri* to *Pieris brassicae* because the incidence of
infection by the microsporidian in the cabbageworm was closely associated with the parasitization by the wasp. Others have confirmed
this observation. *Thelohania ephestiae* is transmitted by *Bracon
hebetor* to *Anagasta kühniella* (Payne, 1933); *Nosema polyvora* by
Apanteles glomeratus to *Pieris brassicae* (Blunck, 1954); and to
Aporia crataegi (Lipa, 1963); *Perezia mesnili* by *A. glomeratus* to
Pieris rapae (Tanada, 1955); *Nosema aporiae* by *A. glomeratus* to
Aporia crataegi (Lipa, 1957, 1963); *Thelohania mesnili* by *A. glom-
eratus* in *P. brassicae* (Lipa, 1963). According to Hostounský (1970),
P. mesnili, *P. legeri*, and *N. polyvora* are nonspecific, and morpho-

logical variations are caused by the different hosts. *Nosema* sp. is transmitted by *Macrocentrus ancylivorus* to *Gnorimoschema operculella* (Allen, 1954); *Nosema* sp. by *Apanteles marginiventris* to *Spodoptera mauritia* (Laigo and Tamashiro, 1967); *N. heliothidis* by *Campoletis sonorensis* and *Cardiochilis nigriceps* to *Heliothis zea* and *H. virescens* (Brooks and Cranford, 1972; Brooks, 1973).

Most of the above hymenopterous vectors are infected by the microsporidians of the host insects (see section, Persistence). On the other hand, Brooks (1973) reports that the mechanical transmission by contaminated ovipositor is the most often reported type, but only a few thorough studies have demonstrated that this is the case. Lipa (1963) reported that *Nosema aporiae* was transmitted by *Apanteles glomeratus* to *Aporia crataegi*, but the transmission appeared to be mechanical because there was no development of the microsporidian in the wasp, even though spores were found in the egg, larva, pupa, and adult wasp. A careful study by Laigo and Tamashiro (1967) revealed that *Apanteles marginiventris* was not infected by the *Nosema* sp. of the insect host, *Spodoptera mauritia*. The transmission was at random depending upon the site, speed, and depth of penetration of the ovipositor and on individual variations in host susceptibility. They observed that when uninfected and *Nosema*-infected larvae were exposed together, the parasite seemed to prefer infected hosts, but the difference was not statistically significant.

IV. HOST POPULATION

Several decades ago, microsporidians were believed to be highly host specific and new species were established mainly on their discovery in a new host. At present, many microsporidians are known to have alternate hosts; some with a wide host spectrum of different families and orders. Accordingly, certain protozoologists (Kramer, 1968a; Weiser, 1969; Hazard and Lofgren, 1971) decry some of the recent practices in species identification where extensive studies have not been made in cross infection, pathology, and life cycles in alternate hosts, since the microsporidian may vary in morphology and in pathology in different hosts. There is a need to develop additional methods and techniques, e.g., those given in the section on Virulence and Infectivity.

The susceptibility of insects to microsporidians may vary with the different larval instars and occasionally with the different stages, i.e., larva, pupa, and adult. In general, the younger are more susceptible to infection than the older larvae, which in some cases may be refractory. However, evidence for such resistance has been supported, thus far, only by a few quantitative studies. Milner (1973a) conducted bioassays on the different larval ages of *Tribolium castaneum* with the microsporidian, *Nosema whitei*. The LD_{50} for mortality after 20 days increased consistently from the first (1.8 X 10^6 spores/g) to the fifth instar (1.0 X 10^{10} spores/g). There was a consistent increase in the slopes of the probit lines (from b=1.1 to b=3.1) with the age of the larvae. Milner (1973b) also tested the comparative pathogenicity of *N. whitei* for four stored-product insects, *Tribolium castaneum*, *T. confusum*, *Orizaephilus surinamensis*, and *T. anaphe*. The susceptibility of the first three species was similar, but *T. anaphe* was at least 100 X more susceptible. This was probably associated with the longer developmental time of this species (28 days at 25°C) compared to that of the other three species (20 days at 25°C). George (1971) studied the effects of malnutrition on the growth and mortality of *Tribolium castaneum* infected by *Nosema whitei*. Deficiencies in cholesterol and protein enhanced the death rate of microsporidian-infected larvae, however the increased death rate was not due to an increased susceptibility to infection but to the stress of diet deficiency. Moreover, the fourth-instar larvae were highly resistant to infection, and malnutrition had no effect on their resistance. Wilson (1974) investigated the dosage mortality of *Nosema fumiferanae* on the larvae of the spruce budworm. He reported an increase in larval mortality as the spore dosage increased, and a decrease in susceptibility with an increase in larval age.

There are certain races of the domesticated insects, honey bee and silkworm, that are more resistant to microsporidians (Tanada, 1963; Weiser, 1969). Weiser (1969) reported that such races also occurred in *Antherea pernyi* and *Platysamia cecropia*. The more susceptible race had larger larvae which consumed more food and regenerated their tissues more slowly than those of the less susceptible race. Aside from these examples, there seems to be no other reports of resistant races or varieties in insects. Frye and Olson (1974) speculated that a different biotope of the European corn borer, *Pyrausta nubilalis*, might occur in southwestern part of the state of North Dakota because collections from this area had no larvae infected with *Perezia pyraustae*, whereas all collections from the southeastern part had infected larvae.

The physical and physiological characteristics of the host may affect the invasion of microsporidians. Weiser (1969) has enumerated three factors: (*i*) failure of spores to germinate in the digestive tract because of the rate of flow, pH, enzymes, and the inadequate digestion of the seal covering the polar filament; (*ii*) host tissues are not susceptible to the microsporidian; (*iii*) host resists infection by actively destroying the microsporidian during its migration to susceptible tissues or by eliminating infected cells and regenerating tissues. The extrusion of the polar filaments of the spores of *Bombyx mori* (Ohshima, 1964) and of *N. fumiferanae* (Ishihara, 1967) are affected by the pH and the presence of certain cations. In *Phormia regina*, 100% of the spores of *Octosporea muscaedomesticae* do not germinate, but the excreted ungerminated spores, when fed to other adults, germinate and produce infection (Kramer, 1968a). During the migration of the microsporidian within the host, the temperature plays an important role in the development of the disease.

Cellular immunity has been observed in hosts infected with micro-sporidians (Weiser, 1969; Brooks, 1971). Cellular immunity is mani-fested in phagocytosis, inflammation, and encapsulation to form giant cells or nodules that may be infiltrated with hemocytes and may be melanized. In spite of the cellular response, the host in-sect generally succumbs to the microsporidian. Brooks (1971) con-cluded that severe cellular response occurred in alternate hosts and that such response is usually absent in the habitual or primary host of the microsporidian, but individual variations may occur. Based on this assumption, Brooks (1970) suggested that even though *Nosema sphingidis* was first discovered in *Manduca sexta*, this insect might not be the habitual host. Recently, severe cellular responses have been detected in stored-product insects infected with *Nosema invadens* (Kellen and Lindegren, 1973) and in mosquito infected with *Pleistophora milesi* (Pillai, 1974).

There is very little evidence, if any, of humoral immunity to microsporidian infections (Weiser, 1969). According to Weiser (1969), humoral response is suggested by the production of polyphenols and of lysins after nodule formation. However, there is no evidence of antibody-like substances, actively or passively acquired, against microsporidians.

A benign microsporidian infection occurs in *Culiseta inornata* in-fected with *Pleistophora caecorum* (Chapman and Kellen, 1967). This microsporidian infects the gastric caeca and is not lethal to any stage and does not affect the fecundity or longevity of the adult mosquito.

A very important observation on the microsporidian-mosquito rela-tionship was made by Kellen *et al.* (1965), who studied the associa-tion of species of *Thelohania* with 16 species of mosquitoes in California. They separated the relationships into four basic types based on the tissue specificity, the sporogonic cycle to the sex of the mosquito, and the expression of patent infection. In 1966, they obtained additional evidence confirming their classification (Kellen *et al.*, 1966a). In Louisiana, Chapman *et al.* (1966) also reported that the species of *Thelohania* collected from 13 species of mosqui-toes had microsporidian-mosquito relationships that conformed to the four types. Kellen *et al.* (1966b) believed that the relationship types to which the thelohanians belong were not indicative of phylo-genetic relationships as these "types" were probably evolved inde-pendently in each mosquito-microsporidian association. The importance of the host-pathogen relationship in persistence, dispersal, and transmission has already been discussed.

In some cases where peroral transmission apparently is absent or occurs rarely, the microsporidian appears to be perpetuated in the mosquito population by transovarial transmission. This is a per-plexing problem, especially if the infection creates a stress or destroys some of the infected individuals. In such cases, peroral transmission would be expected for the survival of the microspori-dian. However, Chapman *et al.* (1967) concluded that the 17% infected eggs of *A. quadrimaculatus* and 6% of the eggs of *Culex salinarius* were adequate to account for the low levels of infection in the aquatic stages when the principal mode of transmission is transovarial. On the other hand, when both sexes, such as in *Culiseta inornata,* were patently infected, the peroral transmission was probably the chief mode of transmission in the field.

Alternate hosts in the ecosystem serve in the persistence, dispersal, and transmission of the microsporidian. Weiser (1957a, 1971a, 1963) stressed the importance of such hosts in microsporidian infections in the field. He (1961a) presented the following characteristics of the biocoenose which connected the hosts of a given microsporidan: (*i*) the taxonomic relationships of the host species, (*ii*) a common life habit, through which the hosts contaminated their food with spores, and (*iii*) a common food indicating a uniformity of the digestive process (enzymes, pH, microflora, etc.). Weiser came to these conclusions from studies on the microsporidians of *H. cunea, E. chrysorrhoea, P. dispar,* and other Lepidoptera. Kaya (1973) reported on a similar situation where *Pleistophora schubergi* infected seven species of Lepidoptera on forest trees. *Nosema algerae* infected perorally several *Anopheles, Culex,* and *Aedes* spp. (Vávra and Undeen, 1970; Undeen and Maddox, 1973). This also may be the case with other microsporidians infecting mosquitoes (Chapman *et al.,* 1969). *Nosema oryzaephili* infected five species of beetles and three species of moths involving five insect families of stored-product insects (Burges *et al.,* 1971). Different species of grasshoppers occurring in the same field were susceptible to *Nosema locustae* (Henry and Oma, 1974). Similar examples may occur in the ecosystems of many insect pests.

Alternate hosts in the ecosystem may vary in their susceptibility to the same microsporidian. Hall (1954) observed that the fiery skipper was more susceptible to infection by *Nosema infesta* than *Crambus bonifatellus.* Weiser (1963) reported that the dosage-mortality curves varied between *Hyphantria cunea* and *Porthetria dispar* fed spores of *Nosema muscularis;* and between *Euproctis chrysorrhoea* and *Malacosoma neustria* infected with *Thelohania hyphantriae.* *Nosema algerae* caused heavy infections in *Anopheles stephensi* and *Anopheles albimanus,* and lighter and less common infections in *Anopheles quadrimaculatus, Culex pipiens,* and *Aedes aegypti,* and did not infect *Anopheles atroparvus* (Vávra and Undeen, 1970; Undeen and Maddox, 1973). Maddox (1973) observed that although closely related hosts might occur in the same location, one host would have a high incidence of microsporidiosis, while the other had a very low incidence, even though both species were equally susceptible in the laboratory. He speculated that the difference in the incidence of infection might be due to host behavioral differences. The situation becomes highly complex when susceptible hymenopterous parasites and hyperparasites are involved together with their habitual and alternate hosts (Brooks, 1973; McNeil and Brooks, 1974).

Microsporidian infections in the host and its parasites may cause deviations in their biological activities, e.g., diapause (Issi and Maslennikova, 1964).

Insect pathogens are considered to be a host-density-dependent mortality factor, but when the pathogens are widely dispersed in the host environment, they may act as a density-independent factor. In the case of the microsporidia, there is very little quantitative data in this area. There are numerous data on the incidence of infection covering a total period of a month, season, or year, but such cumulative data are usually inadequate for density-dependent studies. Weiser (1961a) has concluded that the microsporidians are density-dependent-mortality factor and play an important role in population regulation. He (1963) has reported that microsporidians initially occur in small foci and then spread out in the field. The incidence of infection in 1963 by *Octosporea muscaedomesticae* in the black blow fly, *Phormia regina,* increased at a steady rate with the progression of the season, while the fly population declined over the same period (Kramer, 1967). In 1964, however, the rate followed no discernible pattern, probably because of host scarcity for the entire period following heavy spring rains. An epizootic of *Melolontha melolontha* caused by *Nosema melolonthae* continued to develop and spread during the 3 years under observation from an incidence of 2.5 to 20% (in some plots as high as 50-60%) (Hurpin, 1965). In populations of *Choristoneura fumiferana* there was a higher incidence of infection by *Nosema fumiferanae* toward the end of the budworm season (Wilson, 1973). Since there were more sixth-instar larvae being infected, Wilson (1973) speculated that some light infection might have been overlooked in younger larvae. This may have been the case, but as pointed by Chapman (1974a), care should be taken in estimating incidence of microsporidian infections, especially in older larvae, since the infections prolong larval development beyond that of the uninfected larvae. Thus the high incidence will be based mainly on the infected larvae.

In his discussion of enzootic diseases of insects, Burges (1973) selected the microsporidian, *Nosema whitei,* to illustrate some of the principles of disease outbreaks in stored-product insects. He has concluded that enzootic diseases are much more important in insects occurring in the field, particularly when the pathogen is transmitted transovarially and is well synchronized with the pest's life cycle. It is less important in stored-product insects because unloading of the products or chemical insect control usually limits the infection to the enzootic state.

V. ENVIRONMENTAL FACTORS

Inasmuch as the environmental factors affect the microsporidian, the host, and transmission, their effects can be complex. Some of

these factors have already been discussed in the areas of persistence, dispersal, and transmission. Among the physical factors,
temperature is most important for microsporidian infections (Maddox,
1973). Although the microsporidian spores can tolerate a wide range
of temperatures (Weiser, 1961a, 1965; Maddox, 1973), this may not
be the case with the infectious process. The optimum temperature
of most microsporidian infections is 20-30°C and no development occurs below 10°C (Maddox, 1973). Kramer (1968b) exposed the black
blowfly to spores of *O. muscaedomesticae* at temperatures from 12°
to 32±2°C. There was no infection at 12°C apparently because the
spores failed to germinate. When infection occurred, the harmful
effects were directly proportional to the rise in temperature. At
each temperature, the longevity of the infected flies was about one
half that of the uninfected flies. On the other hand, the pathogenicity of *Nosema whitei* for *Tribolium castaneum* decreased as the
temperature was increased from 25°C (LD_{50}=4.2 X 10^6 spores/g)
through 30°C (LD_{50}=1.3 X 10^7 spores/g) to 35°C (LD_{50}=3.2 X 10^8
spores/g) (Milner, 1973a). The stress of very high or very low
temperatures was harmful to the infected host. Kramer (1959) found
that low winter and high summer temperatures killed more European
corn borers infected by microsporidian than uninfected individuals.
Hurpin (1968) observed that the optimum temperature for the development of *Nosema melolonthae* was 20°C, and this was ecologically
important because the larvae of *Melolontha melolontha* lived in the
soil where the temperature was usually below 20°C.

At very high temperatures, generally above 35°C, the microsporidian fails to develop in the host insect, and this knowledge has
been utilized in the thermal therapy of microsporidian infections
(Weiser, 1961a). Such high temperatures may occur in some agri-
cultural areas, but there is no information on whether the microsporidian can survive diurnal fluctuating temperatures that may exceed 35°C during the day.

When an insect host undergoes hibernation or aestivation, the
microsporidian also slows down or ceases its development (Weiser,
1961a, 1963b; Kellen *et al.*, 1965; Maddox, 1973). This aspect has
also been touched upon in the section on Persistence.

Climatological conditions, mainly that of temperature, may govern
the distribution of certain microsporidia. Weiser (1965) reported
that *Nosema serbica* infected the gypsy moth only in Southern Europe
and the subtropics, and was replaced by other species in Central
Europe. He also noted that some microsporidians, e.g., *Nosema
stricklandi* multiplied in the host during the winter, whereas
Pleistophora simulii and *Thelohania* spp. developed mainly in the
summer. Sikorowski and Madison (1968) observed that the highest
incidence of infection in the larvae of the Clear Lake gnat, *Chaoborus astictopus*, occurred in the overwintering population when the
water temperature was low and the larvae were exposed to the microsporidian, *Thelohania corethrae*, for the longest time. The frequency
of infection gradually declined as the water temperature began to

rise and was lowest in the summer months when the gnat completed
its life cycle in the shortest time. There was a gradual increase
in infection rates as the water temperature declined during the
autumn months.

Humidity and moisture may affect the persistence of microsporidian
spores, but there is little known of their effect on the infectious
process. The protozoan diseases of the honey bee, including the
nosema disease, increased in incidence during the wet season in
Venezuela possibly from the unfavorable effect of rain on the pollen
and nectar of flowers (Stejskal, 1959). Goetze and Zeutzschel (1959)
believed that the epizootics of *Nosema apis* in bee colonies increased
chiefly because of unfavorable general conditions, such as poor
weather and honey flow conditions, unsuitable hive sites, and defec-
tive housing. Milner (1973a) observed that the pathogenicity of
Nosema whitei for *Tribolium castaneum* decreased consistently as the
humidity increased from 10, 30, 50, 70 to 90% relative humidity.
Apparently the low humidity stressed the host and increased the
pathogenicity of the microsporidian.

Solar radiation inactivates microsporidian spores and this may
occur within 5 hours (Maddox, 1973) or 3–5 days (Weiser, 1963).
There is no detailed study, especially with regards to the wave
length and radiant energy. Kaya (personal communication) prolonged
the life of spores of *Pleistophora schubergi* by incorporating a UV
protectant in the spray.

In addition to the interaction with the habitual and alternate
hosts and the parasites, predators, and carriers, the microsporidian
is affected by other biotic factors, such as the food of the host
insect. When larvae of *Archips cerasivoranus* infected with *Nosema
cerasivoranus* were fed cherry foliage painted with plant extracts
from 15 plant species, the life spans of the infected larvae were
either shortened or prolonged (Smirnoff, 1967). Larvae fed extracts
of *Virburnum cassinoides, Abies balsamea,* garlic, and onion lived
10, 7, 4, and 4 days longer, respectively than control larvae, while
those fed *Salix perifolia, Picea mariana, Corylus cornuta,* and common mustard died 3–5 days sooner than the controls. Larvae fed
onion-treated foliage gave rise to pupae with the lowest rate of
infection (8%) compared to 70–100% in others. Subsequently, Smirnoff (1974) found that the plant extracts of birch, spruce, and pine
killed the spores of *Thelohania pristiphorae* in 8–15 minutes.

The larvae of European corn borer, *Pyrausta nubilalis,* feeding
on corn varieties resistant to the borer, were less infected by
Nosema pyraustae than larvae feeding on susceptible corn
varieties (Chiang and Holloway, 1960; McLaughlin, 1971).

VI. APPLICATION OF EPIZOOTIOLOGICAL STUDY

The principles of the epizootiology of infectious diseases of pest
insects may be applied: (*i*) to manipulate or enhance the pathogen
population and initiate the development of epizootics, (*ii*) to stress

the host population and increase its susceptibility to the pathogen, (*iii*) to favor or facilitate the transmission of the pathogen, (*iv*) to activate chronic and latent infections to epizootic levels, and (*v*) to predict the outbreak of epizootics. Thus far these applications have not been achieved except for a single study conducted in Germany where epizootics caused by microsporidians have been predicted in an insect population. By means of a systematic study of the health of young larvae, Franz and Huger (1971) were able to predict a general collapse of the green tortrix, *Tortrix viridana*, by microsporidians, primarily *Nosema tortricis*, and thereby canceled the use of chemical control measures. Smirnoff (1973) attempted to utilize the biochemical analysis of insects infected with pathogens, including several species of microsporidians, to diagnose, forecast and prognosticate the future of the insect populations.

VII. MICROBIAL CONTROL

Microbial control can be divided into short-term or temporary control and long-term or permanent (also designated as introduction) control. In order to apply these control measures, the following conditions should be considered: (*i*) the propagation and storage of the pathogens, (*ii*) compatibility with adjuvants and insecticides, (*iii*) method and timing of application, and (*iv*) safety to nontarget organisms, such as vertebrates, plants, parasites, predators, etc. The pathogens should first be evaluated in the laboratory by bioassay for their virulence and pathogenicity and to establish the appropriate dosage for field application.

A. MASS PRODUCTION

There are several comprehensive reviews on the mass production of insect pathogens (Weiser, 1956; Martignoni, 1964; Ignoffo, 1966; Ignoffo and Hink, 1971). Since the microsporidians are obligate pathogens requiring living cells for their development and have not been grown *in vitro*, they have been propagated, thus far, in laboratory-reared or field collected insects. The habitual host is usually used in propagation but occasionally an alternate host which is easier or more economical to rear has been used. Since mosquitoes are small, they would not be favorable for the mass production of microsporidian spores. Undeen and Maddox (1973) mass produced the spores of *N. algerae* by injecting a spore inoculum into *Heliothis zea* larvae and obtained a yield of 2000 times more spores from one *H. zea* larva than from one mosquito. This was equivalent to about 10,000 times the number of spores that was in the injected inoculum. Undeen and Alger (1975) conducted bioassay of spores of *N. algerae* obtained from its habitual host, *A. stephensi*, and from the infected alternate hosts, *H. zea* and *Phormia regina*. The spores produced in *H. zea* were as infective as those from *A. stephensi*, but those from *P. regina* were significantly less infective. As mentioned in the section on Transmission, the pathogenicity of the microsporidian may be lost when propagated on alternate hosts. The host larvae are usually infected with a low dosage, sufficient to produce a chronic or prolonged infection to obtain a massive spore production (Hostounský and Weiser, 1972). A high dose often results in an acute infection, and the host is killed before maximum spore production is obtained.

Occasionally an insect stock culture may become infected with undesirable insect pathogens, e.g., bacteria, virus, protozoa, etc., and a new culture must be started or the contaminating pathogen eliminated from the culture. McLaughlin (1966) has developed a system of "unit integrity" for rearing disease-free cultures of the boll weevil. The "unit" is a homogeneous grouping and is handled as an entity and separated from all other such units to reduce the danger of cross contamination. This system has produced larger numbers of healthy insects more quickly than the selection of progeny from single pairs of weevils. There is a disadvantage in that the system is more susceptible to failure because of its design; nonetheless McLaughlin has succeeded in eliminating protozoan diseases. He believes that the system is applicable also to contamination by pathogens other than protozoa.

Although the use of *Glugea gasti* has succeeded in controlling the boll weevil (McLaughlin *et al.*, 1969), McLaughlin has informed Cross (1973) that the cost of producing the microsporidian is prohibitive and uneconomical (McLaughlin and Bell, 1970). However, as pointed out by Ignoffo (1966), "Laboratory microbial insecticides are inherently expensive and therefore care should be taken not to eliminate a candidate insect pathogen at this stage solely on the basis of projected costs." Carefully planned techniques and programs, even utilizing alternate hosts, may reduce the cost of producing *Glugea gasti*, just as in the case of insect virus production.

Early workers noticed contaminating microsporidians in their insect tissue cultures, but apparently Ishihara and Sohi (1966) were the first to successfully infect such cultures. They succeeded in infecting an ovarian tissue culture of *Bombyx mori* with *Nosema bombycis*. Subsequently, Ishihara (1968) also succeeded with *N. bombycis* in infecting primary cell cultures of rat, mouse, rabbit, and chick embryos, but spore formation was confirmed only with rat embryo cells. These studies are a significant breakthrough in the mass production of microsporidia, however, there are still problems to be considered, such as the pathogenicity of tissue-culture reared microsporidian for the target insect, and the pathogenicity, especially when reared on vertebrate tissues, to vertebrate animals. This aspect of safety to vertebrates will be discussed later.

When an insect pathogen has been mass produced, the purity of the spores may be questioned by government organizations responsible for the safety of the public. Cole (1970) applied the principle of "triangulation" and counter-current distribution used in chromatography for purifying the spores of *Nosema heliothidis* from larval remains of *H. zea*, and the spores of *N. apis* from the adult remains

of *Apis mellifera*. He obtained a 99% purity of the spores. The
microsporidian spores were suited for this method because they were
relatively uniform in size and density, and offered no problems in
wettability as in the case of fungus spores.

A density gradient method was applied by Undeen and Alger (1971)
in purifying the spores of *Nosema algerae* propagated in mosquito
larvae. They prepared a gradient made from Ludox (colloid of 40%
silica in a NaOH solution, manufactured by du Pont). The gradient
was continuous from pure water at the top to 40% silica on the bottom.

As pointed out earlier, serological techniques should be utilized
in identifying microsporidians, and also in their detection in the
host and habitat. A major problem is the disruption of the spores
to obtain a suitable antigen. Conner (1970) investigated several
methods, including sonic ocillation, disintegrator, and freezing-
pressing, and the most effective method was a sequence of freezing,
grinding, and thawing repeated many times until 95% or more of the
spores were disrupted.

B. *STORAGE*

The persistence of the microsporidian has already been touched
upon. There are great variations in the storage capacity of spores
of different microsporidians (Kramer, 1970; Bailey, 1972; Maddox,
1973). Bailey (1972) has concluded that ". . . no very satisfactory
ways have been found of preserving infective spores for long." In
general, microsporidian spores can withstand storage for prolonged
periods when held in an aqueous medium or in cadavers or feces and
held at low temperatures (0-5°C). Temperatures above 35°C are
usually detrimental to the spores. Water is the most important
factor required for maintaining spore viability (Weiser, 1956). In
some cases the spores cannot withstand drying (Alger and Undeen,
1970; Maddox, 1973). In others, the dried spores, when wetted, may
germinate prematurely and die in the absence of susceptible cells
(Kramer, 1970; Maddox, 1973). Lyophilization has been applied successfully for storing the spores of *Nosema pyraustae* (Lewis and Lynch,
1974). The lyophilized spores are stored in an air-tight container
and held at -12°C, and remain viable for 12 months.

The loss in viability of the stored spores is a gradual process,
involving an increasing mortality. Maddox (1973) observed that the
spores of *Nosema necatrix* when stored in water at 5°C for 2 years,
lost their infectivity by 10,000 times. Henry and Oma (1974) tested
the effect of prolonged storage on the spores of *Nosema locustae*.
They reported that fresh spores resulted in higher incidence of infection than spores stored in water at -10°C for 8 months to 3 years
or spores stored in cadavers for 1 year at -10°C. They estimated
that the storage in water at -10°C resulted in about 90% reduction
and in cadavers for 1 year at -10°C in about 99% reduction in activity.

C. COMPATIBILITY

Microsporidians occur commonly in mixed infections with other types of pathogens. The effect of mixed microsporidian infections has already been discussed in the section on Virulence and Infectivity. In some cases the presence of other pathogens has very little effect on the pathogenicity and multiplication of the microsporidian. The effect is dependent on the virulence and pathogenicity of the associated pathogen. Facultative bacteria generally invade the host insect when very high doses of microsporidian spores are fed to the larvae (Weiser, 1961a, 1963). Apparently the abundance of spores causes extensive damage to the midgut cells and enables the bacteria to invade and infect the host. The associated bacterial infection usually kills the host so rapidly that the development and multiplication of the microsporidian are limited. Fungi generally kill the host rapidly and are disadvantageous to the microsporidian. Some viruses are highly virulent and may kill the host in less than a week, others, e.g., some cytoplasmic-polyhedrosis and granulosis viruses, cause prolonged chronic infections that may not have serious effect on the microsporidian.

It is of interest that the presence of microsporidians appear to be unfavorable for the development of the malaria protozoa (Garnham, 1956; Bano, 1958; Fox and Weiser, 1959; Savage et al., 1971). The microsporidians producing such effects are Pleistophora culicis in Anopheles gambiae (Garnham, 1956) and A. stephensi (Garnham, 1956; Bano, 1958), Nosema sp. in A. quadrimaculatus (Savage et al., 1971), and N. algerae in A. stephensi (Ward and Savage, 1972). According to Fox and Weiser (1959), there is no evidence that the microsporidian is physically antagonistic or that it attacks the Plasmodium, but the microsporidian so severely damages the midgut wall that the Plasmodium cannot develop normally.

Microsporidians have been used with adjuvants in sprays or in baits. Weiser (1956) added molasses, milk, and wheat paste to sprays containing microsporidian spores. Kaya (personal communication) incorporated a UV protectant ("Shade") with the spores of Pleistophora schubergi for the control of Anisota senatoria.

There is very little information on the compatibility of microsporidians and insecticides (Benz, 1971). Rosický (1951) tested the effect of insecticides on the weevil, Otiorrhynchus ligustici, infected with Nosema otiorrhynchi. Arsenicals accelerated the death of the infected beetles, and DDT and a fumigant with contact effect accelerated the knockdown and death. The stomach insecticide (arsenical) caused a quicker kill, by about 25% than the contact insecticides. Rosický (1951) speculated that the accelerated effects of insecticides resulted from the malfunction of the malpighian tubes which were heavily infected by the microsporidian. This promising area of synergistic interaction has not been pursued by recent workers.

When Bacillus thuringiensis and DDT were applied to populations of the green tortrix infected with the microsporidian (N. tortricis), the potential of the microsporidian was better preserved in the surviving population with applications of B. *thuringiensis* than with DDT (Franz and Huger, 1971).

D. *METHODS OF APPLICATION*

After the microsporidian spores have been bioassayed for their pathogenicity to the target insects, they are applied in appropriate dosages in the field. The timing of the application and a thorough coverage, especially in the area of the feeding sites of the insects, are important for successful control. The microsporidians should be applied during the period when the insect is most susceptible to infection under field conditions. The application is usually made as sprays. In some cases, baits have resulted in effective control (McLaughlin *et al.*, 1968, 1969; Henry *et al.*, 1973). McLaughlin *et al.* (1968) utilized the bait principle for boll-weevil control. The baits contained: 1.0 X 10^6 spores/ml; water, 65.7%; cotton seed oil, 16.5%; honey, 16.5%; surfactant, 0.6%; thixotropic agent (hydroxy-methyl cellulose), 26.66 g/liter; and a red marker dye, 3.33 g/liter. The bait was applied with a backpack sprayer with an external mix pneumatic nozzle and applied at the terminal buds and squares on caged cotton plants. In subsequent tests, the bait was applied in field plots (McLaughlin *et al.*, 1969). They found that the timing of spray application was important. The bait was most effective in fall when the weevil entered diapause, and in spring when they emerged from hibernation. Applications were not effective during the summer against the F_1 adults and the succeeding generations.

Henry *et al.* (1973) incorporated the spores of *Nosema locustae* into wheat-bran baits for the control of grasshoppers. They considered the following factors: (*i*) the time of applications (four applications spaced over 22 days), (*ii*) the concentration of spores (1, 30, and 900 spores/in^2) and (*iii*) the level of the spore carrier (1 and 4 pounds of wheat bran/acre). The spore concentration was most important in reducing the densities of the grasshoppers. The reduction in grasshopper numbers and the incidence of infection were greater in grasshopper species which readily accepted the wheat bran.

Under certain situations, a dry dust preparation is more effective and economical than a spray for insect control. This is the case for the control of the European corn borer where the use of a granular formulation is much more effective. The dry coarse granules accumulate at the bases of corn leaves where the corn borer enters the plant. Lewis and Lynch (1974) succeeded in lyophilizing (vacuum drying) the spores of *Nosema pyraustae* in infected corn-borer larvae. They believed that the lyophilized preparation would be suitable for a granular formulation of spores.

E.   SAFETY

According to Weiser (1973), "There is no evidence of any transmission of vertebrate microsporidians to insects or insect microsporidians to vertebrates." Nonetheless, Heimpel (1969) points
out, "Certain of the Microsporidia can cause diseases in fish and
mammals, and any protozoan recommended for dissemination in the
field should be rigorously tested for safety to these animals."
This problem became more involved when Ishihara (1968) reported
that *Nosema bombycis* spores infected primary cell cultures of rat,
mouse, rabbit, and chick embryoes. However, when the cultures
were incubated at 37°C, no development occurred in any of the cultures. Ishihara (1968) concluded that this might be one of the
reasons why *N. bombycis* did not infect warm blooded animals. Mammals, of course, have other defense reactions, such as the enzymes
and pH of the digestive tract, and humoral and cellular defenses
that may prevent microsporidian infections. Undeen (1975) succeeded in culturing *Nosema algerae* also in a vertebrate tissue culture (pig kidney cells). The microsporidian completed its life
cycle in the tissue culture held at 26° and 35°C, but at 37°C the
microsporidian died after 3 days and no spores were produced. He
thus confirmed Ishihara's observation that no infection occurred in
cultures held at high temperatures.

Seibold and Fussell (1973) suspected that the microsporidian infection detected in one out of 170 necropsied monkeys (*Callicebus
moloch cupreus*) might have arisen from infected insects eaten by
the monkeys. Since microsporidia, e.g. *Encephalitozoan* and *Thelohania*, have been reported from a wide variety of mammals, Shadduck
(1973) suggested a protocol for testing the host range and potential pathogenicity of insect microsporidian in mammals.

Some hymenopterous parasites are susceptible to the microsporidians
which infect their insect hosts, and others are refractory (see
sections, Transmission and Host Population). A few parasites appear
to be infected by specific microsporidians which do not infect their
hosts (Brooks and Cranford, 1972). Brooks and Cranford (1972) have
considered, however, the possibility that the parasite-specific
microsporidian may infect the other hosts of the parasites.

The microsporidian infection very likely reduces the effectiveness
of the hymenopterous parasites. The significance of such infection
in the parasites will depend on the relative importance of the parasite as compared to that of the microsporidian in the control of the
insect pest.

There appears to be only a few reports of microsporidians infecting
predaceous insects. In coccinellids, Lipa and Steinhaus (1959) described *Nosema hippodamia* from *Hippodamia convergens;* Cali and Briggs
(1968) described *N. tracheophila* from *Coccinella septempunctata*.
There is no information whether these microsporidians also infect the
hosts of the predators, as in the case of the hymenopterous parasites.

VIII. FIELD APPLICATIONS

When compared to applications of viruses, bacteria, and fungi for insect control, there have been very few attempts made with microsporidia, even though some of them are highly pathogenic for insects. Nearly all attempts have been made on terrestrial insects, but recently the use of microsporidians against aquatic pests, primarily mosquitoes, has been discussed in several reviews (Kellen, 1962; Chapman *et al.*, 1970a, 1972; Laird, 1971; Chapman, 1973, 1974a,b).

A. LONG-TERM APPLICATION OR INTRODUCTION

In order for the long-term application or introduction to be successful, the microsporidian must be applied to a host population, in which it has not occurred previously or in which it is temporarily absent at the time of application. McLaughlin *et al.* (1968, 1969) applied *Glugea gasti*, using the bait principle, for the control of the boll weevil. With the attractive baits, they have been able to infect a native fall population and reduce the spring emergence (McLaughlin *et al.*, 1969). If this introduction does not infect the boll weevil in subsequent years, it should not be considered a long-term control. The microsporidian, *Nosema locustae*, was successfully introduced into populations of several grasshopper species (Henry, 1971; Henry and Oma, 1974). The microsporidian spores were incorporated in wheat bran baits at the rates of 0, 50, 100, 200, 400, and 800 spores/in^2 and applied at 2 pounds/acre. The incidence of infected grasshoppers for treatments at 50 to 800 spores/in^2 did not differ significantly from each other, but all were significantly different from the control. The populations consisted predominantly of *Melanoplus sanguinipes*, *M. gladstoni*, and *M. infantilis*, and the incidence of infection increased in all species after spore application. Most of the heavy infections occurred in *M. sanguinipes*, *M. infantilis*, and *Phoetaliotes nebrascensis*. In addition, infection was observed in the miscellaneous species, *M. bivittatus*, *M. dawsoni*, *Trimerotropis campestris*, *Hesperotettix viridis viridis*, and *Hypocllora alba*. No infection was observed in nine other grasshopper species. The reduction in grasshopper densities after treatment with fresh spore baits was similar in a complex with a single species dominating as compared to a mixed species complex, but the incidence of infection was lower in the mixed species complex than in the complex in which one species dominated (Henry and Oma, 1974). The applications of fresh spores reduced the grasshopper densities in both complexes to levels below the economic thresholds. In the use of the microsporidian, Henry and Oma (1974) stressed that the loss of fecundity as well as the mortality of the grasshoppers should be considered. They concluded that the microsporidian will probably be established in the treated area at least through the following season.

Reynolds (1972) introduced *Pleistophora culicis* into the larval population of *Culex pipiens fatigans* in Nauru, an island in the

Pacific. Two years after the initial introduction, the infection
was still present in the wild population, but the infection rate
was low and not high enough to adversely affect the natural
mosquito population. Reynolds (1972) concluded that the infection
rate of 6000 spores/ml of larval breeding water might not have
been high enough or that the local mosquito population might not
be very susceptible.

B.   SHORT-TERM OR TEMPORARY CONTROL

Among the first microsporidian to be mass produced and applied in
the field is *Nosema infesta* (Hall, 1954). It was mass produced in
alternate hosts, *Gnorimoschema operculella* and *Junonia coenia,* and
applied at the rates of 500 million to 8 billion spores/yd^2 of lawn
for the control of the sod webworm, *Crambus bonifatellus*. At the
very high concentration, nearly all of the larvae were infected,
but at the low concentration, only about 2-3.5% of the recovered
larvae were infected.

Weiser and Veber (1955, 1957) sprayed spores of *Thelohania hyphantriae* on fruit trees infested with *Hyphantria cunea*. After 14 days,
about 25% died, and later 100% were infected, followed by the death
of the larvae. The microsporidian also infected other Lepidoptera
which occurred in the same ecosystem, such as *Malacosoma neustria,
Euproctis chrysorrhoea, Hyponomeuta malinella,* and *Nygmia phaeorrhoea*. It could also be mass-produced in *E. chrysorrhoea* and *M.
neustria*. Weiser and Veber (1957) concluded that they succeeded in
short-term control of these pests but long-term control was not obtained because of the poor dispersal (the spores were not excreted
by infected larvae) and the lack of persistence in the ecosystem
(predators and scavengers removed the infected larvae and cadavers
from the biotope). Weiser informed McLaughlin (1971) that *Pleistophora schubergi* was not effective against *Euproctis chrysorrhoea,*
and that this microsporidian and *Nosema serbica* were fairly successful against first-instar larvae of *Porthetria dispar*. The failure
was caused by the removal of the pathogen by rain and their inacti-
vation by sunlight.

Mistric and Smith (1973) applied spores of *Nosema necatrix* on
tobacco at the rate of 3.3 X 10^8 spores/ml and 2.6 quarts/acre with
the use of a power sprayer operating at 60 lbs/in^2. The microsporidian reduced the infestation and crop damage of tobacco budworm,
H. virescens, but the control was less than that obtained with the
standard insecticide, Methomyl, at 0.5 lb/acre.

The microsporidian, *Pleistophora schubergi,* when applied to oak
trees at 2 X 10 spores/ml and with a UV protectant infected 88% of
Anisota senatoria larvae at 4 days after spray application (Kaya,
personal communication). At the rates of 2 X 10 and 2 X 10
spores/ml, 96% and 72%, respectively, of the *A. senatoria* larvae,
and 100% and 100%, respectively of the *Symerista canicosta* larvae
were infected 14 days after application.

IX. CONCLUSIONS

The microsporidians offer promise for the control of insect pests. On the other hand, Burges (1969) has concluded, "Organisms suitable for microbial insecticides are mainly viruses and bacteria, with some possibilities among the fungi and nematodes, but few among the protozoans." Such a viewpoint stems from the general belief that a pathogen must be highly virulent and pathogenic in order to be effective and that the protozoans, including microsporidians, produce chronic and prolonged infections. The selection of a pathogen for microbial control should not be based solely or largely on the pathogenicity or other properties of the pathogen, but the properties of the host and its habitat should also be considered. In many cases, the pest insect and its habitat have determined the type of pathogen most suitable and effective for application. Outstanding examples of pathogens of low pathogenicity which have been successfully applied are the milky-disease bacteria, *Bacillus popilliae*, for the control of the Japanese beetle, and the virus, *Rhabdionvirus oryctes* for the rhinoceros beetle. In the former case, the success of the pathogen is dependent to a large extent on the lcw pathogenicity and the larval habitat (soil), and in the latter, to the low pathogenicity, the loss in fecundity and longevity of the adults, and the efficient dispersal of the virus.

In a few cases, the microsporidians offer promise against insects of low economic threshold, e.g., *Nosema pyraustae* on the European corn borer, and *Glugea gasti* on the cotton boll weevil. In general, they appear most promising against insects of high economic threshold, e.g., insects of forest, lawn, soil, etc., and under this type of ecosystem, the microsporidians have demonstrated long persistence, effective dispersal, and transmission.

The aquatic habitat and stored products offer very favorable environments for microsporidians. There has been a great increase in the number of microsporidians, some of which cause severe epizootics, from insects of these habitats, and the promising microsporidians should be investigated intensely for control purposes.

There is a need for studies on the factors affecting the epizootics of microsporidan diseases. Information derived from such studies may be of value in initiating or enhancing epizootics and also in predicting the natural occurrence of epizootics.

In the future, I anticipate an increased application of microsporidians, particularly in the integrated control programs of pest management.

REFERENCES

Alger, N. E., and Undeen, A. H. (1970). The control of a microsporidian, *Nosema* sp., in an anopheline colony by an egg-rinsing technique. *J. Invertebr. Pathol.* <u>15</u>, 321-327.

Allen, H. W. (1954). *Nosema* disease of *Gnorimoschema operculella*

(Zeller) and *Macrocentrus ancylivorus* Rohwer. *Ann. Entomol. Soc. Amer.*, <u>47</u>, 407–424.

Bailey, L. (1972). The preservation of infective microsporidan spores. *J. Invertebr. Pathol.*, <u>20</u>, 252–254.

Bano, L. (1958). Partial inhibitory effect of *Plistophora culicis* on the sporogonic cycle of *Plasmodium cynomolgi* in *Anopheles stephensi*. *Nature (London)* <u>181</u>, 430.

Benz, G. (1971). Synergism of micro-organisms and chemical insecticides. *In* "Microbial Control of Insects and Mites" (H. D. Burges and N. W. Hussey, eds.), pp. 327–355. Academic Press, New York.

Blunck, H. (1954). Mikrosporidien bei *Pieris brassicae* L., ihren Parasiten und Hyperparasiten schmarotzenden Mikrosporidien. *Trans. 9th Intern. Congr. Entomol. Amsterdam* <u>1</u>, 432–438.

Brooks, W. M. (1970). *Nosema sphingidis* sp. n., a microsporidian parasite of the tobacco hornworm, *Manduca sexta*. *J. Invertebr. Pathol.*, <u>16</u>, 390–399.

Brooks, W. M. (1971). Protozoan infections of insects with emphasis on inflammation. *Proc. Int. Colloq. Insect Pathol.*, *4th*, 1970, pp. 11–27.

Brooks, W. M. (1973). Protozoa: host-parasite-pathogen interrelationships. *Entomol. Soc. Amer. Misc. Publ.* <u>9</u>, 105–111.

Brooks, W. M., and Cranford, J. D. (1972). Microsporidoses of the hymenopterous parasites, *Campoletis sonorensis* and *Cardiochiles nigriceps*, larval parasites of *Heliothis* species. *J. Invertebr. Pathol.* <u>20</u>, 77–94.

Burges, H. D. (1969). Insect control by micro-organisms. *Atti Accad. Naz. Lincei* <u>128</u>, 189–202.

Burges, H. D. (1973). Enzootic diseases of insects. *Ann. New York Acad. Sci.*, <u>217</u>, 31–49.

Burges, H. D., Canning, E. U., and Hurst, J. A. (1971). Morphology, development, and pathogenicity of *Nosema oryzaephili* n.sp. in *Oryzaephilus surinamensis* and its host range among granivorous insects. *J. Invertebr. Pathol.*, <u>17</u>, 419–432.

Cali, A., and Briggs, J. D. (1968). The biology and life history of *Nosema tracheophila* sp.n. [Protozoa: Cnidospora: Microsporidea] found in *Coccinella septempunctata* Linnaeus (Coleoptera: Coccinellidae). *J. Invertebr. Pathol.* <u>9</u>, 515–522.

Cameron, J. W. M. (1963). Factors affecting the use of microbial pathogens in insect control. *Annu. Rev. Entomol.* <u>8</u>, 265–286.

Canning, E. U. (1971). Transmission of Microsporidia. *Proc. Int. Colloq. Insect Pathol.*, *4th*, 1970, pp. 415–424.

Chapman, H. C. (1973). Assessment of the potential of some pathogens and parasites of biting flies. *Proc. Symp. Univ. Alberta*, 1972, DR 217. *Defense Research Board*, pp. 71–77.

Chapman, H. C. (1974a). Biological control of mosquito larvae. *Annu. Rev. Entomol.* <u>19</u>, 33–59.

Chapman, H. C. (1974b). Pathogens against mosquitoes. *Proc. Ann. Tall Timbers Conf. Ecol. Anim. Contr. by Habitat Man.* No. 5, pp. 43–47.

Chapman, H. C., Clark, T. B., and Peterson, J. J.   (1970a).   Proto-
    zoans, nematodes, and viruses of anophelines. *Misc. Pub.*
    Entomol. Soc. Amer. 7, 134–139.
Chapman, H. C., Clark, T. B., Peterson, J. J., and Woodard, D. B.
    (1969). A two-year survey of pathogens and parasites of
    Culicidae, Chaoboridae, and Ceratopogonidae in Louisiana.
    Proc. 56th Ann. Meet. New Jersey Mosquito Extermination Assoc.,
    1969.
Chapman, H. C., and Kellen, W. R.   (1967). *Plistophora caecorum*
    sp.n., a microsporidian of *Culiseta inornata* (Diptera: Culi-
    cidae) from Louisiana. *J. Invertebr. Pathol.* 9, 500–502.
Chapman, H. C., Peterson, J. J., and Fukuda, T.   (1972). Predators
    and pathogens for mosquito control. *Amer. J. Trop. Med. Hyg.*
    21, 777–781.
Chapman, H. C., Woodard, D. B., Clark, T. B., and Glenn, F. E. Jr.
    (1970b). A container for use in field studies of some patho-
    gens and parasites of mosquitoes. *Mosquito News* 30, 90–93.
Chapman, H. C., Woodard, D. B., Kellen, W. R., and Clark, T. B.
    (1966). Host-parasite relationships of *Thelohania* associated
    with mosquitoes in Louisiana (Nosematidae: Microsporidia).
    J. Invertebr. Pathol. 8, 452–456.
Chapman, H. C., Woodard, D. B., and Peterson, J. J.   (1967). Path-
    ogens and parasites in Louisiana. Culicidae and Chaoboridae.
    Proc. 54th Ann. Meet. New Jersey Mosquito Extermination Assoc.,
    1967.
Chiang, H. C., and Holdaway, F. G.   (1960). Relative effectiveness
    of resistance of field corn to the European corn borer, *Pyrausta*
    nubilalis, in crop protection and in population control. *J.*
    Econ. Entomol. 53, 918–924.
Cole, R. J.   (1970). The application of the "triangulation" method
    to the purification of *Nosema* spores from insect tissues. *J.*
    Invertebr. Pathol. 15, 193–195.
Conner, R. M.   (1970). Disruption of microsporidian spores for
    serological studies. *J. Invertebr. Pathol.* 15, 138.
Cross, W. H.   (1973). Biology, control, and eradication of the boll
    weevil. *Annu. Rev. Entomol.* 18, 17–46.
Dutky, S. R.   (1959). Insect microbiology. *Advan. Appl. Microbiol.*
    1, 175–200.
Fowler, J. L., and Reeves, E. L.   (1974a). Detection of relation-
    ships among microsporidan isolates by electrophoretic analysis:
    hydrophobic extracts. *J. Invertebr. Pathol.* 23, 3–12.
Fowler, J. L., and Reeves, E. L.   (1974b). Detection of relation-
    ships among microsporidan isolates by electrophoretic analysis:
    hydrophilic extracts. *J. Invertebr. Pathol.* 23, 63–69.
Fox, R. M., and Weiser, J.   (1959). A microsporidian parasite of
    Anopheles gambiae in Liberia. *J. Parasitol.* 45, 21–30.
Franz, J. M.   (1961a). Biologische Schädlingsbekämpfung. *In*
    "Handbuch der Pflanzenkrankheiten" (H. Richter, ed.), 2nd ed.,
    No. 3, 6, 1–302. Paul Parey, Berlin.

Franz, J. M.   (1961b).   Biological control of pest insects in Europe.
    Annu. Rev. Entomol. <u>6</u>, 183-200.
Franz, J. M., and Huger, A. M.   (1971).   Microsporidia causing the
    collapse of an outbreak of the green tortrix (*Tortrix viridana*
    L.) in Germany.   *Proc. 4th Intern. Colloq. Insect Pathol.*, pp.
    48-53.
Frye, R. D., and Olson, L. C.   (1974).   Fecundity and survival in
    populations of the European corn borer infected with *Perezia
    pyraustae*.   *J. Invertebr. Pathol.* <u>24</u>, 378-379.
Garnham, P. C. C.   (1956).   Microsporida in laboratory colonies of
    Anopheles.   *Bull. World Health Organ.* <u>15</u>, 845-847.
George, C. R.   (1971).   The effects of malnutrition on growth and
    mortality of the red rust flour beetle *Tribolium castaneum*
    (Coleoptera: Tenebrionidae) parasitized by *Nosema whitei*
    (Microsporidia: Nosematidae).   *J. Invertebr. Pathol.* <u>18</u>, 383-
    388.
Goetz, G., and Zeutzschel, B.   (1959).   Nosema disease of honeybees,
    and its control with drugs--review of research work since 1954.
    Bee World <u>40</u>, 217-225.
Günther, S.   (1956).   Zur Infektion des Goldafters (*Euproctis
    chrysorrhoea* L.) mit *Plistophora schubergi* Zwölfer (Microspori-
    dia).   *Z. angew. Zool.* <u>43</u>, 397-405.
Günther, S.   (1959).   Über die Auswirkung auf die Infektiosität
    bei der Passage insekten pathogener Mikrosporidien durch den
    Darm von Vögeln und Insekten.   *Nachrbl. deut. Pflanzenschutz-
    dienst (Berlin)*, [*N.F.*] <u>13</u>, 19-21.
Hall, I. M.   (1954).   Studies of microorganisms pathogenic to sod
    webworm.   *Hilgardia* <u>22</u>, 535-565.
Hall, I. M.   (1963).   Microbial control. *In* "Insect Pathology an
    Advanced Treatise" (E. A. Steinhaus, ed.), <u>2</u>, 477-517.   Aca-
    demic Press, New York.
Hazard, E. I., and Lofgren, C. S.   (1971).   Tissue specificity and
    systematics of a *Nosema* in some species of *Aedes, Anopheles,*
    and *Culex*.   *J. Invertebr. Pathol.* <u>18</u>, 16-24.
Heimpel, A. M.   (1969).   Microbial control of insects. *In* "Insect-
    Pest Management and Control." <u>3</u>, 165-195.   Publication 1695.
    National Acad. Sci. National Res. Council, Washington, D.C.
Henry, J. E.   (1971).   Experimental application of *Nosema locustae*
    for control of grasshoppers.   *J. Invertebr. Pathol.* <u>18</u>, 389-
    394.
Henry, J. E., and Oma, E. A.   (1974).   Effect of prolonged storage
    of spores on field applications of *Nosema locustae* (Microsporida:
    Nosematidae) against grasshoppers.   *J. Invertebr. Pathol.* <u>23</u>,
    371-377.
Henry, J. E., Tiahrt, K., and Oma, E. A.   (1973).   Importance of
    timing, spore concentrations, and levels of spore carrier in
    applications of *Nosema locustae* (Microsporida: Nosematidae) for
    control of grasshoppers.   *J. Invertebr. Pathol.* <u>21</u>, 263-272.
Hostounský, Z.   (1970).   *Nosema mesnili* (Paill.), a microsporidian

of the cabbageworm, *Pieris brassicae* (L.), in the parasites *Apanteles glomeratus* (L.), *Hyposoter ebeninus* (Grav.) and *Pimpla instigator* (F.). *Acta Entomol. Bohemoslovaca* 67, 1-5.

Hostounský, Z., and Weiser, J. (1972). Production of spores of *Nosema plodiae* Kellen *et* Lindegren in *Mamestra brassicae* L. after different infective dosage, I. *Vestn. Cesk. Spolecnosti Zool.* 36, 97-100.

Hurpin, B. (1965). An epizootic caused by *Nosema melolonthae* (Krieg) in the larva of the cockchafer *Melolontha melolontha* (Linnaeus). *J. Invertebr. Pathol.* 7, 39-44.

Hurpin, B. (1968). The influence of temperature and larval stage on certain diseases of *Melolontha melolontha*. *J. Invertebr. Pathol.* 10, 252-262.

Ignoffo, C. M. (1966). Possibilities of mass-producing insect pathogens. "Proceedings International Colloquium Insect Pathology and Microbial Control," pp. 91-117. North-Holland Publ., Amsterdam.

Ignoffo, C. M., and Hink, W. F. (1971). Propagation of arthropod pathogens in living systems. *In* "Microbial Control of Insects and Mites" (H. D. Burges and N. W. Hussey, eds.), pp. 541-580. Academic Press, New York.

Ishihara, R. (1967). Stimuli causing extrusion of polar filaments of *Glugea fumiferanae* spores. *Can. J. Microbiol.* 13, 1321-1332.

Ishihara, R. (1968). Growth of *Nosema bombycis* in primary cell cultures of mammalian and chicken embryos. *J. Invertebr. Pathol.* 11, 328-329.

Ishihara, R., and Sohi, S. S. (1966). Infection of ovarian tissue culture of *Bombyx mori* by *Nosema bombycis* spores. *J. Invertebr. Pathol.* 8, 538-540.

Issi, I. V., and Maslennikova, V. A. (1964). The effect of microsporidiosis upon the diapause and survival of *Apanteles glomeratus* L. (Hymenoptera, Braconidae) and *Pieris brassicae* L. (Lepidoptera, Pieridae). *Entomol. Obozvrenie* 43, 112-117.

Kaya, H. K. (1973). Pathogenicity of *Pleistophora schubergi* to larvae of the orange-striped oakworm and other lepidopterous insects. *J. Invertebr. Pathol.* 22, 356-358.

Kaya, H. K. Persistence of spores of *Pleistophora schubergi* [Cnidospora, Microsporida] in the field, and their application in microbial control. (Personal communication)

Kellen, W. R. (1962). Microsporidia and larval control. *Mosquito News* 22, 87-95.

Kellen, W. R., Chapman, H. C., Clark, T. B., and Lindegren, J. E. (1965). Host-parasite relationships of some *Thelohania* from mosquitoes (Nosematidae: Microsporidia). *J. Invertebr. Pathol.* 7, 161-166.

Kellen, W. R., Chapman, H. C., Clark, T. B., and Lindegren, J. E. (1966a). Transovarian transmission of some *Thelohania* (Nosematidae: Microsporidia) in mosquitoes of California and Louisiana. *J. Invertebr. Pathol.* 8, 355-359.

Kellen, W. R., Clark, T. B., and Lindegren, J. E. (1967). Two previously undescribed *Nosema* from mosquitoes of California (Nosematidae: Microsporidia). *J. Invertebr. Pathol.* 9, 19–25.

Kellen, W. R., Clark, T. B., Lindegren, J. E., and Sanders, R. D. (1966b). Development of *Thelohania californica* in two hybrid mosquitoes. *Exp. Parasitol.* 18, 251–254.

Kellen, W. R., and Lindegren, J. E. (1969). Host-pathogen relationships of two previously undescribed microsporidia from the Indian-meal moth, *Plodia interpunctella* (Hübner), (Lepidoptera: Phycitidae). *J. Invertebr. Pathol.* 14, 328–335.

Kellen, W. R., and Lindegren, J. E. (1971). Modes of transmission of *Nosema plodiae* Kellen and Lindegren, a pathogen of *Plodia interpunctella* (Hübner). *J. Stored Prod. Res.* 7, 31–34.

Kellen, W. R., and Lindegren, J. E. (1973). *Nosema invadens* sp.n. (Microsporida: Nosematidae), a pathogen causing inflammatory response in Lepidoptera. *J. Invertebr. Pathol.* 21, 293–300.

Kellen, W. R., and Lipa, J. J. (1960). *Thelohania californica* n. sp., a microsporidian parasite of *Culex tarsalis* Coquillett. *J. Insect Pathol.* 2, 1–12.

Kellen, W. R., and Wills, W. (1962). The transovarian transmission of *Thelohania californica* Kellen and Lipa in *Culex tarsalis* Coquillett. *J. Insect Pathol.* 4, 321–326.

Kramer, J. P. (1959). Observations on the seasonal incidence of microsporidiosis in European corn borer populations in Illinois. *Entomophaga* 4, 37–42.

Kramer, J. P. (1967). An octosporeosis of the black blowfly, *Phormia regina*: incidence rates of host and parasite. *Z. Parasitenkunde* 30, 33–39.

Kramer, J. P. (1968a). On microsporidian diseases of noxious invertebrates. *Proc. Joint U.S.–Japan Sem. Microbial Control Insect Pests, Fukuoka,* 1967, pp. 135–138.

Kramer, J. P. (1968b). An octosporeosis of the black blowfly *Phormia regina*: effect of temperature on the longevity of diseased adults. *Texas Rep. Biol. Med.* 26, 199–204.

Kramer, J. P. (1970). Longevity of microsporidian spores with special reference to *Octosporea muscaedomesticae* Flu. *Acta Protozool.* 8, 217–224.

Laigo, F. M., and Tamashiro, M. (1967). Interactions between a microsporidian pathogen of the lawn armyworm and the hymenopterous parasite *Apanteles marginiventris*. *J. Invertebr. Pathol.* 9, 546–554.

Laird, M. (1971). Microbial control of arthropods of medical importance. *In* "Microbial Control of Insects and Mites" (H. D. Burges and N. W. Hussey, eds.), pp. 387–406. Academic Press, New York.

Lewis, L. C., and Lynch, R. E. (1974). Lyophilization, vacuum drying, and subsequent storage of *Nosema pyrausta* spores. *J. Invertebr. Pathol.* 24, 149–153.

Lipa, J. J. (1957). Observations on development and pathogenicity of the parasite of *Aporia crataegi* L. (Lepidoptera) – *Nosema aporiae* n.sp. *Acta Parasitol. Polonica* 5, 559–584.

Lipa, J. J. (1963). Studia inwazjólogiczne i epizootiologiczne nad kilkoma gatunkami pier wotniaków z rzędu Microsporidia pasozytującymi w owadach. *Prace Naukowe Instytutu Ochrony Roślin* 5, 103–165.

Lipa, J. J., and Steinhaus, E. A. (1959). *Nosema hippodamia* n.sp., a microsporidian parasite of *Hippodamia convergens* Guérin (Coleoptera, Coccinellidae). *J. Insect Pathol.* 1, 304–308.

Maddox, J. V. (1973). The persistence of the Microsporida in the environment. *Entomol. Soc. Amer. Misc. Publ.* 9, 99–104.

Martignoni, M. E. (1964). Mass production of insect pathogens. *In* "Biological Control of Insect Pests and Weeds" (P. DeBach and E. I. Schlinger, eds.), pp. 579–609. Chapman and Hall, London.

McLaughlin, R. E. (1966). Laboratory techniques for rearing disease-free insect colonies: Elimination of *Mattesia grandis* McLaughlin, and *Nosema* sp. from colonies of boll weevils. *J. Econ. Entomol.* 59, 401–404.

McLaughlin, R. E. (1971). Use of protozoans for microbial control of insects. *In* "Microbial Control of Insects and Mites" (H. D. Burges and N. W. Hussey, eds.), pp. 151–172. Academic Press, New York.

McLaughlin, R. E. (1973). Protozoa as microbial control agents. *Entomol. Soc. Amer. Misc. Publ.* 9, 95–98.

McLaughlin, R. E., and Bell, M. R. (1970). Mass production *in vivo* of two protozoan pathogens, *Mattesia grandis* and *Glugea gasti*, of the boll weevil, *Anthonomus grandis*. *J. Invertebr. Pathol.* 16, 84–88.

McLaughlin, R. E., Cleveland, T. C., Daum, R. J., and Bell, M. R. (1969). Development of the bait principle for boll weevil control. IV. Field tests with a bait containing a feeding stimulant and the sporozoans *Glugea gasti* and *Mattesia grandis*. *J. Invertebr. Pathol.* 13, 429–441.

McLaughlin, R. E., Daum, R. J., and Bell, M. R. (1968). Development of the bait principle for boll-weevil control. III. Field-cage tests with a feeding stimulant and the protozoans *Mattesia grandis* (Neogregarinida) and a microsporidian. *J. Invertebr. Pathol.* 12, 168–174.

McNeil, J. N., and Brooks, W. M. (1974). Interactions of the hyper-parasitoids *Catolaccus aeneoviridis* [Hym.: Pteromalidae] and *Spilochalis side* [Hym.: Chalcididae] with the microsporidans *Nosema heliothidis* and *N. campoletidis*. *Entomophaga* 19, 195–204.

Milner, R. J. (1973a). *Nosema whitei*, a microsporidan pathogen of some species of *Tribolium*. IV. The effect of temperature, humidity and larval age on pathogenicity for *T. castaneum*. *Entomophaga* 18, 305–315.

Milner, R. J. (1973b). *Nosema whitei*, a microsporidan pathogen of some species of *Tribolium*. V. Comparative pathogenicity and host range. *Entomophaga* 18, 383–390.

Mistric, W. J., Jr., and Smith, F. D. (1973). Tobacco budworm: control on flue-cured tobacco with certain microbial pesticides. *J. Econ. Entomol.* 66, 979–982.

Ohshima, K. (1964). Stimulative or inhibitive substance to evaginate the filament of *Nosema bombycis* Nägeli. I. The case of artificial buffer solution. *Japan. J. Zool.* 14, 209–229.

Paillot, A. (1933). "L'infection chez les insectes." G. Patissier, Trévoux.

Payne, N. M. (1933). A parasitic hymenopteron as a vector of an insect disease. *Entomol. News* 44, 22.

Pillai, J. S. (1974). *Pleistophora milesi*, a new species of Microsporida from *Maorigoeldia argyropus* Walker (Diptera: Culicidae) in New Zealand. *J. Invertebr. Pathol.* 24, 234–237.

Reynolds, D. G. (1972). Experimental introduction of a microsporidan into a wild population of *Culex pipiens fatigans* Wied. *Bull. WHO* 46, 807–812.

Rosický, B. (1951). Nosematosis of *Otiorrhynchus ligustici*. II. The influence of the parasitization by *Nosema otiorrhynchi* Weiser 1951 on the susceptibility of the beetles to insecticides. *Vestn. Česk. Společnosti Zool.* 15, 219–234.

Savage, K. E., Lowe, R. E., Hazard, E. I., and Lofgren, C. S. (1971). Studies of the transmission of *Plasmodium gallinaceum* by *Anopheles quadrimaculatus* infected with a *Nosema* sp. *Bull. WHO* 45, 845–847.

Seibold, H. R., and Fussell, E. N. (1973). Intestinal microsporidiosis in *Callicebus moloch*. *Lab. Ani. Sci.* 23, 115–118.

Shadduck, J. A. (1973). Possible hazards of Protozoa to non-target animals and man. *WHO VBC/WP/73.4*, 4 pp.

Sikorowski, P. P., and Madison, C. H. (1968). Host-parasite relationships of *Thelohania corethrae* (Nosematidae: Microsporidia) from *Chaoborus astictopus* (Diptera: Chaoboridae). *J. Invertebr. Pathol.* 11, 390–397.

Smirnoff, W. A. (1967). Effects of some plant juices on the uglynest caterpillar, *Archips cerasivoranus*, infected with microsporidia. *J. Invertebr. Pathol.* 9, 26–29.

Smirnoff, W. A. (1968). Adaptation of the microsporidian *Thelohania pristiphorae* to the tent caterpillars *Malacosoma disstria* and *Malacosoma americanum*. *J. Invertebr. Pathol.* 11, 321–325.

Smirnoff, W. A. (1973). Biochemical exploration in insect pathology. *In* "Current Topics Comparative Pathobiology" (T. C. Cheng, ed.), 2, 89–106. Academic Press, New York.

Smirnoff, W. A. (1974). Adaptation of *Thelohania pristiphorae* on ten species of Diprionidae and Tenthredinidae. *J. Invertebr. Pathol.* 23, 114–116.

Steinhaus, E. A. (1949). "Principles of Insect Pathology." McGraw-Hill, New York.

Steinhaus, E. A. (1954). The effects of disease on insect populations. *Hilgardia* 23, 197–261.

Steinhaus, E. A. (1957). Microbial diseases of insects. *Ann. Rev. Microbiol.* 11, 165-182.

Stejskal, M. (1959). Correlation entre les maladies des abeilles et les conditions atmosphériques. *Bull. Apicole* 2, 103-106.

Tanabe, A. M. (1971). The pathology of two Microsporida in the armyworm, *Pseudaletia unipuncta* (Haworth) (Lepidoptera, Noctuidae). Ph.D. thesis, University of California, Berkeley.

Tanada, Y. (1955). Field observations on a microsporidian parasite of *Pieris rapae* (L.) and *Apanteles glomeratus* (L.). *Proc. Hawaii. Entomol. Soc.* 15, 609-616.

Tanada, Y. (1959). Microbial control of insect pests. *Ann. Rev. Entomol.* 4, 277-302.

Tanada, Y. (1963). Epizootiology of infectious diseases. *In* "Insect Pathology an Advanced Treatise" (E. A. Steinhaus, ed.), 2, 423-475. Academic Press, New York.

Tanada, Y. (1964). Epizootiology of insect diseases. *In* "Biological Control of Insect Pests and Weeds" (P. DeBach and E. I. Schlinger, eds.), pp. 548-578. Chapman and Hall, London.

Tanada, Y. (1967). Microbial pesticides. *In* "Pest Control Biological, Physical, and Selected Chemical Methods" (W. W. Kilgore and R. L. Doutt, eds.), pp. 31-88. Academic Press, New York.

Tanada, Y., and Omi, E. M. (1974). Persistence of insect viruses in field populations of alfalfa insects. *J. Invertebr. Pathol.* 23, 360-365.

Thomson, H. M. (1958). Some aspects of the epidemiology of a microsporidian parasite of the spruce budworm, *Choristoneura fumiferana* (Clem.). *Can.J. Zool.* 36, 309-316.

Undeen, A. H. (1975). Growth of *Nosema algerae* in pig kidney cell cultures. *J. Protozool.*, 22, 107-110.

Undeen, A. H., and Alger, N. E. (1971). A density gradient method for fractionating microsporidian spores. *J. Invertebr. Pathol.* 18, 419-420.

Undeen, A. H., and Alger, N. E. (1975). The effect of the microsporidian, *Nosema algerae* in *Anopheles stephensi*. *J. Invertebr. Pathol.* 25, 19-24.

Undeen, A. H., and Maddox, J. V. (1973). The infection of non-mosquito hosts by injection with spores of the microsporidan *Nosema algerae*. *J. Invertebr. Pathol.* 22, 258-265.

Vávra, J., and Undeen, A. H. (1970). *Nosema algerae* n.sp. (Cnidospora, Microsporida) a pathogen in a laboratory colony of *Anopheles stephensi* Liston (Diptera, Culicidae). *J. Protozool.* 17, 240-249.

Ward, R. A., and Savage, K. E. (1972). Effects of microsporidian parasites upon anopheline mosquitoes and malarial infection. *Basic Res. Malaria, Spec. Issue, Proc. Helminthol. Soc. Washington* 39, 434-438.

Weiser, J. (1956). Protozoäre Infektionen im Kampfe gegen Insekten. *Z. Pflanzenkrankh. (Pflanz npath.) Pflanzenschutz.* 63, 625–638.

Weiser, J. (1957a). Mikrosporidien des Schwammspinners und Goldafters. *Z. Angew. Entomol.* 40, 509–521.

Weiser, J. (1957b). Možnosti biologického boje s přastevníčkem americkým (*Hyphantria cunea* Drury)-III. *Cesk. Parasitol.* 4, 359–367.

Weiser, J. (1961a). Die Mikrosporidien als Parasiten der Insekten. *Monographien Z. Angew. Entomol.* 17, 149 pp.

Weiser, J. (1961b). A new microsporidian from the bark beetle *Pityokteines curvidens* Germar (Coleoptera, Scolytidae) in Czechoslovakia. *J. Insect Pathol.* 3, 324–329.

Weiser, J. (1963). Sporozoan infections. *In* "Insect Pathology an Advanced Treatise" (E. A. Steinhaus, ed.), 2, 291–334. Academic Press, New York.

Weiser, J. (1965). Influence of environmental factors on protozoan diseases of insects. *Proc. 12th Intern. Cong. Entomol.*, p. 726.

Weiser, J. (1966). "Nemoci Hmyzu." Academia, Prague.

Weiser, J. (1969). Immunity of insects to Protozoa. *In* "Immunity to Parasitic Animals" (G. J. Jackson, R. Herman, and I. Singer, eds.), 1, 129–147. Appleton-Century-Crofts, New York.

Weiser, J. (1970). Recent advances in insect pathology. *Annu. Rev. Entomol.* 15, 245–256.

Weiser, J., and Veber, J. (1955). Možnosti biolgického boje s přastevníčkem americkým (*Hyphantria cunea* Drury)-II. *Cesk. Parasitol.* 2, 191–199.

Weiser, J., and Veber, J. (1957). Die Mikrosporidie *Thelohania hyphantriae* Weiser des weissen Bärenspinners und anderer Mitglieder seiner Biocönose. *Z. Angew. Entomol.* 40, 55–70.

Wilson, G. G. (1973). Incidence of Microsporida in a field population of spruce budworm. *Bi-monthly Res. Notes Environ. Can. Forestry Serv.* 29, 35–36.

Wilson, G. G. (1974). Effects of larval age at inoculation, and dosage of microsporidan (*Nosema fumiferana*) spores, on mortality of spruce budworm (*Choristoneura fumiferana*). *Can. J. Zool.* 52, 993–996.

Methods in Microsporidiology

JIŘÍ VÁVRA

DEPARTMENT OF PROTOZOOLOGY
INSTITUTE OF PARASITOLOGY
CZECHOSLOVAK ACADEMY OF SCIENCES
PRAHA 2, VINCINO 7
CZECHOSLOVAKIA

AND

J. V. MADDOX

SECTION OF ECONOMIC ENTOMOLOGY
ILLINOIS NATURAL HISTORY SURVEY
URBANA, ILLINOIS 61801

I. INTRODUCTION

The purpose of this chapter is to inform the reader (at all levels of experience with microsporidian research) of the methods most commonly used by microsporidiologists. In addition to the classical methods that have been used for many years, more sophisticated techniques, utilizing many different scientific disciplines, are increasingly being employed in the study of microsporidia. We believe that a working knowledge of this methodology should be possessed by workers in the field of microsporidology. We realize that old methods are constantly being modified and new methods developed. Consequently, this chapter will be out of date soon after it is finished. In any event, we hope it will help microsporidologists expand the scope of their research.

II. FIELD COLLECTIONS

When the investigator is simply interested in determining whether a microsporidian infection occurs in an animal population, any collection technique that is most productive can be used. Southwood (1966) describes many collection techniques for invertebrate animals. Large numbers of the animals can be collectively pulverized in a blender or homogenizer, strained through a medium mesh cheesecloth to remove the large debris, and centrifuged at 1,000 g for 10 minutes. The bottom layer of the resulting sediment is then examined under a compound microscope for the presence of microsporidian spores. If no microsporidian spores are found after examining several hundred individuals in this manner, one may assume the animal population either is free from microsporidian infections or the incidence of infection is so low there is very little chance of finding individually infected animals.

Even when microsporidian spores are found in this sediment, it does not necessarily mean a microsporidian infection exists in that animal population. Predators and scavengers often ingest other animal species which are infected with microsporidia and these spores may remain in the digestive tract for some time. If spores are found in the composite sample, individually infected animals of that species should be collected and active infections of the host confirmed. A few individuals of the host population should be preserved for identification.

When the investigator is sampling populations to determine not only the presence of a microsporidian infection, but also the incidence of the infection in the population, the choice of a sampling technique becomes more important. Animals infected with microsporidia often exhibit behavioral or activity differences that cause certain sampling techniques to bias the selection of infected individuals. For example, a number of workers (Kudo, 1921, 1922; Kramer, 1965; Savage and Lowe, 1970) observed that

infected insects are often less active than healthy ones. Kudo
(1921) was able to capture infected copepods with a pipette but
was unable to capture healthy ones, and others have had the same
experience with infected mosquito larvae. Therefore, any type of
collection technique which allows the more active, healthy
individuals to escape while capturing a larger percentage of the
slower, more inactive, infected individuals would produce a biased
sample, giving results which would indicate a higher percentage
infection than actually exists in the host population. Sweepnets,
aquatic dredge nets, and individual hand collections could produce
such biased results.

Another bias, but in the opposite direction, often results when
using various types of traps which attract the animals. If these
traps require the animal to move for a considerable distance, and
if infected hosts are weakened and, therefore, not as capable of
movement as healthy individuals, these traps will capture a
smaller percentage of infected individuals than is actually
present in the host population. *Chironomus californicus,* adults
of the aquatic midge, infected with a *Gurleya* sp. were unable to
fly (Hunter 1968). Kramer (1968) thought that his estimate of
Octosporea muscaedomesticae infections in black blow fly populations had a downward bias because the weaker infected flies
were not as likely to enter his bait traps as were the healthy
flies. We have found that this sampling error occurs when light
traps are used to collect adults of the buff colored sod webworm
moth, *Crambus trisectus*. Light traps placed over 100 yards from
sod containing the sod webworm population trapped only 6% infected adults. Traps placed 100 ft from this sodded area trapped
over 20% infected adults and collections made by hand directly
from the sodded area contained 60% infected adults (Maddox,
unpublished results).

It is therefore very important, when the instance of a microsporidian infection within a host population is significant, that
any activity or behavioral differences on the part of infected
hosts be taken into consideration when designing the sampling
technique. If the effects of the microsporidian on its host are
not known, it may be desirable to use more than one type of
sampling procedure.

A third type of bias may result from a higher susceptibility of
infected animals to environmental changes during the subsequent
handling of collected samples. This may occur when samples of
living planctonic organisms are transported under unfavorable
conditions such as high temperature and lack of oxygen. Under
these conditions the infected animals die first and decompose
quickly, causing an apparent reduction in the percentage of
infected animals in the sample (Vavra, unpublished results).

III. SELECTING HEALTHY AND DISEASED ANIMALS

The ability to distinguish between healthy individuals and those
with microsporidian infections is largely dependent on the pathogenicity of the microsporidian species, the host tissues infected
by that microsporidian, and the cellular response of the host.
Many animals with microsporidian infections appear normal. The
differences between healthy and infected animals can be largely
classified as either morphological or behavioral differences.

A. MORPHOLOGICAL DIFFERENCES

Many microsporidian infections cause deformities in their hosts,
such as the large cysts in fish (Kudo, 1924), the molting abnormalities in larval insects, deformed shells in snails (Mickelson,
1963), larvaeform appearance of insect pupae, and twisted wings of
infected insect adults. Microsporidian infections sometimes
produce color differences and infected individuals often appear
milky-white. This is especially true of animals with transparent
or translucent exoskeletons, such as mosquito larvae, chironomid
larvae, copepods, and *Daphnia,* and is usually the result of an
infected tissue such as the fat body being enlarged and filled
with microsporidian spores (Kudo, 1924: Hunter, 1968). Some
animals infected with microsporidia develop colors other than the
milky white color described above. Blue crabs infected with a
Nosema sp. are pale greenish (Sprague 1965), and Simulid larvae
infected with *Caudospoa simuli* have large red pigmented cysts
(Weiser 1964). Size differences are often noted between infected
and healthy animals. Some microsporidian infections cause their
hosts to be stunted in growth whereas other microsporidian infections cause their hosts to delay molting and continue growth
until their size exceeds that of the normal healthy individuals
(Kudo 1924, Fisher 1961).

B. BEHAVIORAL DIFFERENCES

Animals infected with microsporidia are often more sluggish than
healthy animals. They may walk or swim slowly or with difficult
uncoordinated movement and heavily infected adult insects are
sometimes unable to fly at all (Kramer, 1965; Hunter, 1968).
Infected animals sometimes take on an unusual posture or abnormal
body movements such as the twitching of legs and spontaneous
muscular contractions (Savage and Lowe, 1970). Although few
observations have been made in this area, there is an indication
that some animals infected with microsporidia respond differently
to such environmental stimuli as light and temperature. For
example, during sunny days *Daphnia hyalina* infected with
Pleistophora schafernai assemble in large masses in shallow, un-
shaded parts of ponds. This distribution is maintained until

sunset when the infected individuals quickly disperse and mix with the rest of the population (Vavra, unpublished results).

From the diverse symptoms produced by the different microsporidian infections, it is obvious that one cannot always depend on external appearance to distinguish between infected and uninfected animals. Many infected animals have no external symptoms and those external symptoms displayed by animals infected with microsporidia are not exclusive to animals infected with microsporidia. These symptoms, however, may be very helpful in separating healthy from diseased animals if their limitations are understood.

IV. EXAMINATION OF DISEASED HOSTS

When the animal to be examined is small, such as a mosquito or a copepod, the simplest method for determining the presence of a microsporidian infection is to place the animal in a small drop of water on a microscope slide and cover it with a cover glass. If the epidermis is transparent, the intact animal can be examined under a compound microscope and the tissues infected by the microsporidian determined. The use of Zernike phase-contrast or Nomarski interference-contrast greatly facilitates identification of spores and vegetative forms of the microsporidian. Some animals have their cuticle more transparent at the ventral side (black fly larvae, mosquito larvae). However, when these animals are put into a drop of water on a slide, they immediately turn with their ventral side down. They should be placed into a drop of water on a cover slip and inverted rapidly on the slide. The pressure between the cover slip and the slide will hold them securely in the desired position. If the cuticle of the animal being examined is not transparent, the animal can be squashed with slight pressure on the cover glass. If the vegetative forms of the microsporidian are to be observed, measured, or photographed, physiological saline or insect tissue culture fluid should be substituted for the drop of water placed on the slide. In water, the vegetative forms swell and burst as a result of osmotic pressure.

In larger invertebrates individual tissues can be removed and examined under a cover slip on a microscope slide. For example, large insect larvae are pinned ventral side up in a small wax-bottom dish and the body cavity opened with fine surgical scissors from head to the anus along a med-ventral longitudinal line. The body wall is then pulled open, pinned to the wax dish, and the dish flooded with invertebrate saline. The individual tissues of the larva are then removed with fine pointed tweezers, rinsed in a separate container of invertebrate saline and squashed gently between a glass microscope slide and cover slip. This slide can then be examined under a compound microscope. When possible, observations on the individual host tissues should be supplemented with observations of serially sectioned infected hosts.

It is often desirable to determine the presence of a micro-sporidian infection in a living host without sacrificing the host. When part of the digestive tract of the host is infected by the microsporidian, the presence of a microsporidian infection can frequently be determined by examining the fecal material for microsporidian spores. The animal in question can be held in an individual container for a short period of time and the resulting fecal material examined. Care must be taken not to overlook the possibility that this host did not simply ingest portions of another infected animal. The previous history of the animal being examined (field collected, laboratory reared, etc.) should obviously be considered. Microsporidian infections that do not involve the digestive tract can frequently be diagnosed without sacrificing the animal by clipping off a leg, collecting a small amount of hemolymph, and examining this hemolymph for the presence of microspridia. The removal of an arthropod leg usually does not interfere with normal development of the animal.

V. EXTRACTION AND PURIFICATION OF SPORES FROM INFECTED HOSTS

Microsporidian spores can be extracted from small invertebrate hosts by the following procedure. Infected animals are homogenized in sterile water in a blender, tissue grinder, or other similar apparatus. To depress melanosis of host hemolymph, a volume of 0.01 M solution of the sodium salt of diethyldithiocarbamic acid equal to the host volume may be added to the blender prior to trituration (Fowler and Reeves, 1974a). Ascorbic acid (0.005 M solution in 0.135 M NaCl or Krebs-Ringer saline) may also be used for this purpose. This solution is used for the first washing of the spores. The solution is progressively diluted in each sub-sequent washing (i.e. 1:2, 1:4 etc.) until the material is transferred into distilled water (Cerkasovova, unpublished re-sults).

It is important to estimate during the disruption procedure the actual percentage of damaged spores. When observed with a phase-contract microscope spores damaged by the disruption pro-cess are no longer refractive. A more convenient method is to make a permanent smear with the bacteriological ink ("Burri ink"). The ink penetrates into spores that were open by disruption and stains them grey. Undamaged spores appear as bright spots surrounded by a dark halo of the ink.

After disruption, the homogenate is strained through a double thickness of cheesecloth, a fine mesh screen, or any similar filter which will allow the microsporidian spores to pass through but will filter out the larger body particles of the host. This filtrate is then centrifuged slowly until a pellet of spores is produced. Undeen and Alger (1971) recommend centrifuging at 170 g for 20 minutes, but we have found that centrifuging at greater speeds (20,000 g) for shorter periods of time does not reduce the

viability of most microsporidian spores (Maddox, unpublished
results). The supernatant is examined for the presence of
microsporidian spores, and if no spores are present, the supernatant is discarded. The pellet usually contains two layers,
a white bottom layer and a darker upper layer. The white bottom
layer consists primarily of mature spores whereas the dark, upper
layer contains some mature spores, immature spores, and debris.
The upper layer is removed with a pasteur pipette and discarded
along with the supernatant. The centrifuging process can be
repeated several times to further purify the spores. With minor
modifications, this routine is the most common that has been
used to extract microsporidian spores from small invertebrate
hosts (McLaughlin and Bell, 1970; Cole, 1970; Henry, 1971;
Alger and Undeen, 1971; Ignoffo and Hink, 1971).

Sometimes the homogenization procedure described above does
not adequately separate microsporidian spores and some of these
spores tend to occur in clumps. The clumps of spores are often
removed by the filtering process and, therefore, lost, or if they
are separated in the spore pellet, they may interfere if the
suspension is later counted in a bacterial counter. These clumps
can be broken apart by sonicating the homogenate before filtration,
but care must be taken not to sonicate for too long or at too
high wattage. Twenty watts for ten minutes does not destroy the
viability of most microsporidian spores, but over 50 watts for
three minutes greatly reduces viability (Maddox, unpublished
results). The effect of sonication on each microsporidian species
should be determined before using sonication as a part of the
purification process.

The spores of some microsporidia, such as *Nosema whitei*,
extrude their filaments when dried spores are placed in a water
suspension, and the procedure described above is not applicable
for the extraction or preparation of these spores. This procedure
is discussed later.

For most uses, the purity of the spores obtained from the
above procedure is sufficient. For certain studies, however,
additional purification methods are necessary. For example, very
pure preparations are required for serological and biochemical
studies of microsporidian spores, for injection into animals,
and introduction into tissue cultures. Cole (1970) achieved
levels of purity greater than 99% using a method based on the
principles of "triangulation" and counter current distribution
chromatography. This method requires no specialized equipment
and does not expose the spores to any chemical other than water.

The method for obtaining extremely pure microsporidian spores
for protein analysis (Fowler and Reeves, 1974a) is a modified
Cole's procedure. However, before final purification the crude
spore sample is subjected to osmotic shock treatment with a high
ionic strength salt solution (58 g NaCl; 37.2 g Na-EDTA; 12 g
tris(hydroxymethyl)ammomethane base; 100 ml distilled water).

This treatment disrupted osmotically sensitive immature stages of the pathogen and host cell, minimized spore clumping, and released adhering materials from the exterior of the spores. Bioassay of spores subjected to osmotic shock indicated little loss of viability.

Undeen and Alger (1971) obtained very pure *Nosema algerae* spores using a density gradient method. The density gradient was made from Ludox (a colloid of 40% silica in a sodium hydroxide solution with a pH of 9.8 and a specific gravity of 1.303, du Pont). A continuous gradient from 40% silica on the bottom to almost pure water on the top was established. Mosquitoes were crushed in a tissue grinder, strained through an 80 mesh copper screen, and centrifuged at 170 g for 20 minutes. The resulting residue was resuspended in one ml of distilled water, carefully layered on top of the gradient and centrifuged in a swinging bucket head at 16,300 g for 20 minutes at 4°C. The spore fraction was drawn off and washed twice with distilled water to remove the silica and sodium hydroxide. A high yield of spores infective to the first instar *Anopheles stevensi* larvae was obtained by this method.

McLaughlin and Bell (1970) inactivated microbial contaminants in a *Glugea gasti* spore suspension by treating with a concentrated solution of quarternary ammonium salt (Zephiran, 1 to 500 dilution) for fifteen minutes. Spores were then removed from this concentration of Zephiran by centrifugation and resuspended in a Zephiran solution (1 to 1000 dilution). Such treatment eliminated microbial growth when spores were applied to the surface of the host (boll weevil) diet.

VI. QUANTITATING SPORE SUSPENSIONS AND SPORE DOSAGES

For many experiments the concentration of spores in a spore suspension or the number of spores administered to a host must be known. Some type of counting chamber is almost universally used for this purpose. In order to obtain meaningful results with a counting chamber, it must be used correctly and enough counts taken to make the standard error as low as possible. At least 400 spores should be counted. Burgess and Thompson (1971) have described the correct procedures for using a counting chamber to determine concentrations of microorganisms in suspension.

The suspension can be dispensed or fed with a syringe, micro-liter pipette, or calibrated wire loop. It is very important, however, that the spores remain uniformly suspended while aliquots are being dispensed or fed. If a syringe is being used, some method must be used to prevent the spores from settling to the bottom of the syringe barrel. McLaughlin (1967) used a 2% aqueous solution of hydroxyethyl cellulose for suspending spores of *Mattesia grandis* and this works well for microsporidian spores. The 2% solution is autoclaved and passed through a

coarse fritted-glass filter before use. If one is concerned
about the addition of the hydroxyethyl cellulose, a magnetic
stirring device can be used to prevent the settling of spores in
the syringe (Angus, 1964). A small steel ball-bearing is
placed in the barrel of the syringe and the rotation of a motor-
driven magnet directly above the syringe causes the steel ball
to oscillate within the barrel of the syringe. Even when these
methods are used, it is good practice to occasionally check the
number of spores being dispensed by the syringe to insure that
spore distribution remains uniform. When aliquots of the spore
suspension are drawn from a standing container, the container
must be constantly agitated to maintain even spore distribution.

VII. EXPERIMENTAL INFECTION

In many cases the investigator may simply want to establish a
microsporidian infection in a host and is not concerned with the
number of spores ingested by the host. When the number of spores
ingested by a host is not an important consideration, any feeding
method that will cause the host to ingest a large enough number
of spores to initiate an infection is satisfactory. Placing
animals in containers previously occupied by infected hosts is
often sufficient. The host's natural food plant may be dipped
into or sprayed with a suspension containing microsporidian
spores, or spores may be mixed with the food of animals such as
stored grain pests or incorporated into artificial dietary
mixtures. Infected tissues may be fed directly to the hosts and
with aquatic insects, such as mosquitoes, the macerated bodies of
infected hosts may be added to rearing containers.

When ingested in large numbers, some microsporidia cause a
bacterial septicemia that is often fatal to the host before the
microsporidian has had time to complete its development. It is,
therefore, desirable, even when the exact spore dosage is not
important, to feed at least two different spore concentrations
to the host if both heavy and light concentrations of spores are fed
the possibility of the host dying of bacterial septicemia as a result of excessive spore dosages will be reduced. For example, when
second instar larvae of the fall webworm, *Hypantria cunea*, are fed
100,000 or more spores of the microsporidian *Nosema necatrix*, over
90% mortality occurs within four days after feeding, before the
microsporidian has completed its development (Nordin 1971). Feeding
a high and a low spore dose reduces the possibility of killing all
the hosts with an excessive spore dosage and likewise reduces the
possibility of feeding too few spores to infect the host.

It is often essential that the number of spores ingested by the
host be known. This is obviously a necessity for bioassay or
dosage mortality studies, but the number of spores ingested also
influences many of the host-parasite relationships between the
microsporidian and its host. Larval growth and development,

deformities, fecundity, activity, the extent of transovarial transmission and the generation time of the microsporidian are all influenced by the spore dosage.

Actively feeding terrestrial animals that ingest solid food are most easily fed known spore dosages. Known quantities of spores can be applied to small pieces of the host's natural food and these small pieces of food offered to the host for a predetermined period of time. Those hosts that entirely consume their food have ingested the entire spore dose and those animals not consuming the entire piece of food can be discarded from the experiment. Maddox (1968) applied this method by using small pieces of corn leaves to feed known dosages of *Nosema necatrix*, to the armyworm, *Pseudaletia unipuncta*. Henry (1967) used small lettuce discs to feed known numbers of *Nosema acridophagus* spores to grasshoppers.

When spores with identifiable morphological characters are to be selected for infection, the isolation technique described by Fowler and Reeves (1974c) can be used. This procedure requires the spreading of a spore suspension over a slide coated with agar and the removal of the desired spore(s) by cutting out a small agar disc from the agar layer with a Darley isolator. The agar disk is then fed to the host animal together with its natural food.

Known spore dosages can often be administered to predatory animals by applying the spore dose to the body of the prey and then feeding the prey to the predator. For example, spores may be applied to the abdomen of small flies that can then be fed to praying mantids. If the mantid consumes the entire fly, it has ingested the entire spore dosage. Spore suspensions can be fed directly to some animals. Henry (1967) was able to feed spore suspensions of *N. acridophagus* directly to grasshoppers by placing the spore suspension on the mouthparts. We have been able to use this method for feeding spore suspensions directly to lepidopteran larvae but some larvae will often refuse to ingest the spore dosage directly and must be discarded from the experiment. This method is also very time consuming. Some adult flies, such as the black blowfly, *Phormia reginia*, can be fed spore suspensions directly if a small amoutn of sucrose is added to the spore suspension and the flies are not watered 24 hours prior to a calibrated platinum wire loop for feeding. This holding device consists of a vacuum source attached to a small glass medicine dropper by a flexible rubber tube. The flies are knocked down with CO_2, the vacuum cut off by squeezing the flexible rubber tubing and the glass medicine dropper touched to the dorsal thorax of the fly. The pressure on the rubber tube is released and the vacuum holds the fly to the medicine dropper. After feeding, the glass medicine dropper is inserted into the fly cage, the flexible rubber tube pinched shut, and the fly falls into the cage (Maddox, unpublished).

Phytophagous insects with sucking mouthparts present special difficulties in feeding known spore dosages. We have had considerable difficulty feeding known spore dosages of a microsporidian from the green stink but, *Acrosternum hilarie*, to its host and to other hemipterans. The stink bug can be fed spore suspensions through a membrane but the spores settle out quickly, making spore dosage estimates very difficult. After starving for one day, stink bugs can often be induced to feed by forcing the beak into a small capillary tube containing a known quantity of spore suspension. Known spore dosages can be fed to hemipterans in this manner, but it is a very time-consuming process and many individuals must be discarded because they refuse to drink the entire suspension (Maddox, unpublished results).

Spore dosages are often determined in a relative manner by allowing animals to feed on a medium containing known concentrations of spores. This is the method most often used with stored grain insects (Milner, 1972a; Burgess *et al.*,1971). The insects may be allowed to feed on this diet for a given period of time, then removed and placed in a medium containing no spores. If the average food consumption of that insect and the concentration of spores per unit of diet are known, the approximate number of spores ingested by the insect can be calculated. In many cases, however, the insects are simply placed in a medium containing a known concentration of spores and allowed to develop in that medium for the duration of the experiment. In this case, the spore dosage is usually stated in number of spores per gram of diet rather than actual number of spores ingested by the insect. This type of quantitating procedure differs from methods described earlier in that the hosts are constantly ingesting spores over a long period of time rather than receiving a single spore dose.

It is usually difficult to determine how many spores are ingested by small aquatic invertebrates. Mosquito larvae can be infected with some microsporidia by adding spores to water in larval rearing dishes (Canning and Hulls, 1970; Undeen and Maddox, 1973). Known numbers of spores can be added to known volumes of water, but the spores settle to the bottom of the dish, and the number of spores per unit area of the bottom of the rearing container is probably a more accurate way of stating spore concentration than number of spores per volume of water. Bioassays and dosage mortality studies can be conducted with some mosquito microsporidia by exposing mosquito larvae to known concentrations of spores for specific periods of time (Undeen, personal communication), but the results are more variable than when spores are incorporated into a solid diet. The spores are not homogenously distributed on the bottom of the rearing dishes. Aquatic insects feed in various ways: some are bottom feeders, some are surface feeders, and some are filter feeders. This makes it extremely difficult to determine the number of spores ingested per host and increases the varability in the number of spores ingested per host. It may be possible to incorporate spores of microsporidia infecting aquatic insects into small diet pellets that could be fed to individual larvae, but so far this procedure has not been sucessfully utilized. One of the problems in formulating

pellets containing spores is that spores of many aquatic insects
cannot withstand drying and this is often necessary for formulating
a pellet that does not disintegrate in water.

Many animals can be force fed by inserting a blunt needle into
the buccal cavity (Martouret, 1962). This procedure is much
easier and produces less shock in larger animals. Care must be
taken not to pucture the walls of the gut. When the gut is
badly punctured, the insect will usually die from bacterial
septicemia before the microsporidian has a chance to develop.

Burgess and Thompson (1971) discussed the practical aspects of
feeding known dosages of pathogens. They cautioned that larvae of
a species that are cannibalistic or eat dead bodies must be kept
singly and that when artificial media are being used to rear the
host the stability of the microsporidian in the medium must be
checked carefully. Any antibiotics or preservatives may be
omitted if they affect the microsporidian. We have found that
starvation prior to feeding causes some insects to be more
susceptible to microsporidian infections. The LC_{50} of *Nosema*
necatrix is lower in armyworm larvae starved for 24 hours prior
to feeding than in larvae that have not been starved (Maddox,
unpublished results). This is probably because when the midgut
lumen is empty, ingested spores have a much greater chance of
extruding filaments through epithelial cells of the digestive
tract than when the gut is filled with food. Animals with
microsporidian infections involving the midgut must be kept singly
if the duration of the experiment exceeds the generation time of
the microspridian. When animals with such infections are held in
a common cage or container, one infected animal can spread the
infection to the others, making bioassay or dosage mortality
studies meaningless.

Transmission can be accomplished experimentally in the laboratory by transplanting infected tissue (Fisher and Sanborn, 1959)
or injecting purified forms of the microsporidian (Undeen and
Maddox, 1973) into the hemocoel of the host. Insects can be
infected by injecting sterile spore suspensions into the hemocoel
if the spores extrude their filaments into the hemolymph. If
filaments are not extruded into the hemocoel, some pretreatment
of the spores to extrude the polar filament is necessary before
injection. The suspension injected into the hemocoel must be
sterile, otherwise the insect will die from bacterial septicemia.
Undeen and Maddox (1973) were able to infect many different
arthropod hosts with *Nosema algerae,* a microsporidian from
mosquitoes, by injecting sterile spore suspensions into the
hemocoel of these arthropods. The spore suspension was purified
by a density gradient method (Undeen and Alger, 1971) described
earlier. One hundred units of penicillin, 100 milligrams of
streptomycin sulfate, and 0.25 milligrams of fungizone were added
per milliliter of spore suspension.

Injections can be made with a 27-gauge or smaller hypodermic
needle mounted on a glass syringe. The needle is pushed through
the insect's integument into the hemocoel without puncturing the

alimentary canal. In insect larvae, little bleeding will occur if
the needle is pushed through a proleg. By injecting microsporidia
into the hemocoel it is frequently possible to infect a wide range
of hosts that are not susceptible to that microsporidian administered *per os* (Fisher and Sanborn, 1962; Undeen and Maddox, 1973).
Care must be taken when comparing microsporidian infections transmitted to insects by injection *per os*. When spores of *Nosema
mesnili* were injected into the hemocoel of *Pieris brassicae* on the
ovipositer of Hymenoptera, the usual sequence of tissue invasion
seen in *per os* infections was reversed (Hostounsky, 1970). Large
quantities of microsporidian spores can often be obtained by injecting the microsporidian into a host that is considerably larger
than its natural host. Undeen and Maddox (1973) were able to obtain as many *N. algerae* spores from one infected *Heliothis zea*
larva as were produced by 2,000 infected mosquitoes.

Infections can often be transmitted from one host to another
by injecting blood from an infected host into the hemocoel of a
noninfected host. Because the blood is already sterile and
contains vegetative forms of the microsporidian, the purification
and extrusion treatments necessary before spores can be injected
into the hemocoel are not necessary when blood from an infected
host is used.

In some kinds of hosts the invasion route of the microsporidian
during the experimental infection may be determined by a ligaturing
technique (Abdel-Malek and Steinhaus, 1948). In this method, the
host larva is allowed to feed on infected material and then
ligatured into several body segments. Later, it is determined
in which segment and in which organ the infection develops. The
technique is, of course, limited to hosts that can withstand
ligaturing for a period of time sufficient for the development
of the microsporidian.

VIII. MAINTENANCE OF MICROSPORIDIAN INFECTIONS IN THE LABORATORY

In order to maintain microsporidian infections in the laboratory,
one must first be able to rear the host. For methods on maintaining
laboratory cultures of insects the reader is referred to Smith
(1966).

A. *NOSEMA WHITEI*

Nosema whitei can be easily maintained in laboratory cultures of
the stored grain pest *Tribolium castaneum* (Fisher 1961, Milner
1972a). Healthy cultures of these beetles are reared in a medium
containing plain flour and dried yeast mixed in a 12 to 1 ratio that
may be autoclaved before use. At 30°C these beetles complete a
generation in about 30 days.

T. castaneum colonies can be infected by rearing in medium
containing 10^4 spores per gram. Spore counts much higher than
this cause high mortality of early instars of the beetle and are
not satisfactory for maintaining infected cultures. The spore

mixture is prepared by grinding dry diseased cadavers in a mortar. A weighed aliquot of this finely ground spore mixture is mixed with a known volume of water and the number of spores determined with a bacteria counter. The number of spores per gram in the dry cadaver mixture can then be calculated and diluted with the rearing medium to give a final spore concentration of 10^4 spores per gram. Approximately 100 grams of the above mixture is placed in a container and 50 to 100 *T. castaneum* adults introduced. This infected colony can be maintained for several months by periodically removing excess adults and adding fresh sterile food. However, in order to insure continued production of infected individuals, an infected colony should be set up every 60 days as described above.

These infected colonies should be checked periodically and the dead, diseased larvae removed with a sieve and stored as dry cadavers at 5°C until needed. Dry *Nosema whitei* spores cannot be mixed with water before being added to the dietary medium because most of the polar filaments are extruded when dry spores are wet.

B. *OCTOSPOREA MUSCAEDOMESTICAE*

Octosporea muscaedomesticae, an intestinal parasite of Calypterate flies, is not easily maintained as a continuously infected culture, but it is easy to maintain the infection in the laboratory by periodic transmission from diseased to healthy adults.

The black blow fly, *Phormia regina*, is a common host of *O. muscaedomesticae* and easily reared in the laboratory. Adult flies are caged in one-pint cardboard containers covered with an inverted petri dish bottom. Glass shell vials containing food, water, and an ovipositional site are inserted through holes in the pint container. The flies are fed a dry 1:1 mixture of sucrose and powdered milk in one of the shell vials. Another shell vial is filled with water and plugged with a cotton stopper, and the third shell vial contains a small piece of pork liver as an ovipositional site. The eggs are placed on pork liver contained in a small aluminum tray. This tray is placed in a gallon cardboard container, the bottom of which is covered with 2 inches of sawdust. As the fly larvae mature, they crawl out of the aluminum pan and pupate in the sawdust. The pupae are removed from the sawdust and allowed to emerge in the adult cages described above.

O. muscaedomesticae spores can be introduced into the adult fly cages by a number of methods, but we have found that the simplest way to infect 50-100 adult flies is to introduce two or three heavily infected blow fly adults into the cage containing healthy adults. Within one week, most of the healthy flies will be infected. This method eliminates having to extract the spores from infected flies and prepare a spore inoculum. Infected flies live for about three weeks at 27°C, so if flies are held at this

temperature, the above procedure should be repeated every three
weeks in order to have a constant supply of infected *Phormia
regina* adults (Maddox, unpublished results).

C. *NOSEMA NECATRIX*

N. necatrix is a microsporidian that is very pathogenic and not
transovarilly transmitted. Since the infection is confined to the
fat body, spores are not transmitted with fecal material. The
infection must be transmitted from one host to another by ex-
tracting spores from an infected host and feeding them orally to
uninfected larvae. Although the procedure described here is
strictly for the maintenance of *N. necatrix*, this is the basic
procedure we use for maintaining a number of different microsporidian infections in Lepidoptera (Maddox, unpublished results).

N. necatrix has a very wide host range and will infect many
lepidopteran larvae but we have found the woolly bear, *Diacrisia
virginica*, and the salt marsh caterpillar, *Estigmene*, to be
convenient hosts for maintaining *N. necatrix* infections in the
laboratory. Larvae of both these insects are maintained on an
artificial medium described by Yearian *et al.*(1966). The head
and midgut are removed from heavily infected larvae and the
microsporidian spores extracted and purified according to the
preliminary purification method described earlier.

Reusable glass vials, 20 x 50 ml, with plastic snap-on lids
are filled approximately one-half full of the same artificial
medium used to rear the larvae and 10,000 *N. necatrix* spores from
the purified aqueous suspension applied to the surface of the diet.
At least 20 ul of this suspension are needed to obtain a uniform
distribution over the entire diet surface. The suspension is
quantitated and adjusted so that the quantity of fluid applied to
the diet surface contains 10,000 spores. The material is applied
with a 100 µl syringe. The surface of the diet is air dried and
one fourth-instar larva placed in the vial. A piece of filter
paper (one in x one in) is inserted between the neck of the vial
and the plastic cap to prevent excessive moisture build-up within
the vial and to allow some air circulation.

After one to two weeks, depending on the temperature at which the
host is held, the larva will be heavily infected with the microsporidian and can be sacrificed for the extraction of spores.

Modifications of this procedure can be used to maintain laboratory infections of many entomophilic microsporidians. With some
microsporidia such as *N. necatrix*, the spore dosage is critical
because if spore dosage is much in excess of the recommended
dosage, the larvae will die from bacterial septicemia before the
microsporidian infection has a chance to develop. With other
microsporidians such as *Nosema trichoplusiae* and *Pleistophora
schubergi*, the spore dosage is not so critical since very high
spore dosages of these microsporidia do not cause bacterial

septicemia in their hosts. Another problem that is often encountered when adding spore suspensions to artificial media used
to rear insects is the development of bacterial and fungal contaminants on the surface of the medium. This is seldom a problem
on the Yearian diet because the low pH of this diet inhibits the
growth of most microorganisms. When such contamination problems
occur, the spore suspension added to the diet surface must be
subjected to one of the additional purification methods described
previously in order to eliminate bacterial and fungal contaminants.

D. *NOSEMA ALGERAE*

Infections of *N. algerae* can be maintained in the laboratory
by feeding spores to mosquito larvae, or by injection of spores
into non-mosquito hosts.

Uninfected mosquito larvae are maintained in white enamel pans
with glass covers at 26°C with a light cycle of 16 hrs light and
eight hrs dark. Larvae are daily fed a small amount of powdered
rat chow. About ten infected adult mosquitoes are ground in a
glass tissue grinder and added to an enamel pan containing 500-
1,000 eggs or first-instar larvae from the uninfected colony.
These larvae are reared as described above. After the larvae
pupate they are removed and placed in a nylon mesh cage where
they emerge as infected adults. These adults are gound up and
used as the inoculum or the spores are separated according to the
preliminary purification technique described earlier and stored
at 50°C. Spores can be stored at this temperature at least one
year without complete loss of viability (Undeen, personal communication).

N. alterae can also be maintained in the laboratory by injecting
a sterile spore suspension into the hemocoel of other arthropods
(Undeen and Maddox, 1973). This procedure was described above.

E. *NOSEMA HELIOTHIDIS*

N. heliothidis can be maintained continuously in a laboratory
colony of *Heliothis zea*. The larvae of *H. zea* are cannibalistic
and must be reared individually. For specific rearing procedures
the reader is referred to Smith (1966). *N. heliothidis* is
transovarially transmitted and no special methods are necessary
to insure passage from one generation to another. Brooks
(personal communication) has maintained small infected colonies
for five or six generations and suggests that the addition of
healthy adults to the colony should allow the colony to continue
for an extended period.

F. *ENCEPHALITOZOON CUNICULI*

E. cuniculi is the only vertebrate microsporidian that has
been successfully maintained in the laboratory. Maintenance

can be achieved either by serial passage of ascitic fluid or tissue of infected mice at three-five week intervals (Nelson, 1962, 1967; Lainson *et al.*, 1964) or more conveniently by the cultivation of the parasite in tissue culture of rabbit choroid plexus (Shadduck, 1969; Vavra *et al.*, 1972; Montrey *et al.*, 1973). Because many rabbits are latently infected with *Encephalitozoon*, great care should be exercised in selecting the animal that is used for the isolation of the primary, noninfected tissue culture. On the other hand, the method can be used for isolation of new strains of the parasite either when tissue culture is started from a spontaneously infected animal or when material containing parasites (e. g. macrophages from infected mice) is added to the choroid plexus cell culture. Rabbit choroid plexus cells are conveniently maintained in Minimal Essential Medium (MEM) supplemented with 10% calf serum, 100 units of penicillin, and 100 µg of streptomycin per ml of the final medium. Amphotericin B (Fungizone, 2 mg/ml) may be added for the inhibition of fungal contamination with no apparent effect on the parasite (Vavra *et al.*, 1972).

IX. STORAGE OF MICROSPORIDIAN SPORES

A. *HOST CADAVERS*

Microsporidia which extrude their polar filaments when exposed to wetting agents can best be stored in dried host cadavers. Larval and adult *Tribolium castaneum* cadavers infected with *Nosema whitei* should be placed in small glass vials and held at about 4°C until needed. Spores may be stored in this manner for at least two years. Milner (1972b) found that *N. whitei* spores stored in flour at 4°C lost no viability after 15 months storage.

B. *AQUEOUS MEDIA*

Most microsporidian spores can be stored in water at temperatures slightly above freezing. The length of time microsporidian spores can be stored in this manner as reported by a number of different workers has varied from several months to ten years. The species of microsporidian involved, the freedom of the microsporidian suspension from other microorganisms, and the temperature at which the suspension is stored greatly influence the length of time the microsporidian spores will remain viable. Kramer (1970) has reviewed the works on longevity of microsporidian spores.

Most microsporidian spores can be stored for at least several months in a water suspension at 5°C if the spores are cleaned by the preliminary purification method previously described. If bacterial or fungal growth becomes a problem, 100 units of penicillin, 100 milligrams of streptomycin sulfate, and 0.25 milligrams Fungizone per milliliter should be added to the spore suspension.

C. SUBFREEZING TEMPERATURES

Spores stored at temperatures slightly below freezing (-5 to
-15°C) will not remain viable for long periods of time. We have
been unable to store spores for extended periods at these temperatures. Bailey (1972) stored whole bees infected with *Nosema
apis* at -20°C for 24 months, but at the end of 24 months,
viability of these spores was 7.5 times less than the viability
of fresh spores. We have been able to store spores of 15 different
species of microsporidia in liquid nitrogen for extended periods of
time with very little loss of viability. Those microsporidia we
have been able to bioassay (*Nosema necatrix, N. trichoplusiae,
and Octosporea muscaedomesticae*) have lost only 2-3% viability
after storage in liquid nitrogen for over seven years (Maddox,
unpublished results). Storage in liquid nitrogen requires no
special preparation. The spore suspension is placed in glass
tubes that are sealed and dropped directly into the liquid
nitrogen container. We routinely store half of our spores in
water and half in a 50-50 glycerol-water mixture. The addition
of glycerol slightly increases the viability of spores stored in
liquid nitrogen. When the spore suspensions are needed, they are
removed from the liquid nitrogen container, warmed to room
temperature as quickly as possible, and fed to the host insect at
the desired dosages.

All the microsporidia we have recovered from terrestrial
insects can be successfully stored in liquid nitrogen. However,
spores of *Nosema algeri* (Undeen, personal communication) could
not be successfully preserved in liquid nitrogen. It is possible
that spores of microsporidia infecting aquatic insects have some
characteristic(s) that prevents their being successfully stored
in liquid nitrogen.

The mammalian microsporidian *Encephalitozoon cuniculi* is
another species that can be stored in liquid nitrogen when frozen
together with the rabbit choroid plexus cells (Bedrnik and Vavra,
1971).

D. LYOPHILIZATION

Bailey (1972) successfully lyophilized abdomens of bees infected with *Nosema apis*. Abdomens were cooled to -20°C and held
for 18 hrs over P_2O_5 at 10-20 microns Hg. Abdomens were then
placed in glass tubes and evacuated over P_2O_5 at 2-5 microns Hg
for 7 hrs before being sealed. The viability of lyophilized
spores was reduced very little immediately after lyophilization,
but the length of time spores remained viable after being
lyophilized has not yet been determined.

Lewis and Lynch (1974) successfully lyophilized and vacuum-
dried *Nosema pyraustae* spores. Intact infected larvae were
lyophilized by freezing at -12°C and then lyophilized at 5 μm
Hg for 16 hr. Vacuum drying was accomplished by omitting the

freezing process. Spores survived vacuum drying better than
lyophilization. Lyophilization initially reduced infectivity
approximately 50% whereas vacuum drying did not significantly
reduce viability. However, significant additional viability of
both vacuum-dried and lyophilized spores was lost after six months
storage at 22-24°C.

We have been able to successfully lyophilize purified spore
preparations of *Nosema necatrix* but were unable to lyophilize
spores of *Octosporea muscaedomesticae*. *N. necatrix* spores were
lyophilized in a 20% sucrose medium. When less than 20% sucrose
was used, viability of the lyophilized spores was greatly reduced.
The sucrose medium containing the spores was placed in glass
tubes, frozen in an acetone dry ice bath, and subjected to four
microns Hg for eight hours before being sealed. *O. muscaedomesticae*
did not survive this lyophilization process (Maddox, unpublished
results).

Although *N. necatrix* spores survived lyophilization with very
little loss of viability, this lyophilization process did not
improve the storage properties of *N. necatrix* spores. The
viability of lyophilized *N. necatrix* spores at 21°C decreased at
about the same rate as that of *N. necatrix* spores stored in water
suspensions (Maddox, unpublished results). It is possible that
the lyophilization of other microsporidian spores or the use of
other lyophilization procedures such as the ones described by
Bailey (1972) or Lewis and Lynch (1974) may be useful for preserving viability of microsporidian spores.

We recommend liquid nitrogen storage for the long-term preservation of those microsporidia which withstand this process. For
shorter storage periods and for those microsporidians that are
unable to withstand freezing temperatures, storage of spores in a
clean aqueous suspension at 5°C is recommended. Microsporidia
such as *Nosema whitei* that extrude their filaments when dry spores
are placed in water should be stored as dry infected cadavers at
5°C.

X. USE OF TISSUE CULTURE IN THE STUDY OF MICROSPORIDIA

Several microsporidian species have been successfully maintained in tissue culture. In addition to the entomophilic
species that are mentioned below, the mammalian microsporidian
Encephalitozoon cuniculi can be maintained indefinitely in tissue
cultures of rabbit choroid plexus and canine-embryo cells (see
section "Maintenance of Microsporidian Infections in the Laboratory").
This microsporidian once established *in vitro* has little specificity
as far as the type of host cell is concerned. *Encephalitozoon* can
be grown (although less successfully) in HeLa cells, L cells,
pork kidney cells, hamster kidney cells, chick embryo kidney
cells, primary glial cells from rabbits, mice and hamsters, primary kidney cells from rabbits, mice and hamsters, rabbit cornea
cells and mouse fibroblasts (Vavra *et al.*, 1973). It can also

infect fat head minnow, *Timephales promeles*, cell line, but is
unable to grow in cell culture MOS-55 derived from *Anopheles
gambiae* (Bedrnik and Vavra, 1972).

Susceptible insect tissues can be infected by introducing
spores that have been previously treated to extrude polar filaments. Ishihara and Sohi (1966) infected four- to five-day
cultures of *Bombyx mori* ovarian sheath with *Nosema bombycis* by
introducing *N. bombycis* spores previously treated with 0.1 *M*
KOH for 40 minutes. The microsporidian completed its development
and after 21 days at 28°C, the host cells were filled with spores.
The authors did not indicate how many spores were added to the
tissue culture and this would presumably influence the length of
time required for complete infection to occur. Using the same
method, Ishihara (1968) infected rat embryo cells and chick
embryo cells with *N. bombycis*, but confirmed spore formation
only in the rat embryo cells. Recently, Undeen (1975) introduced
spores of *Nosema algerae* from *Anopheles stephensi* into pig kidney
cell culture maintained in the Minimum Essential Medium. Spores
extrude in the cultivation medium without any further activation
and the microsporidian completes the whole development within the
pig kidney cells.

When introducing microsporidian spores into a tissue culture,
the spore suspension obviously must be as pure as possible and
free from microbial contaminants. This may be accomplished by
one of the purification methods previously described. The treatment of microsporidian spores for extrusion of the polar filament
will vary with the microsporidian species involved and is covered
in another section.

Development of microsporidian infections in insect organ cultures
can be obtained by infecting insects prior to the explanation of
organs. Sen Gupta (1964) fed fourth-instar larvae of *Pieris
brassicae* spores of *Nosema mesnili;* 24 hr after feeding, the gut
and fat body were removed, placed in roll tubes containing the
growth medium, and incubated at 26°C. After seven days, the
tissues were filled with mature spores identical in size and shape
to those obtained from living hosts.

We have obtained development of the microsporidian *N. necatrix*
in organ cultures of *Pseudaletia unipuncta* fat body using the
following methods (Maddox, unpublished results). Twenty-four hours
after molting to the sixth-instar, armyworm larvae were fed one
million spores by oral injection. These larvae were held at 26°F
for 48 hr, after which they were surface sterilized in an alcohol-
Hyamine solution, air-dried, and pinned in a sterile dissecting
dish. Small pieces of fat body were removed with sterile dissecting
instruments and passed through two washes of invertebrate saline
containing 200 units of penicillin G per milliliter and 200 µg of
streptomycin sulphate per ml. The pieces of fat body were left
in each of the two washes for ten minutes and then were transferred
to Grace's tissue culture medium containing 100 units of penicillin

G per milliliter and 100 µg of streptomycin sulphate per ml. This medium was incubated at 26°F. Four days after transferring the fat body to the tissue culture medium, many fat body cells were heavily infected with *N. necatrix* spores. These spores appeared normal and produced normal infections when fed back to armyworm larvae.

Although little work has been published concerning the growth of entomophilic microsporidians in tissue cultures, some microsporidia are able to infect tissue cultures by introducing spores that have been previously treated to extrude the filament and some microsporidia are capable of infecting a number of different cell lines (Fisher and Sanborn, 1959; Ishihara, 1968). With an increasing number of invertebrate cell lines available (Hink, 1972), the use of tissue culture as an experimental tool will undoubtedly increase. Studies on mechanisms of host and tissue specificity, and the development, physiology, and nutrition of microsporidia could be facilitated by the use of tissue culture.

XI. LABELING MICROSPORIDIAN SPORES WITH RADIOACTIVE COMPOUNDS

Techniques involving the use of radioactive compounds have seldom been used for studying microsporidia, though these techniques offer many possibilities. Microsporidian spores labeled with a radioisotope could provide much useful information that would otherwise be difficult if not impossible to obtain. For example, the distribution of labeled spores when introduced into a real or simulated ecosystem could be determined by measuring the radio-activity of samples taken from various locations within the ecosystem. This would be especially helpful in aquatic ecosystems where microsporidian transmission from one aquatic host to another is poorly understood. When the nuclear material of the microsporidian sporeplasm within the spore is labeled with a radioactive compound, the temporal relationships and location of sporeplasms within the body of the host could be quantitatively determined by counting and audio-radiographic techniques. Tracer techniques would also be helpful in studying the physiology, metabolism, and development of microsporidia in living hosts or in tissue culture. The following techniques are based on preliminary experiments involving isotope labeling of microsporidian spores.

Sixth-instar *Pseudaletia unipuncta* larvae were injected with 1.6 µCi of the sodium salt of $[1-^{14}C]$ in sterile distilled water. Twenty-four hours later, these larvae were fed one million *Nosema necatrix* spores. Twenty-four hours after spores were fed to the armyworm larvae, the larvae were injected a second time with 1.6 µCi $[1-^{14}C]$ acetate solution. These larvae were held for ten days at 80°F, after which they were sacrificed and the spores were purified as described above. After purification, spores were washed five more times to insure that all radioactive material was removed. The last wash was saved and checked later for radioactivity. The spores were smeared on microscope slides, dried, and audioradiographs prepared by the method described by Gude (1965). Labeled spores were easily identified by the presence of black silver grains in the emulsion surrounding the spores. Radioactivity was also detected in a liquid scintillation counter, but the radiation emitted per spore was not determined (Maddox, unpublished results).

XII. RECORDING OF MICROSPORIDIAN SPORES

The shape and the size of microsporidian spores are useful taxonomic characters. Similarly the size and the shape of the posterior vacuole, the thickness of the spore membrane, the presence or absence of exosporal appendages or of the mucus layer may be used for the characterization of individual species. However, the recording of such spore characters is by no means a simple task. Microsporidian spores are not only very small, but are also highly refractile. When in suspension, they are easily translocated by the Brownian movement. When they are pressed in clumps or squeezed among pieces of host tissue, they overlap and their exact shape cannot be estimated. Therefore, immobilization of freely dispersed spores is necessary for accurately recording spore characters. Spores are recorded preferably when fresh. In some species spores stored in cold water suspensions can be used. Dried and rehydrated spores are unsuitable.

A. OBTAINING SPORE MONOLAYERS

Single layers of spores undisturbed by the Brownian movement can be obtained according to the technique of Vavra (1964a). A small drop of a thick suspension of spores on a cover slip is inverted upon a drop of paraffin oil lying on a microscope slide. Water having better affinity for glass than the oil, spreads in a thin layer on the cover slip causing spores to become trapped one by one in this layer. The "agar cushion method," a modification of a technique for obtaining spore monolayers originally devised for the observation of trypanosomes by Ormerod et al. (1963), is recommended for microsporidian spores (Vavra, 1964a, Lom and Weiser, 1969). A large drop of melted agar (1.5%, w/v, or the thinnest solution that will settle firmly when cooled to room temperature) is placed upon a slide and allowed to cool. The surface of the drop must be smooth and slightly convex. A cover slip with a small drop of spore suspension is then applied to the surface of the agar drop causing spores to be slightly compressed between the cover slip and the agar. The agar technique is for phase-contrast microscopy; paraffin oil is not suitable for phase-contrast microscopy.

B. STORAGE OF SPORE MONOLAYERS

Preparations obtained by both methods mentioned above can be
stored from several days to several weeks in the refrigerator.
Dessication can be prevented by framing the cover slip with
Canada balsam. Monolayers of spores fixed in ten percent formalin
can be preserved for longer periods (Vavra, 1964b).

C. PHOTOGRAPHIC RECORDING

Photomicrography is ideally suited for exact recording of
different structural characters. The greatest advantage of
photography is that spores of individual species can be conveniently compared. A standard technique such as the following should
be used: (1) Use only freshly prepared spore monolayers; (2)
use high-contrast, fine-grain film. e. g., phototechnical film
for reproduction of line drawings ORWO F 05 (ORWO, Wolfen, GDR)
gives satisfactory results; the negative should be developed in a
high-contrast repro-type of developer; (3) photographs should be
taken at a standard calibrated magnification; (4) the negative
should be printed on a contrast glossy paper with magnification
accurately controlled.

D. DEMONSTRATING THE PRESENCE OF THE MICROSPORIDIAN MUCUS

A mucous layer is present around spores of many microsporidian
species. The presence of mucus is revealed by the addition of
India ink to the spore suspension (Lom and Vavra, 1962); the
mucus appears as a white halo around the spore. Normal India ink
for drawing should be used. The special bacteriological ink for
negative staining ("Burri ink") has smaller particles that penetrate the microsporidian mucus and fail to reveal it.

E. DEMONSTRATING THE PRESENCE OF SPORE APPENDAGES

Spores of many microsporidian species are equipped with appendages.
Some are easily observed in light optics, especially phase-contrast.
Thinner appendages are revealed in negatively stained preparations
with India or bacteriological ink (Vavra, 1963). Some types of
appendages can only be observed in the electron microscope.

F. MEASURING MICROSPORIDIAN SPORES

Freshly prepared spore monolayers are best suited for precise
spore measurements. High refractivity of the spores makes
measuring spores a difficult task, especially if one uses an
eyepiece micrometer with an engraved scale or a filar micrometer.
It is difficult to judge the exact superposition of the scale
divisions with the spore rim. If very precise measurements are
required, spores on suitable enlarged and exactly calibrated

photomicrographs may be measured. The best and most accurate method for measuring spores involves the use of the image splitting eyepiece (Vickers Instruments Ltd.) (Kramer 1964).

XIII. PHYSIOLOGICAL TECHNIQUES WITH MICROSPORIDIAN SPORES

A. *SPORE STIMULATION FOR EXTRUSION*

Generally, microsporidian spores react to a number of stimuli (see Kudo, 1924) by extrusion of the polar filament. However, no universal method for polar filament extrusion exists and different microsporidian species vary considerably in their readiness for polar tube evagination. Some spores discharge their filaments easily and under a number of stimuli; others do not. Pressure on spores contained in a water suspension between a microscope slide and cover slip will evoke response but this method often results in a less than complete discharge of the filament (including the germ). Some spores discharge filaments upon drying and rewetting (Kramer, 1960). Other spores react to the change in the ionic strength of the medium. Such spores can sometimes be discharged in a drop of water to which a few small crystals of NaCl are added. Convection currents which occur upon the dissolution of the salt expose spores to changing concentrations of NaCl (Vavra, unpublished). Hydrogen perixide (5%, v/v) also extrudes some spores. Addition of gelatin and saccharose to such a solution causes slow extrusion, suitable for cinematography (Lom and Vavra, 1963). *Nosema apis* spores readily extrude their filaments when suspended in Ringer's saline mixed with an equal volume of glycerin-gelatin to which 0.5-4% of catalase is added (Steche, 1965). *Nosema algerae* spores in distilled water will extrude their filaments when transferred to a medium having a pH of 9.5-10 and containing various salts (Undeen, unpublished results). Spores of most microsporidia infecting lepitopterans can best be extruded by a two-step process (Undeen, unpublished results): (1) Activate spores by pretreating for 30 min in a 0.1 M KCl solution (pH 10.5-12); and (2) transfer spores to a 0.1 M KCl solution of lower pH. The pH optima required for extrusion differ with various species.

The method of Ohshima (1937), modified by Ishihara and Hayashi (1968) was devised for activating spores of *Nosema bombycis.* A concentrated sample of spores was incubated in 0.1 N KOH for 40 min and was transferred into four volumes of silkworm serum (Hemolymph heated to 60°C for 15 min and centrifuged at 23,000 g for 15 min). More than 80% of the spores extruded their filaments within 10 min after transfer into serum. Weidner (1972) successfully activated spores of *Ameson (syn. Nosema) michaelis,* parasite of the blue crab *Callinectes sp.* The spores were incubated in Michaelis veronal acetate buffer at pH 10 for 30-45 min. The buffer was decanted and, the spores were resuspended in tissue culture medium. Spore discharge occurred immediately after placement into the medium.

B. SPORE DISRUPTION

Microsporidian spores are difficult to disrupt. Several methods were evaluated by Conner (1970), Cerkasovova and Vavra (1972), and Weidner (this monograph). The usual disruption methods, such as French pressure treatment, sonication, mortar grinding with glass powder, repeated freezing and thawing, and homogenization in a tissue grinder are not effective for disrupting microsporidian spores. The most widely used method is to spin spores at 2,000-4,000 rpm with very fine glass beads (ca. 0.02-0.1 mm diameter) for 30-60 sec (Cerkasovova and Vavra, 1972). The detailed procedure for disruption with glass beads has been described by Fowler and Reeves (1974a). For enzymatic studies it is necessary to use glass beads that contain no lead. Unfortunately, many batches of beads are manufactured from lead crystal glass to give high refractivity. A disadvantage of using glass beads is that a great quantity of material becomes absorbed to the surface of the beads and is lost during further separation of the spore debris from the beads. Separating the cellular particles from the beads and glass chips is difficult (Conner 1970). Precaution also should be taken to keep the sample cool. If the disruption device filled with spore suspension and the glass beads is precooled to about 0°C, the temperature of the sample will not rise above 10°C during disruption, which usually takes no more than 1 minute (Cerkasovova, personal communication). After disruption, phase-contrast microscopy can be used to distinguish disrupted and undamaged spores. Undamaged spores are bright whereas disrupted spores are dark. Another method is to make a dry smear stained with bacteriological ink ("Burri ink"). The ink penetrates damaged spores, and they can be easily recognized under oil immersion.

C. ISOLATION OF SPORE PROTEINS FOR ELECTROPHORETIC ANALYSIS

Polyacrylamide gel electrophoresis for determining the relationships of various microsporidia was recently described by Fowler and Reeves (1974a, b). This technique, previously used in phylogenetic studies of other organisms, is a novel approach to the taxonomy and physiology of microsporidia. The method requires careful cleaning of spores, disruption, and protein extraction. Hydrophobic proteins can be extracted by phenol-glacial acetic acid-distilled water; hydrophilic proteins can be extracted from phosphate buffer extracts by the addition of ammonium sulphate. and subsequent dialysis. Proteins are separated by disc electrophoresis in polyacrylamide gel and the resulting bands compared. Hydrophobic protein spectra are stable when (1) two different genera of hosts are used for spore propagation, (2) hosts are reared at a variety of temperatures, (3) protein is extracted

from spores harvested at different stages of sporogenesis. On the
other hand hydrophilic spore proteins were unstable under the
conditions (1) and (2) mentioned above and when spore incubation
period and storage was different.

XIV. IMMUNOLOGICAL TECHNIQUES

Immunological techniques have been used for detection of infections and species identification.

A. DETECTION OF INFECTIONS

Techniques based on the occurrence of specific antibodies in
infected animals have been used only for the detection of
Encephalitozoon cuniculi infections in laboratory reared rodents.
Indirect fluorescent antibody test (IFAT) and the skin test are
suitable for this purpose. The IFAT was developed by Chalupsky
et al. (1971, 1973) and independently by Jackson *et al.* (1973).
A similar principle was used by Cox *et al.* (1972) for the demo-
stration of microsporidia in diseased rabbits. Spores of the
parasite, preferably obtained from tissue cultures, are used as
antigen. If spores for antigen are obtained from infected animals,
the reaction is usually less sqecific because antibodies may have
adsorbed to them *in vivo*. When spores from infected animals
must be used as antigen, the specificity of the reaction can be
improved by washing the antigen with 0.1 *M* citrate, 0.1 *M* phosphate
buffer, pH 2.0 for five minutes followed by thorough washing in
phosphate buffered saline (Cox *et al.*, 1972). The test itself is
performed according to routine immunofluorescence procedures. The
IFAT can distinguish noninfected grown infected rabbits (Chalupsky
et al., 1973) and guinea pigs. Its value for detecting latent
Encephalitozoon infections in laboratory rats and mice is presently under investigation (Chalupsky *et al.*, personal communication, the allergic skin test (Pakes *et al.*, 1972) requires
intradermal injection of rabbits by disintegrated *Encephalitozoon
cuniculi* spores ("Encephalitozoonin"). In positive animals,
induration and erythema develop 24-72 hr after administration.
To date, the test has been used only in rabbits.

B. IDENTIFICATION OF MICROSPORIDIAN SPECIES

Immunological techniques are also useful in microsporidian
taxonomy (Kalalova and Weiser, 1973; Weiser, this monograph).
Rabbits injected with a suspension of purified microsporidian
spores develop species-specific antibodies. Sera from such rabbits
can be reacted with unidentified spores. This technique would be
of a great value to microsporidian taxonomists if a bank of
immune species-specific sera could be developed.

XV. CYTOLOGICAL AND HISTOLOGICAL TECHNIQUES

Most currently used cytological and histological techniques can be applied to microsporidia. Microsporidiologists should be well acquainted with these methods because the resulting preparations are not only a valuable source of information but can also be used as type material (see Erickson, this monograph). The most commonly used methods are briefly discussed below.

A. *FIXATION AND STAINING*

Three techniques can be used in preparing material for fixation and staining: dry smears, wet smears, and *in toto* fixation.

The dry smear technique is the most commonly used, probably because of its simplicity. It also flattens the fixed objects and renders them more transparent. However, dry smears do not accurately preserve the size or shape of the fixed objects and they produce many artefacts. It is, therefore, unfortunate that many investigators use the dry smear technique exclusively. To prepare a dry smear, the material is smeared (usually in a small drop of saline) on a clean slide and allowed to dry.

For wet smears, the material is smeared on a cover slip and is fixed while wet by floating the cover slip (first smear side down, later the cover slip is turned over with the smear side up) in fixative. Because wet smears preserve the shape and the internal structure of the fixed objects they should be considered a basic method for handling microsporidian materials.

In toto fixation is used in material that is to be sectioned. It is indispensable for determining the three dimensional shape of a parasite as well as its location in the host tissue(s).

Common histological fixatives can be used for microsporidia. Frequently used fixatives are methanol (for dry smears with subsequent Giemsa staining), Carnoy, Schaudin's fluid, Zenker's fluid, Bouin, Bouin-Dubosq-Brazil, Bouin-Hollande (Bouin's fluid with $CuCl_2$). Vapors of osmic acid can be used for fixing dry smears. However, they can also be used for fixation of specimens *in toto* if the fixation is performed in a small drop of saline directly above the surface of OsO_4. In such a way, even bulk objects (e.g., whole cyclopoid copepode) can be satisfactorily preserved in just a few minutes.

Several stains are useful for fixed material. The periodic acid-Schiff reagents reveal the "polar cap" which is typical of microsporidia (Vavra, 1959; Huger, 1960).

The gram stain (or any of its numerous modifications) is useful for revealing mature microsporidian spores that are usually gram-positive. This character is particularly useful in distinguishing mammalian microsporidia from other tissue parasites (e.g., *Toxoplasma gondi*) that are gram negative. Also, the Goodpasture-Perrin stain (see Appendix) is very reliable for staining encephalitozoa in tissue sections.

B. PERMANENT SPORE PREPARATIONS

Negative staining, using bacteriological ink ("Burri ink"), is the simplest method for permanent preparations of spore material. A drop of the unfixed spore suspension is mixed with a drop of the bacteriological ink. This suspension is then smeared on a slide and dried. Structural aspects of the spores are relatively well preserved and spore appendages, if present, are revealed. The technique is also useful in demonstrating spore arrangement.

Giemsa staining is the most popular among microsporidiologists. It can be used for both smears and sections. Giemsa staining after acid hydrolysis (Piekarski, 1937) is a useful method for revealing nuclei in microsporidian spores if nuclei are obscured by the dense spore content after normal staining. Giemsa staining after hydrolysis (for details see appendix) is not always specific for DNA but usually gives more satisfactory results than Feulgen's reaction. Application of the classical Feulgen's nucleal reaction to microsporidian material was first described by Jirovec (1932). However, because microsporidian nuclei are very small and the DNA content is low, application of this stain to microsporidia is difficult.

Haematoxylin staining.--Various types of haematoxylin stains have been used for staining microsporidia. The best is Heidenhain's iron haematoxylin. This stain is applicable for wet smears as well as for sections. Unfortunately, Heidenhain's stain is not used frequently by most researchers because it is time consuming and difficult.

Wheatley's modified Gomori trichrome stain introduced (see Alger, 1966) is excellent for localizing mature microsporidian spores in tissues (Vavra and Undeen, 1970). A modification of Claudius stain has been useful for determining the presence of microsporidian spores in honeybees (Fyg, 1963).

Semithin sections of material embedded in epoxy or polyester resins for electron microscopy, provide an excellent material for light microscope observations. Such material is very well preserved and can be sectioned easily at 0.5-3 um. Staining such sections is, however, difficult and few stains are available.

XVI. ELECTRON MICROSCOPE TECHNIQUES

A. FIXATION

Most of the principle fixatives have been used for microsporidian material with various successes. These include buffered osmium tetroxide (Vavra, 1965), glutaraldehyde buffered with either cacodylate or phosphate buffer and followed by postosmication, Dalton's chrome-osmium fixative after glutaraldehyde fixation (Sprague et al., 1968), permangante fixative (Gassouma and Ellis, 1973), and osmic vapors alone (Vavra, unpublished results). All these fixatives give moderately satisfactory results depending on

the material and handling during fixation. However, it must be
stressed that there is no single ideal fixative for preserving
microsporidian ultrastructure. Microsporidia are more sensitive
to osmotic effects than the surrounding tissues. Consequently,
the toxicity of the fixative must be carefully adjusted for good
preservation of fine structure. Addition of sucrose to the
veronal-acetate buffered oxmium has given consistently good
results for many years (Vavra, unpublished results).

B. DEHYDRATION

Dehydration procedures routinely used for electron microscopy
are satisfactory for microsporidia. Uranyl acetate is often added
to dehydration ethanol for stabilization purposes.

C. EMBEDDING

All commonly used types of embedding media have been used for
microsporidia. Developmental stages are easily infiltrated, but
infiltration into spores is very difficult. To achieve good
spore infiltration, Weidner (1970) subjected spores to a pressure
of 3,000-5,000 psi in a French press. This method collapsed the
spore and disrupted the spore contents, allowing a rather uniform
infiltration of the fixative and embedding medium.

D. SECTIONING AND STAINING

Blocks containing microsporidian spores are difficult to section.
Spores are usually not properly infiltrated with the embedding
medium in the region of the posterior vacuole. This phenomenon
interferes with sectioning and reduces stability of the sections
in the electron beam. Thin sections of microsporidian material
are stained according to routine procedures. Double staining
with uranyl acetate followed by lead citrate is very reliable.

E. SPECIAL TECHNIQUES

Polysaccharides can be detected at the ultrastructural level by
the application of Seligman's periodic acid-thiocarbohydrazide
(or thiosemicarbazide) reagents (Vavra, 1972). Glycoproteins can
be detected by the application of Rambourg's (1967) silver-
methenamine method (Walker and Hinsch, 1972; Percy, 1973) or by
Wright and Lumsden's (1968) modification of the same technique
(Weidner, 1972). Other methods for detecting glycoproteins include
Luft's (1971) ruthenium violet method and Nicholson and Singer's
(1971) procedure using ferritin-conjugated Concanavalin A (Weidner,
1972). Premeability of the pansporoblast membrane was demonstrated
by lanthanum hydroxide (Overstreet and Weidner, 1974).

F. *SCANNING ELECTRON MICROSCOPY (SEM)*

Surface patterns of microsporidian spores are revealed either
by carbon replication (Vernick *et al.*, 1969) or by scanning electron microscopy (Lom and Weiser, 1972; Frost and Nolan, 1972;
Vavra, unpublished results). For SEM, the spores are carefully
cleaned, fixed, mounted on stubs, and freeze-dried (critical
point drying method has not yet been successfully applied to
microsporidia). Osmium fixatives are preferred because the
impregnation of spores with osmium reduced charging during
SEM. Lom and Weiser (1972) successfully used Parduca's fluid
for fixation. Carbon and gold or gold-palladium alloy is best (2
parts of 2% sublimate and 6 parts of 2% osmic acid) for specimen
coating. Frost and Nolan (1972) were able to observe spores
formerly preserved in lactophenol.

G. *FREEZE-ETCHING*

Valuable data on the fine structure of microsporidia have been
obtained by freeze-etching techniques (see Structure of Microsporidia, this monograph, for a discussion of these methods).

XVII. INDUCING AND CONTROLLING MICROSPORIDIAN INFECTIONS

Artifically inducing latent microsporidian infections for
research purposes has so far been used only for the mammalian
microsporidian, *Encephalitozoon cuniculi*. Cortisone, given
weekly at the rate of 2.5-5 mg per animal has been used for
inducing latent encephalitozoonosis in mice (Innes *et al.*, 1962;
Bismanis,1970). Kaneda (1969) used the antitumor drug, Endoxan
(cyclohexamide), for a similar purpose. The basic principles for
the control of microsporidian infections are discussed in the
monograph of Weiser (1961) include the selection of healthy animals
for culture, a technique introduced by Pasteur (1870). A similar
principle has been used by McLaughlin (1966) and by Jenkins
et al. (1970) for the elimination of two microsporidian species
from a laboratory colony of boll weevils. Another physical method
is the application of thermal stress either to the infected
host (Lotmar, 1944) or to the infected eggs of the host. The
latter method was widely used in the silkworm industry as well as
by Allen and Brunson (1947) for eliminating *Nosema destructor*
from laboratory colonies of the potato tuberworm, *Gnorimoscheme
operculella*.

Several chemical compounds with anti-microsporidian activity
have been developed for the control of nosematosis in the honey-
bee (see Fritzsch, 1970 for a review). One of these compounds is
"Nosemack" (2-aethylmercurymercaptobenzoxazol-5 sodium) of
Gontarski and Wagner (1954). The antibiotic Fumagilin, isolated
from *Aspergillus fumigatus* (Katznelson and Jamieson, 1952) and
distributed under the commercial name Fumidil B (Abbott) or

Fumagilin DCH (Chinoin, Budapest) has also been widely used for the control of bee nosematosis and for the control of *Nosema pyraustae* in colonies of the European corn borer (Lynch and Lewis, 1971). Recently, a promising antimicrosporidian agent was found by Hsiao and Hsiao (1973). These authors apparently succeeded in eliminating *Nosema* sp. from a laboratory colony of the alfalfa weevil, *Hypera postica*, fed on a diet containing a systemic fungicide benomyl [methyl-1-(butylcarbamoyl)-2-benzimidazole carbamate] (Benlate, du Pont).

APPENDIX: SELECTED METHODS FOR STAINING MICROSPORIDIAN MATERIALS

Giemsa Staining for Histological Sections (Shortt and Cooper, 1948)

1. Fix material in Carnoy, embed in paraffin.
2. Stain for one hour or longer in Giemsa, 10 ml; acetone, 10 ml; methanol 10 ml, distilled water, 100 ml.
3. Rinse in tap water.
4. Differentiate in colophonium, 15 g; acetone, 100 ml; differentiation should be controlled under the microscope.
5. Wash in acetone, 70 ml; xylol, 30 ml. Repeat several times.
6. Clear in several baths of xylene.
7. Mount with a synthetic resin, e.g., Euparal and Caedax.

Goodpasture-Perrin's method for Staining Encephalitozoa (According to Lillie, 1965, modified)

1. Fix in Zenker fixative.
2. Embed in paraffin.
3. Stain with Goodpasture's anilin-carbolfuchsine (basic fuchsine, 0.39 g; aniline, 1 ml; crystalline phenol, 1 g; 30% of ethanol, 100 ml) for 10 min at room temperature. In the original recipe, staining is performed at 70°C for 5 min.
4. Rinse in distilled water.
5. Differentiate in 40% formaldehyde for 10-20 min.
6. Rinse in distilled water.
7. Counterstain in a saturated solution of picric acid for 1 min.
8. Differentiate in 95% ethanol.
9. Dehydrate in 100% ethanol followed by several baths of xylene.
10. Mount with synthetic resin, e.g. Caedax.

Giemsa Staining after Hydrolysis (Piekarski, 1937, Modified)

1. Fix in osmic vapor, methanol, Schaudin's fixative, and others.
2. Wash well in distilled water.
3. Hydrolyze for 10 min. in 1 N HCl at 60°C.
4. Wash several times in distilled water.
5. Stain in Giemsa diluted 1:20 with buffered water at pH 7.0-7.2.
6. Rinse in tap water.
7. Clear in acetone-xylene (1:1, v/v) or let dry from water directly
8. Mount with Caedax.

REFERENCES

Abdel-Malek, A., and Steinhaus, A. (1948). Invasion route of
   Nosema sp. in the potato tuberworm, as determined by
   ligaturing. *J. Parasitol.* 34:

Alger, N. (1966). A simple, rapid, precise stain for intestinal
   protozoa. *Amer. J. Clin. Pathol.* 45: 361-362.

Allen, H. V., and Brunson, M. H. (1947). Control of *Nosema*
   disease of potato tuberworms, a host used in the mass production of *Macrocentrus ancylivorus*. *Science* 105: 394.

Angus, T. A. (1964). A magnetic stirring device for syringes.
   J. Invertebr. Pathol. 6: 126.

Bailey, L. (1972). The preservation of infective microsporidian
   spores. *J. Invertebr. Pathol.* 20: 252-254.

Bedrnik, P., and Vavra, J. (1971). Cryopreservation of the
   mammalian microsporidian *Nosema cuniculi*. *J. Protozool.*
   18 (Suppl.): 47.

Bedrnik, P., and Vavra, J.(1972). Further observations on the
   maintenance of *Encephalitozoon cuniculi* in tissue culture.
   J. Protozool. 19 (Suppl.): 75.

Bismanis, J. E. (1970). Detection of latent murine nosematosis
   and growth of *Nosema cuniculi* in cell cultures. *Canad. J.
   Microbiol.* 16: 237-242.

Burges, H. D., Canning, E. U., and Hurst, J. A. (1971). Morphology
   development, and pathogenicity of *Nosema oryzoephili N.* sp.
   in *Oryzaephibes surinamensis* and its host range among granivorous
   insects. *J. Invertebr. Pathol.* 17: 319-332.

Burges, H. D., and Thompson, E. M. (1971). Standardization and
   assay of microbial insecticides. In "Microbial Control of
   Insects and Mites" (H. D. Burges and N. W. Hussey, eds.).
   Academic Press, New York.

Canning, E. U., and Hulls, R. (1970). A microsporidian infection
   of *Anopheles gambia* Gibs, from Tanzania, interpretation of its
   mode of transmission and notes on *Nosema* infections in
   mosquitoes. *Protozool.* 17: 531-539.

Cerkasovova, A., and Vavra, J. (1972). Disintegration of microsporidian spores for physiological studies. SIP Newsletter
   4: 21.

Chalupsky, J., Bedrnik, P., and Vavra, J. (1971). The indirect
   fluorescent antibody test for *Nosema cuniculi*. *J. Protozool.*
   18 (Suppl.): 47.

Chalupsky, J., Vavra, J., and Bedrnik, P. (1973). Detection of
   antibodies to *Encephalitozoon cuniculi* in rabbits by the
   indirect immunofluorescent antibody test. *Folia Parasitol.*
   (Praha) 20: 281-284.

Cole, R. J. (1970). The application of the "triangulation" method
   to the purification of *Nosema* spores from insect tissues.
   J. Invertebr. Pathol. 15: 193-195.

Conner, R. M. (1970). Disruption of microsporidian spores for serological studies. *J. Invertebr. Pathol.* <u>15</u>: 138.

Cox, J. C., Walden, N. B., and Nairn, R. C. (1972). Presumptive diagnosis of *Nosema cuniculi* in rabbits by immunofluorescence. *Res. Vet. Sci.* <u>13</u>: 595-597.

Fischer, F. M., and Sanborn, R. C. (1959). Pathogenicity of a sporozoan parasite analyzed by tissue culture. Abstract Fed. Amer. Soc. Expt. Biol. Proc. <u>18</u>: 45.

Fischer, F. M. (1961). Interactions between a sporozoan and its insect hosts. Ph.D. thesis, Department of Zoology, Purdue University.

Fowler, J., and Reeves, E. (1974a). Detection of relationships among microsporidian isolates by electrophoretic analysis: Hydrophobic extracts. *J. Invertebr. Pathol.* <u>23</u>: 3-12.

Fowler, J. and Reeves, E. (1974b). Detection of relationships among microsporidian isolates by electrophoretic analysis: Hydrophilic extracts. *J. Invertebr. Pathol.* <u>23</u>: 63-69.

Fowler, J. L., and Reeves, E. L. (1974c). Spore dimorphism in a microsporidian isolate. *J. Protozool.* <u>21</u>: 538-542.

Fritzsch, W. (1970). Erprobung eines Heilmittels gegen Nosematose. *Arch. Exp. Vet. Med.* <u>24</u>: 951-984.

Frost, S., and Nolan, R. A. (1972). The occurrence and morphology of *Caudospora* spp. (Protozoa: Microsporida) in Newfoundland and Labrador blackfly larvae (Diptera: Simuliidae). *Canad. J. Zool.* <u>50</u>: 1363-1366.

Fyg, W. (1963). Eine einfache Methode zur elektiven Farbung von Mikroorganismen in Ausstrichen und Gewebeschnitten. *Z. Bienen.-Forsch.* <u>6</u>: 179-183.

Gassouma, M.S.S., and Ellis, D. S. (1973). The ultrastructure of sporogonic stages and spores of *Thelohania* and *Plistophora* (Microsporida, Nosematidae) from *Simulium ornatum* larvae. *J. Gen. Microbiol.* <u>74</u>: 33-43.

Gontarski, H., and Wagner, O. (1954). Quantitative Versuche zur chemotherapeutischen Bekampfung von *Nosema apis* Z. bei der Honigbiene. *Arzneim.-Forsch.* 4: 161-168.

Gude, W. D. (1968). Autoradiographic Techniques. Prentice-Hall., Inc. Englewood Cliffs, N. J. 113 pp.

Henry, J. E. (1967). *Nosema acridophagus* sp. N, a microsporidian isolated from grasshoppers. *J. Invertebr. Pathol.* <u>9</u>: 331-341.

Henry, J. E. (1971). Experimental application of *Nosema locustae* for control of grasshoppers. *J. Invertebr. Pathol.* <u>18</u>: 389-394.

Hink, W. F. (1972). A catalog of invertebrate cell lines. *In* Invertebrate Tissue Culture Volume Two, (C. Vago ed.) Academic Press, New York.

Hostounsky, Z. (1970). *Nosema mesnili* (Paill.), a microsporidian of the cabbage-worm, *Pieris brassicae* (L.) in the parasites *Apanteles glomeratus* (L.), *Hyposoter ebenius* (Grav.) and *Pimpla instigator* (F.). *Acta. Entomol. Bohemoslov* <u>67</u>: 1-5.

Hsiao, T. H., and Hsiao, C. (1973). Benomyl: a novel drug for controlling a microsporidian disease of the alfalfa weevil. *J. Invertebr. Pathol.* <u>22</u>: 303-304.

Huger, A. (1960). Electron microscope study on the cytology of a microsporidian spore by means of ultrathin sectioning. *J. Insect Pathol.* 2: 84-105.

Hunter, D. K. (1968). Response of populations of *Chironomus californicus* to a microsporidian *(Gurleya* sp.). *J. Invertebr. Pathol.* <u>10</u>: 387-389.

Ignoffo, C. M., and Hink, W. F. (1971). Propagation of arthropod pathogens in living systems. *In* "Microbial Control of Insects and Mites" (H. D. Burges and N. W. Hussey, eds.). Academic Press, New York.

Innes, J.R.M., Zeman, W., Frenkel, J. K., and Borner, G. (1962). Occult endemic encephalitozoonosis of the central nervous system of mice (Swiss-Bagg-O"Grady strain). *J. Neuropathol. Exp. Neurol.* <u>21</u>: 519-533.

Ishihara, Ren. (1968). Growth of *Nosema bombycis* in primary cell cultures of mammalian and chicken embryos. *J. Invertebr. Pathol.* <u>11</u>: 328.

Ishihara, R., and Hayashi, Y. (1968). Some properties of ribosomes from the sporoplasm of *Nosema bombycis*. *J. Invertebr. Pathol.* <u>11</u>: 377-385.

Ishihara, Ren, and Sohi, S. S. (1966). Infection of ovarian tissue cultures of *Bombyx mori* by *Nosema bombycis* spores. *J. Invertebr. Pathol.* <u>8</u>: 538-540.

Jackson, S. J., Solorzano, R. F., and Middleton, C. C. (1973). An indirect fluorescent antibody test for antibodies to *Nosema cuniculi (Encephalitozoon)* in rabbits. Proc. Annual Meeting U.S. Animal Health Association 1973, 77th, pp. 478-490.

Jenkins, J. N., McLaughlin, R. E., Parrott, W. L., and Wouters, C.J.J. (1970). Eliminating *Glugea gasti* (Protozoa: Microsporidia) from genetic stocks of the boll weevil. *J. Econ. Entomol.* <u>63</u>: 1638-1639.

Jirovec, O. (1932). Ergebnisse der Nuclealfarbung an den Sporen der Microsporidien nebst einigen Bemerkungen uber *Lymphocystis*. *Arch. Protistenk* <u>77</u>: 379-390.

Kalalova, S., and Weiser, J. (1973). Identification of microsporidia by indirect fluorescent antibody tests. Abst. Int. Conf. Insect Pathol., Fifth, Oxford, England; p. 111.

Kaneda, Y. (1969). Studies on the effect of endoxan, an antitumor substance, to promote the growth of *Nosema cuniculi in vivo* and *in vitro*. *Jap. J. Parasitol.* <u>18</u>: 294-303.

Katznelson, H., and Jamieson, C. A. (1952). Control of *Nosema* disease of honey bees with fumagillin. *Science* 115: 70-71.

Kramer, J. P. (1960). Observations on the emergence of the microsporidian sporoplasm. *J. Insect Pathol.* <u>2</u>: 433-439.

Kramer, J. P. (1964). *Nosema kingi* sp. n., a microsporidian from *Drosophila willistoni* Sturtevant, and its infectivity for other muscoids. *J. Insect Pathol.* 6: 491-499.

Kramer, J. P. (1965). Effect of an Ostosporeosis locomotor activity of adult *Phormia regina* (Meigen) (Dipt. Calliphoridae). *Entomophaga* 10: 339-342.

Kramer, J. P. (1968). An Octosporeosis of the black blowfly, *Phormia regina:* Incidence rates of host and parasite. *A. fur Parasitenk* 30: 33-39.

Kramer, J. P. (1970). Longevity of microsporidian spores with special reference to *Octosporea muscaedomesticae* Flu. *Acta. Protozool.* 8: 217-224.

Kudo, R. (1921). Microsporidia Parasitic in Copepods. *J. Parasitol.* 7: 137-143.

Kudo, R. (1922). Studies on microsporidia parasitic in mosquitoes. II. On the effect of the parasite upon the host body. *J. Parasitol.* 8: 70-77.

Kudo, R. (1924). A biologic and taxonomic study of the Microsporidia. Illinois Biol. Monogr. IX, Nos. 1 and 2. 268 pp.

Lainson, R., Garnham, P.C.C., Killick-Kendrick, R., and Bird, R. G. (1964). Nosematosis, a microsporidial infection of rodents and other animals, including man. *Brit. Med. J.* ii: 470-472.

Lewis, L. C., and Lynch, R. E. (1974). Lyophilization, vacuum drying, and subsequent storage of *Nosema pyraustae* spores. *J. Invertebr. Pathol.* 24: 149-153.

Lillie, R. D. (1965). Histopathologic technic and practical histochemistry. McGraw-Hill Book Co., New York, Toronto, Sydney, London.

Lom, J., and Vavra, J. (1962). Mucous envelopes of spores of the subphylum Cnidospora (Doflein 1901). Vest. Cs. Spol. Zool. 27: 4-6.

Lom, J., and Vavra, J. (1963). The mode of sporoplasm extrusion in microsporidian spores. *Acta. Protozool.* 1: 81-89.

Lom, J., and Weiser, J. (1969). Notes on two microsporidian species from *Silurus glanis* and on the systematic status of the genus *Glugea* Thelohan. *Folia Parasit.* (Praha) 16: 193-200.

Lom, J., and Weiser, J. (1972). Surface pattern of some microsporidian spores as seen in the scanning electron microscope. *Folia Parasitol.* (Praha) 19: 359-363.

Lotmar, R. (1944). Uber den Einfluss der Temperatur auf den Parasiten *Nosema apis*. *Schweiz. Bienen.-Z.* 67: 17-19.

Luft, J. H. (1971). Ruthenium red and violet. 1. chemistry, purification, methods of use for electron microscopy and mechanism of action. *Anat. Rec.* 171: 347-368.

Lynch, R. E., and Lewis, L. C. (1971). Reoccurrence of the microsporidan *Perezia pyraustae* in the European corn borer, *Ostrinia nubilalis*, reared on diet containing Fumidil B. *J. Invertebr. Pathol.* 17: 243-246.

Maddox, J. V. (1968). Generation time of the microsporidian, *Nosema necatrix* in larvae of the armyworm, *Pseudaletia unipuncta*. *J. Invertebr. Pathol.* 11: 90-96.

Martouret, D. (1962). Etude pathologiques sur le mode d'action de *Bacillus thuringiensis*. Int. Congr. Ent., Twelth, Vienna, 1960. 2: 849-855.

McLaughlin R. E. (1966). Laboratory techniques for rearing disease-free insect colonies: Elimination of *Mattesia grandis* McLaughlin, and *Nosema* sp. from colonies of boll weevils. *J. Econ. Entomol.* 59: 401-404.

McLaughlin, R. E., Bell, M. R., and Daum, R. J. (1967). Suspension of microorganisms in a thixotropic solution. *J. Insect. Pathol.* 9: 35-39.

McLaughlin, R. E., and Bell, M. R. (1970). Mass production *in vivo* of two protozoan pathogens, *Mattesie grandis* and *Glugea gasti* of the boll weevil, *Anthonomus grandis*. *J. Invertebr. Pathol.* 16: 84-88.

Michelson, E. H. (1963). *Plistophore husseyi*, sp. n., a microsporidian parasite of aquatic pulmonate snails. *J. Invertebr. Pathol.* 5: 28-38.

Milner, R. J. (1972a). *Nosema whitei*, a microsporidian pathogen of some species of *Tribolium*. 1. Morphology, life cycle, and generation time. *J. Invertebr. Pathol.* 19: 231-238.

Milner, R. J. (1972b). The survival of *Nosema whitei* spores stored at 4°C. *J. Invertebr. Pathol.* 20: 256-257.

Montrey, R. D., Shadduck, J. A., and Pakes, S. P. (1973). *In vitro* study of host range of three isolates of *Encephalitozoon* (Nosema). *J. Infect. Dis.* 127: 450-454.

Nelson, J. B. (1962). An intracellular parasite resembling a microsporidian associated with ascites in Swiss mice. Proc. Soc. Exp. Biol. Med. 109: 714-717.

Nelson, J. B. (1967). Experimental transmission of a murine microsporidian in Swiss mice. *J. Bacteriol.* 94: 1340-1345.

Nicholson, G. L., and Singer, S. J. (1971). Ferritin-conjugated plant agglutinins as specific saccharide stains for EM: application to saccharides bound to cell membranes. Proc. Nat. Acad. Sci. (U.S.) 68: 942-945.

Nordin, G. L. (1971). Studies on a nuclear polyhedrosis virus and three species of microsporidia pathogenic to the fall webworm, *Hyphantria cunea* (Drury). Ph.D. thesis, Department of Entomology, University of Illinois, Urbana.

Ohshima, K. (1937). On the function of the polar filament of *Nosema bombycis*. *Parasitology* 29: 220-224.

Ormerod, W. E., Healey, P., and Armitage, P. (1963). A method of counting trypanosomes allowing simultaneous study of their morphology. *Exp. Parasit.* 13: 374-385.

Overstreet, R. M., and Weidner, E. (1974). Differentiation of microsporidian sporetails in *Inodosporus spraguei* gen. et sp. n. *Z. Parasitenk.* 44: 169-186.

Pakes, S. P., Shadduck, J. A., and Olsen, R. G. (1972). A diagnostic skin test for encephalitozoonosis (nosematosis) in rabbits. Lab. Anim. Sci. 22: 870-877.

Percy, J. (1973). The intranuclear occurrence and fine structural details of schizonts of *Perezia fumiferanae* (Microsporida: Nosematidae) in cells of *Choristoneura fumiferana* (Clem.) (Lepidoptera: Tortricidae). *Canad. J. Zool.* 51: 553-554.

Piekarski, G. (1937). Cytologische Untersuchungen an Paratyphus und Colibakterien. *Arch. Mikrobiol.* 8: 428-438.

Rambourg, A. (1967). An improved silver methenamine technique for the detection of periodic acid-reactive complex carbohydrates with the electron microscope. *J. Histochem. Cytochem.* 15: 409-412.

Savage, K. E., and Lowe, R. E. (1970). Studies of *Anopheles quadrimaculatus* infected with a *Nosema* sp. Proc. Int. Colloq. on Insect Pathol., Fourth, College Park, Maryland.

Sen Gupta, K. (1964). Cultivation of *Nosema mesnili* Paillot (Microsporidia) *in vitro. Cur. Sci.* 33: 407-408.

Shadduck, J. A. (1969). *Nosema curiculi: in vitro* isolation. *Science* 166: 516-517.

Shortt, H. E., and Cooper, W. (1948). Staining of microscopical sections containing protozoal parasites by modification of McNamara's method. *Trans. R. Soc. Trop. Med. Hyg.* 41: 427-428.

Smith, C. N. (ed.). (1966). "Insect Colonization and Mass Production. Academic Press, New York.

Southwood, T.R.E. (1966). Ecological methods with particular reference to the study of insect populations. London: Methuen.

Sprague, Victor. (1965). *Nosema* sp. (Microsporidia, Nosematidae) in the musculature of the Crab, *Callinectes sopidus. J. Protozool.* 12: 66-70.

Sprague, V., Vernick, S. H., and Lloyd, B. J. Jr. (1968). The fine structure of *Nosema* sp. Sprague, 1965 (Microsporida, Nosematidae) with particular reference to stages in sporogony. *J. Invertebr. Pathol.* 12: 105-117.

Steche, W. (1965). Zur Ontologie von *Nosema apis* Zander in Mitteldarm der Arbeitsbiene. Bull, Apicole 8: 181-212.

Undeen, A. H. (1975). Growth of *Nosema algerae* in pig kidney cell cultures. *J. Protozool.* 22: 107-110.

Undeen, A. H., and Alger, N. E. (1971). A density gradient method for fractionating microsporidian spores. *J. Invertebr. Pathol.* 18: 419-420.

Undeen, A. H., and Maddox, J. V. (1973). The infection of non-mosquito hosts by injection with spores of the microsporidian *Nosema algerae. J. Invertebr. Pathol.* 22: 258-265.

Vavra, J. (1959). Beitrag zur Cytologie einiger Mikrosporidien. *Vest. Cs. Zool. Spol.* 23: 347-350.

Vavra, J. (1963). Spore projections in Microsporidia. *Acta Protozool.* 1: 153-155.

Vavra, J. (1964a). Recording microsporidian spores. *J. Insect Pathol.* 6: 258-260.

Vavra, J. (1964b). Some recent advances in the study of microsporidian spores. Proc. Int. Congr. Parasitol., First, Roma, 1964, 1: 443-444.

Vavra, J. (1965). Etude au microscope electronique de la morphologie et du developpement de quelques Microsporidies. *C. R. Acad. Sci. Paris.* 261: 3467-3470.

Vavra, J. (1972). Detection of polysaccharides in microsporidian spores by means of the periodic acid-thiosemicarbazide-silver proteinate test. *J. Microscopie* 14: 357-360.

Vavra, J., and Undeen, A. H. (1970). *Nosema algerae* n. sp. (Cnidospora, Microsporida), a pathogen in a laboratory colony of *Anopheles stephensi* Liston (Diptera, Culicidae). *J. Protozool.* 17: 240-249.

Vavra, J., Bedrnik, P., and Cinatl, J. (1972). Isolation and *in vitro* cultivation of the mammalian microsporidian *Encephalitozoon cuniculi*. *Folia parasit.* (Praha) 19: 349-354.

Vernick, S. H., Tousimis, A., and Sprague, V. (1969). Surface structure of the spores of *Glugea weissenbergi*. Proc. Annual EMSA. Twenty seventh.

Walker, M. H., and Hinsch, G. W. (1972). Ultrastructural observations of a microsporidian protozoan parasite in *Libinia dubia* (Decapoda). I. Early spore development. *Z. Parasitenk* 39: 17-26.

Weidner, E. (1970). Ultrastructural study of microsporidian development. I. *Nosema* sp. Sprague, 1965 in *Callinectes sapidus* Rathbun. *Z. Zellforsch.* 105: 33-54.

Weidner, E. (1972). Ultrastructural study of microsporidian invasion into cells. *Z. Parasitenk.* 40: 227-242.

Weiser, J. (1961). Die Mikrosporidien als Parasiten der Insekten. Monographien zur angew. Entomol. Nr. 17. Verlag Paul Parey, Hamburg und Berlin. 149 pp.

Weiser, J. (1964). Parasitology of black flies. Bull. W.H.O. 31: 483-485.

Weiser, J. (1969). Immunity of insects to protozoa. *In* "Immunity to Parasitic Animals" (G. J. Jackson, R. Herman, and I. Singer, eds.), 1: 129-147. Appleton-Century-Crofts, New York.

Wright, R. D., and Lumsden, R. D. (1968). Ultrastructural and histochemical properties of the acanthocephalan epicuticle. *J. Parasitol.* 54: 1111-1123.

Yearian, W. C., Gilbert, K. L., and Warren, L. O. (1966). Rearing the fall webworm, *Hyphantria cunea* (Lepidoptera: Arctiidae) on a wheat germ medium. *J. Kans. Ent. Soc.* 39: 495-499.

The International Protozoan Type Slide Collection: Its Origin and Goals

BURDETTE W. ERICKSON, JR.

DIVISION OF CANCER TREATMENT
NATIONAL CANCER INSTITUTE
NATIONAL INSTITUTES OF HEALTH
BETHESDA, MARYLAND

I. AN HISTORICAL PERSPECTIVE

At the First International Conference on Protozoology held in
Prague, 1961, Dr. Jaroslav Weiser urged protozoologists around
the world to consolidate their slide collections, publish the
contents, and deposit type materials in centralized locations.
Between 1961 and 1970, the single strongest force for organized
invertebrate collections was the founder of the Society for
Invertebrate Pathology (S.I.P.), the late Dr. Edward A. Steinhaus.
In June, 1965, he was instrumental in the formation of the
Registry of Tumors in Lower Animals, a joint venture of the
National Cancer Institute and the Smithsonian Institution. By
July, 1968, he had established the Center for Pathobiology under
the auspices of the University of California at Irvine. In an
editorial to the Society (1968), Dr. Steinhaus stressed the need
for centers around the world to serve, among other purposes, as
repositories for type materials of infectious agents.

When the Fourth International Colloquium on Insect Pathology
convened at the University of Maryland in August, 1970, the newly-
formed Division on Microsporidia of the S.I.P. echoed Weiser and
Steinhaus. At that time the author volunteered to locate a
depository for Microsporidian type specimens in the Washington
area. By Summer, 1971, three institutions had been approached:
the National Animal Parasite Laboratory at Beltsville, Md.; the
American Type Culture Collection at Rockville, Md.; and the
National Museum of Natural History at the Smithsonian in
Washington, D.C. Whereas all three expressed a willingness to
cooperate with the Division, only the Smithsonian seemed well-
suited for the task. The National Animal Parasite Laboratory is
primarily helminth-oriented and the American Type Culture
Collection handles only viable material in culture. In August a
letter recommending the Smithsonian as the deposition site was
sent to Dr. Jiri Vavra, Chairman of the Division. This report
drew a letter of encouragement from Dr. Weiser who had been
painstakingly building an extensive "working" collection. Unfortunately, Dr. Weiser could not contribute any of his material
due to state regulations.

Simultaneously, Dr. John Briggs of the S.I.P., while trying to
create an efficient information exchange system for invertebrate
pathology, became aware of the urgent need for specimen central-
ization. Having contacted the National Animal Parasite Laboratory
and the Smithsonian, he personally solicited the opinions of
Dr. Alois Huger, Dr. Jerzy Lipa, Dr. John Corliss, Dr. Weiser,
and others. By Fall, 1972, these eminent investigators had
responded enthusiastically. Dr. Briggs, discovering the efforts
of the author, decided not to pursue his own any farther. In
January, 1972, Dr. Corliss of the University of Maryland had
deposited his International Collection of Ciliate Type Specimens
at the Smithsonian. It was to form the nucleus of an expanded

International Protozoan Type Slide Collection. One year later, after concluding a series of discussions on services and regulations with Dr. Klaus Reutzler of the Smithsonian, the author submitted the first announcement of the Collection to the S.I.P. Newsletter (Erickson, 1973).

II. FUNCTIONS OF A TYPE COLLECTION

Type specimens serve as standard comparatives for similar organisms. They are invaluable for new species descriptions, taxonomic revisions, and monographic studies. Their most important role is resolving taxonomic controversies caused by conflicting evidence or insufficient documentation. Weiser (1964) remarked that new techniques frequently give confusing data with respect to ultrastructure, sexuality, and infectivity on individuals within a single species or closely related species. The problem of identity is greatly compounded if the relevant type material has become misplaced or accidentally discarded. The purpose of a type slide collection is to centralize and preserve such specimens. This activity requires a coordinated effort to locate types, replace lost ones, publicize those available (Table 1), and make them accessible to investigators in the field. If successful, a well-documented baseline for comparing morphologic, developmental, and biochemical characteristics among species can be established. Additional stability can be achieved by placing paratype preparations in a number of different centralized depositories.

The terminology associated with designation of type specimens and its application to protozoologic material are discussed at length elsewhere (Corliss, 1972; Smith and Williams, 1970; Stoll *et al.*, 1964). For the reader's convenience, a short glossary is appended.

III. A PLAN OF ACTION

To establish definite standards of comparison for future research in Protozoology, particularly for microsporidia, the Standing Committee on Type Slide Collections has initiated a program to contact investigators with laboratory or personal collections urging them to deposit their material in the International Protozoan Type Slide Collection. Specimens need not be type specimens to be entered in the Collection. Suitable preparations of any protozoologic material are desired and their deposition is encouraged. In addition, the Committee plans to expand its publicity of the Collection and coordinate the formation of taxonomic advisory groups to aid the Museum.

Long-range goals of the Committee are based on the report of Irwin *et al.* (1973) to the Association of Systematics Collections (A.S.C.) outlining a national plan to develop collections as a

Table 1

Published Location of Some Microsporidian Type Specimens

Specimen	Author(s)/Year	Type[1]	Collection Location[2]
Caudospora alaskensis	Jamnback (1970)	H&P	New York State Museum
Caudospora brevicauda	Jamnback (1970)	H&P	New York State Museum
Caudospora nasiae	Jamnback (1970)	H&P	New York State Museum
Caudospora pennsylvanica	Beaudoin & Wills (1965)	H	Center for Pathobiol., Univ. of Calif., Irvine, Calif.
Coccospora brachynema	Richards & Sheffield (1970)	P	W. Kellen, R. Kudo, J. Weiser
		H	Center for Pathobiol., Univ. of Calif., Irvine, Calif.
Glugea bychowskyi	Gasimagomedov & Issi (1970)	S?	All-Union Inst. Plant Protection, Lenningrad, U.S.S.R.
Glugea dogieli	Gasimagomedov & Issi (1970)	S?	All-Union Inst. Plant Protection, Lenningrad, U.S.S.R.
Glugea gasti	McLaughlin (1969)	S	E.R.D., A.R.S., U.S.D.A., State College, Mississippi & Plant Industry Stat., U.S.D.A., Beltsville Md.
Glugea schulmani	Gasimagomedov & Issi (1970)	S?	All-Union Inst. Plant Protection, Lenningrad, U.S.S.R.
Gurleya sokolovi	Issi & Lipa (1968)	H&P	Authors
Inodosporus spraguei	Overstreet & Weidner (1974)	S	Nat. Mus. Natural History, Smithsonian, Wash., D.C.
Nosema bioloviesiana	Lipa (1966)	H	Author
		P	J. Weiser
Nosema campoletidis	Brooks & Cranford (1972)	H&P	Nat. Mus. Natural History, Smithsonian, Wash., D.C.
Nosema cardiochilis	Brooks & Cranford (1972)	H&P	Nat. Mus. Natural History, Smithsonian, Wash., D.C.

Table 1 (Cont.)

Specimen	Author(s)/Year	Type	Collection Location
Nosema chapmani	Kellen *et al.* (1967)	H	Div. Insect Pathol., Univ. of Calif., Berkeley, Calif.
		P	Authors, J. Lipa, J. Weiser
Nosema cuneatum	Henry (1971)	H&P	E.R.D.,A.R.S.,U.S.D.A., Montana State Univ., Bozeman
Nosema heterosporum	Kellen & Lindegren (1969)	H&P	Nat. Mus. Natural Hist., Helm. Coll., Smithsonian
Nosema juli	Wilson (1971)	S	Nat. Mus. Natural Hist., Smithsonian, Wash., D.C.
Nosema legeri	Dollfus (1912)	H?	Mus. Nat. d'Hist. Naturelle, Paris, France
Nosema leptinotarsae	Lipa (1968a)	H	Author
Nosema lepturae	Lipa (1968b)	H	Author
Nosema lunatum	Kellen *et al.* (1967)	H	Div. Insect Pathol., Univ. of Calif., Berkeley, Calif.
		P	Authors, J. Lipa, J. Weiser
Nosema necatrix	Kramer (1965	H&P	Illinois Natural History Survey, Urbana, Ill.
Nosema phryganidiae	Lipa & Martignoni (1968)	H&P	Authors
Nosema plodiae	Kellen & Lindegren (1968)	H&P	Nat. Mus. Natural Hist., Smithsonian, Wash., D.C.
Nosema sauridae	Narasimhamurti & Kalavati (1972)	H?	Dept. of Zoology, Andhra Univ., Waltair, India
Nosema sperchoni	Lipa (1962)	H	Author
		P	Div. Insect Pathol., Univ. of Calif., Berkeley, Calif.
Nosema sphingidis	Brooks (1970)	H&P	Center for Pathobiol., Univ. of Calif., Irvine, Calif.
Nosema weiseri	Lipa (1968c)	H	Author
		P	J. Weiser

Table 1 (Cont.)

Specimen	Author(s)/Year	Type	Collection Location
Octosporea effeminans	Bulnheim & Vavra (1968)	H	H. Bulnheim
		H	J. Vavra, J. Weiser
Pleistophora caecorum[3]	Chapman & Kellen (1967)	H	Div. Insect Pathol., Univ.of Calif., Berkeley, Calif.
Pleistophora cependianae	Putz et al. (1965)	P	Authors
		H	Nat. Mus. Natural Hist., Helm. Coll., Smithsonian
Pleistophora chaobori	Rapsch (1950)	H	Author
		P	Zool. Inst. Tech. Hochsch., Braunschweig
Pleistophora chapmani	Clark & Fukuda (1971)	H	Div. Insect Pathol, Univ. of Calif., Berkeley, Calif.
		P	Mosquito Investigation Laboratory, Lake Charles, La.
Pleistophora collessi	Laird (1959)	H	Dominion Museum, Wellington, New Zealand
Pleistophora geotrupina	Lipa (1968d)	P	Author
		H	Author
Pleistophora milesi	Pillai (1974)	P	Zool. Inst., Warsaw; J. Weiser
		H	National Museum, Wellington, New Zealand
Pleistophora mochlonicis	Rapsch (1955)	P	J. Weiser, J. Lipa, M. Laird, Center for Pathobiol.
		H	Author
Pleistophora myotrophica	Canning et al. (1964)	P	Zool. Inst. Tech. Hochsch., Braunschweig
Pleistophora ovalis	Rapsch (1955)	S	Authors; Imperial College, London
		H	Author
		P	Zool. Inst. Tech. Hochsch., Braunschweig

Table 1 (Cont.)

Specimen	Author(s)/Year	Type	Collection Location
Pleistophora salmonae	Putz *et al.* (1965)	H	Nat. Mus. Natural Hist., Helm. Coll., Smithsonian
Pleistophora sauridae	Narasimhamurti & Kalavati(1972)	H?	Dept. of Zoology, Andhra Univ., Waltair, India
Pleistophora scolyti	Weiser (1968)	S	Author
Pleistophora siluri	Gasimogomedov & Issi (1970)	S?	All-Union Inst. Plant Protection, Leningrad, U.S.S.R.
Pleistophora tuberifera	Gasimogomedov & Issi (1970)	S?	All-Union Inst. Plant Protection, Leningrad, U.S.S.R.
Pyrotheca cuneiformis	Murand *et al.*(1972)	H&P	J. Maurand
Stempellia lunata	Hazard & Savage (1970)	H	Insect Laboratory, Gainesville, Fla
		P	J. Weiser
Stempellia milleri	Hazard & Fukuda (1974)	H	Nat. Mus. Natural Hist., Smithsonian, Wash., D.C.
		P	J. Briggs, H. Chapman, J. Weiser
Stempellia moniezi	Jones (1943)	S?	Author; Miller School of Biology, Univ. of Virginia
Thelohania barra	Pillai (1968)	H	Dominion Museum, Wellington, New Zealand
		P	Author, J. Lipa, J. Weiser, R. Kudo, British Museum
Thelohania benigna	Kellen & Wills (1962)	H	Div. Insect Pathol., Univ. of Calif., Berkeley, Calif.
		P	Authors, J. Lipa, J. Weiser, R. Kudo
Thelohania bolinasae	Kellen & Wills (1962)	H	Div. Insect Pathol., Univ. of Calif., Berkeley, Calif.
		P	Authors, J. Lipa, J. Weiser, R. Kudo

Table 1 (Cont.)

Specimen	Author(s)/Year	Type	Collection Location
Thelohania californica	Kellen & Lipa (1960)	H	Div. Insect Pathol., Univ. of Calif., Berkeley, Calif.
Thelohania diazoma	Kramer (1965)	H&P	Illinois Natural History Survey, Urbana, Ill.
Thelohania duorara	Iversen & Manning (1959)	S?	Nat. Mus. Natural Hist., Smithsonian, Wash.,D.C., & Univ. of Miama, Miami, Fla.
Thelohania gigantea	Kellen & Wills (1962)	H	Div. Insect Pathol., Univ. of Calif., Berkeley, Calif.
		P	Authors, J. Lipa, J. Weiser, R. Kudo
Thelohania inimica	Kellen & Wills (1962)	H	Div. Insect Pathol., Univ. of Calif., Berkeley, Calif.
		P	Authors, J. Lipa, J. Weiser, R. Kudo
Thelohania nana	Kellen & Lindegren (1969)	H	Nat. Mus. Natural Hist., Helm. Coll., Smithsonian
Thelohania nepa	Lipa (1966)	H	Author
Thelohania noxia	Kellen & Wills (1962)	H	Div. Insect Pathol., Univ. of Calif., Berkeley, Calif.
		P.	Authors, J. Lipa, J. Weiser, R. Kudo
Thelohania periculosa	Kellen & Wills (1962)	H	Div. Insect Pathol., Univ. of Calif., Berkeley, Calif.
		P	Authors, J. Lipa, J. Weiser, R. Kudo
Thelohania thomsoni	Kramer (1961)	H&P	Illinois Natural History Survey, Urbana, Ill.
Thelohania urica	Kellen & Wills (1962)	H	Div. Insect Pathol., Univ. of Calif., Berkeley, Calif.
		P	Authors, J.Lipa, J.Weiser, R.Kudo
Weiseria sommermanae	Jamnback (1970)	H&P	New York State Museum

Table 1 (Cont.)

[1] Type is indicated by H = holotype, P = paratype, S = syntype; question mark (?) indicates uncertainty.

[2] The current addresses of most individual investigators can be obtained from the 1973-1975 Membership List of the Society for Invertebrate Pathology

[3] *Plistophora* Labbé, 1899, has been shown by Sprague (*J. Invert. Pathol.* 17: 1-2, 1971) to be a junior synonym of *Pleistophora* Gurley, 1893.

natural resource. These include periodic publication of a type
slide directory, formation of an Advisory Committee for Systematic
Recources in Protozoology to the A.S.C., development of centralized
literature centers dealing with specific protozoan groups, and
establishment of an electronic data processing system for Protozoa
to supplement the literature centers and Type Slide Collection.
Regarding the last two items mentioned above, Drs. Canning, Pilley,
and Sprenkel (1975) have developed a data retrieval system for
microsporidia. Furthermore, our British colleagues, headed by
Drs. Curds and Pilley, have founded a paratype collection at the
British Museum. Material for this depository is enthusiastically
solicited. Any investigator who wishes to deposit slides in the
British Museum Protozoan Type Slide Collection is requested to
send his material to Dr. Colin Curds, Protozoan Section, Department
of Zoology, British Museum (Natural History), Cromwell Road,
London SW7 5BD. It is sincerely hoped that more centralized
depositories become available and that they be used for the
distribution of paratypes.

IV. GUIDELINES

   To insure a viable collection, certain rules are necessary for
order and consistency. The procedures outlines here were developed
for slide deposition in the International Protozoan Type Slide
Collection and reported to the Division on Microsporidia of the
S.I.P. These procedures likewise apply to deposition of slides in
the British Museum Protozoan Type Slide Collection. Those materials
should, of course, be forwarded to Dr. Curds (see above).
   Any investigator wishing to contribute material to the International Protozoan Type Slide Collection is requested to:
   1. Forward his slides to Dr. Klaus Reutzler, Division of
       Echinoderms and Lower Invertebrates, National Museum of
       Natural History, Smithsonian Institution, Washington,
       D.C., 20560, U.S.A. Contributors making large depositions
       are asked to notify Dr. Reutzler by mail before shipment
       so adequate preparations can be made. For small depositions,
       a short leter of information may be enclosed with the slides.
       Becklund (1969) suggests slides be individually wrapped in
       paper, then placed in a wooden or flexible plastic box with
       shock-absorbing material between the slides. This protects
       the slides from each other in case of breakage and allows
       recovery of broken pieces for possible reconstruction.
   2. Permanently mount all specimens on 3" X 1" (76 mm X 25 mm)
       glass microscope slides identified with permanent labels.
       Gummed paper slide labels are perfectly acceptable. The
       genus, species, and type should be etched into the reverse
       side in case the label is lost (Figure 1). If mixtures of
       species are present, those specimens belonging to the new
       species should be carefully and permanently indicated.

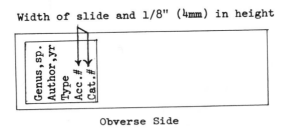

Width of slide and 1/8" (4mm) in height

Obverse Side

Etched into glass with diamond stylus

Reverse Side

Fig. 1. Schematic diagram of slide preparation for deposition.

Fig. 2. Standardized format for data sheet to accompany specimen slide.

International Protozoan Type Slide Collection
National Museum of Natural History
Smithsonian Institution
Washington, D.C., U.S.A.

From: Accession#: _____

Data Sheet for Slide Deposition

Cat.#	Genus and Species	Author and Year	Type	Host	Locality	#Syntypes	Group	Stain

Names of Identifiers (if one or more were consulted):

Special Remarks:

Labels should be hand printed in ink for clarity. Perti-
nent information includes:
  a) Genus, species, author, and year.
  b) Material type (holotype, paratype, etc.).
  c) Space for a seven digit accession number (width
      of the slide and 1/8" or 4 mm in height).
  d) Space for a seven digit catalogue number (same
      as in "c"), particularly in the case of type
      specimens.
3. Submit slides in some predetermined order accompanied by
    three copies of additional information (data sheets). Such
    information might include:
    a) Host, if species is parasitic.
    b) Collection locality.
    c) Stain. Weiser (1964) recommends iron hematoxylin,
        silver impregnation, or other non-deteriorating
        method.
    d) Original number of syntypes.
    e) Identifier, if one is consulted.
    f) Higher classification.
    g) Any pertinent remarks.
  To facilitate this request, the Standing Committee on Type
  Slide Collections of the Division of Microsporida has
  provided a standardized format (Figure 2).
4. Submit an additional data sheet for each type specimen
    deposited. Due to their taxonomic importance, type specimens
    will comprise a separate subcollection receiving special
    care.
5. Include a copy of the paper(s) originally describing any
    type material being deposited. If a reprint is not yet
    available, the paper should have been accepted for publi-
    cation or be in press before deposition is made. To
    enjoy nomenclatural recognition, a new species name must
    be made available to the public in scientific context.
    This procedure guarantees the integrity and continuity of
    the Collection. Specimens which, for some reason, have
    not yet been given a specific designation may be marked sp.,
    author, and date, then submitted. All specimens will be
    filed according to the designation of the original author.
6. Send only microscope slide specimens. While the type slide
    is not the sole source of descriptive data necessary for
    precise identification, the Museum is not equipped to
    handle other supportive materials (e.g., life cycle
    illustrations, electron micrographs, specimen blocks).
  The National Museum of Natural History assumes responsibility
for the International Protozoan Type Slide Collection and agrees
to:

1. Decline acceptance of material in unsatisfactory condition. The Museum requests responsible investigators to refurbish valuable materials that are badly preserved, stained, or mounted before deposition. The Museum does not wish to be responsible for the loss of or damage to original type material.

2. Identify each slide received with a lot accession number reserved for that group of slides. Slides are stored numerically by accession number in "Technicon" slide cabinets with type material housed separately. Weiser (1964) recommends the use of special tapes to mark type material. All materials deposited become the property of the National Museum of Natural History.

3. Make the collection available in part or in full to interested investigators and institutions. Duration of a loan is negotiable, not to exceed one year. Loans are renewable annually upon request with justification. All loaned materials are expected to be carefully maintained.

4. Assign catalogue numbers to type slides, particularly for publication. Although all slides should be catalogued, shortage of personnel does not allow such thoroughness.

The author wishes to extend his sincerest thanks to Dr. Ann Cali of the Armed Forces Institute of Pathology and Dr. Anne Caldwell of the National Library of Medicine for reviewing the text of this chapter and offering their suggestions. Dr. Cali is a member of the Standing Committee on Type Slide Collections.

Special thanks are due Dr. Victor Sprague of the Chesapeake Biological Laboratory, University of Maryland, for sparking the author's interest in the microsporidia and making his excellent facilities available to the author.

REFERENCES

Beaudoin, R., and Wills, W. (1965). A description of *Caudospora pennsylvanica* sp. n. (Caudosporidae, Microsporidia) a parasite of the larvae of the black fly, *Prosimulium magnum* Dyar and Shannon. *J. Invert. Pathol.* 7: 152-155.

Becklund, W. W. (1969). The national parasite collection at the Beltsville Parasitological Laboratory. *J. Parasit.* 55: 375-380.

Brooks, W. M. (1970). *Nosema sphingidis* sp. n., a microsporidian parasite of the tobacco hornworm, *Manduca sexta*. *J. Invert. Pathol.* 16: 390-399.

Brooks, W. M. and Cranford, J. D. (1972). Microsporidioses of the hymenopterous parasites, *Campoletis sonorensis* and *Cardiochiles nigriceps*, larval parasites of *Heliothis* species. *J. Invert. Pathol.* 20: 77-94.

Bulnheim, H. P., and Vavra, J. (1968). Infection by the micro-
    sporidian *Octosporea effeminans* sp. n. and its sex determining
    influence in the amphipod *Gammarus duebeni*. *J. Parasit.*
    54: 241-248.

Canning, E. U., Elkan, E., and Trigg, P. I. (1964). *Plistophora
    myotrophica* spec. nov., causing high mortality in the common
    toad *Bufo bufo* L., with notes on the maintenance of *Bufo*
    and *Xenopus* in the laboratory. *J. Protozool.* 11: 157-166.

Canning, E. U., Pilley, B. M., and Sprenkel, R. K. (1975).
    Computer-based data retrieval system. *Soc. Invert. Pathol.
    Newsl.* 7: 2.

Chapman, H. C., and Kellen, W. R. (1967). *Plistophora caecorum*
    sp. n., a microsporidian of *Culiseta inornata* (Diptera:
    Culicidae) from Louisiana. *J. Invert. Pathol.* 9: 500-502.

Clark, T. B., and Fukuda, T. (1971). *Pleistophora chapmani*
    n. sp. (Cnidospora: Microsporida) in *Culex territans*
    (Diptera;Culicidae) from Louisiana. *J. Invert. Pathol.*
    18: 400-404.

Corliss, J. O. (1972). Current status of the International
    Collection of Ciliate Type-Specimens and guidelines for future
    contributors. *Trans. Amer. Micros. Soc.* 91: 221-235.

Dollfus, R. Ph. (1912). Contribution a l'etude des trematodes
    marins des cotes du Boulonnais. Une meta-cercaire margaritigene
    parasite de *Donax vittatus* Da Costa. *Mem. Soc. Zool. France*
    25: 85-144.

Erickson, B. W., Jr. (1973). Protozoan type slide collection.
    Soc. Invert. Pathol. Newsl. 5: 4.

Gasimagomedov, A. A., and Issi, I. V. (1970). Microsporidia --
    parasites of fishes of the Caspian Sea. *Zool. Zhurn.*
    49: 1117-1125.

Hazard, E. I., and Fukuda, T. (1974). *Stempellia milleri* sp. n.
    (Microsporida:Nosematidae) in the mosquito *Culex pipiens
    quinquefasciatus* Say. *J. Protozool.* 21: 497-504.

Hazard, E. I., and Savage, K. E. (1970). *Stempellia lunata* sp. n.
    (Microsporida:Nosematidae) in larvae of the mosquito *Culex
    pilosus* collected in Florida. *J. Invert. Pathol.* 15: 49-54.

Henry, J. E. (1971). *Nosema cuneatum* sp. n. (Microsporida:
    Nosematidae) in grasshoppers (Orthoptera:Acrididae).
    J. Invert. Pathol. 17: 164-171.

Irwin, H. S., Payne, W. W., Bates, D. M., and Humphrey, P. S.
    (1973). *America's Systematics Collections: A National Plan.*
    Association of Systematics Collections.

Issi, I. V., and Lipa, J. J. (1968). *Gurleya sokolovi* sp. n.,
    a microsporidian parasite of the water mite *Limnochares
    aquatica* L. (Acarina:Hydrachnellae), and a note on a gregarine
    infection in the same mite. *J. Invert. Pathol.* 10: 165-175.

Iversen, E. S., and Manning, R. B. (1959). A new microsporidan
    parasite from the pink shrimp (*Panaeus duorarum*). *Trans. Amer.
    Fish. Soc.* 88: 130-132.

Jamnback, H. A. (1970). *Caudospora* and *Weiseria*, two genera of Microsporidia parasitic in blackflies. *J. Invert. Pathol.* 16: 3-13.

Jones, A. W. (1943). A further description of *Stempellia moniezi* Jones, 1942, a microsporidian parasite (Nosematidae) of cestodes. *J. Parasit.* 29: 373-378.

Kellen, W. R., Clark, T. B., and Lindegren, J. E. (1967). Two previously undescribed *Nosema* from mosquitoes of California (Nosematidae:Microsporidia). *J. Invert. Pathol.* 9: 19-25.

Kellen, W. R., and Lindegren, J. E. (1968). Biology of *Nosema plodiae* sp. n., a microsporidian pathogen of the Indian-meal moth, *Plodia interpunctella* Hb. (Lepidoptera:Phycitidae). *J. Invert. Pathol.* 11: 104-111.

Kellen, W. R. and Lindegren, J. E. (1969). Host-pathogen relationships of two previously undescribed Microsporidia from the Indian-meal moth, *Plodia interpunctella* (Hbn.) *J. Invert. Pathol.* 14: 328-335.

Kellen, W. R. and Lipa, J. J. (1960). *Thelohania californica* n. sp., a microsporidian parasite of *Culex tarsalis* Coquill. *J. Insect Pathol.* 2: 1-12.

Kellen, W. R. and Wills, W. (1962). New *Thelohania* from California mosquitoes (Nosematidae:Microsporidia). *J. Insect Pathol.* 4: 41-56.

Kramer, J. P. (1961). *Thelohania thomsoni* n. sp., a microsporidian parasite of *Muscina assimilis* (Fallen) (Diptera, Muscidae). *J. Insect Pathol.* 3: 259-265.

Kramer, J. P. (1964). *Nosema kingi* sp. n., a microsporidian from *Drosophila willistoni* Sturtevant, and its infectivity for other muscoids. *J. Insect Pathol.* 6: 491-499.

Kramer, J. P. (1965). *Nosema necatrix* sp. n., and *Thelohania diazoma* sp. n., microsporidians from the armyworm *Pseudaletia unipuncta* (Haworth). *J. Invert. Pathol.* 7: 117-121.

Laird, M. (1959). Malayan Protozoa. I. *Plistophora collessi* sp. n. (Sporozoa:Microsporidia), an ovarian parasite of Singapore mosquitoes. *J. Protozool.* 6: 37-45.

Lipa, J. J. (1962). *Nosema sperchoni* n. sp. (Microsporidia), a new parasitic protozoan from the water mite *Sperchon* sp. (Hydracarina, Acarina). *Bull. l'Acad. Polon. Sci.* 10: 435-437.

Lipa, J. J. (1966). Miscellaneous observations on protozoan infections of *Nepa cinerea* Lin. including descriptions of two previously unknown species of Microsporidia, *Nosema bialoviesianae* sp. n. and *Thelohania nepa* sp. n. *J. Invert. Pathol.* 8: 158-166.

Lipa, J. J. (1968a). *Nosema leptinotarsae* sp. n., a microsporidian parasite of the Colorado potato beetle, *Leptinotarsa decemlineata* Say. *J. Invert. Pathol.* 10: 111-115.

Lipa, J. J. (1968b). *Nosema lepturae* sp. n., a new microsporidian parasite of *Leptura rubra* L. (Coleoptera,Cerambycidae). *Acta Protozool.* 5: 269-274.

Lipa, J. J. (1968c). On two microsporidians: *Nosema whitei* Weiser from *Tribolium confusum* and *Nosema weiseri* sp. n. from *Rhizopertha dominica*. *Acta Protozool.* 5: 375-382.

Lipa, J. J. (1968d). *Plistophora geotrupina* sp. n., a microsporidian parasite of dung beetles *Geotrupes* sp. (Coleoptera, Scarabaeidae). *Acta Protozool.* 6: 341-348.

Lipa, J. J. and Martigoni, M. (1960). *Nosema phryganidiae* n. sp., a microsporidian parasite of *Phryganidia california* Packard. *J. Insect Pathol.* 2: 396-410.

Maurand, J., Fize, A., Michel, R., et Fenwick, B. (1972). Quelques donnees sur les microsporidies parasites de copepodes cyclopoides des eaux continentales de la region de Montpellier. *Bull. Soc. Zool. France* 97: 707-717.

McLaughlin, R. E. (1969). *Glugea gasti* sp. n., a microsporidian pathogen of the boll weevil *Anthonomus grandis*. *J. Protozool.* 16: 84-92.

Narasimhamurti, C. C., and Kalavati, C. (1972). Two new species of microsporidian parasites from a marine fish *Saurida tumbil*. *Proc. Indian Acad. Sci.* Sect. B. 76: 165-170.

Overstreet, R. M., and Weidner, E. (1974). Differentiation of microsporidian spore-tails in *Inodosporus spraguei* gen. et sp. n. *Z. Parasitenk.* 44: 169-186.

Pillai, J. S. (1968). *Thelohania barra* n. sp., a microsporidian parasite of *Aedes (Halaedes) australis* Erichson, in New Zealand. *Z. Angew. Entomol.* 62: 395-398.

Pillai, J. S. (1974). *Pleistophora milesi*, a new species of Microsporida from *Maorigoeldia argyropus* Walker (Diptera:Culicidae) in New Zealand. *J. Invert. Pathol.* 24: 234-237.

Putz, R. E., Hoffman, G. L., and Dunbar, C. E. (1965). Two new species of *Plistophora* (Microsporidea) from North American fish with a synopsis of Microsporidea of freshwater and euryhaline fishes. *J. Protozool.* 12: 228-236.

Rapsch, I. (1950). Microsporidien in Larven der Culiciden-Gattung *Chaoborus* Lichtenstein. *Z. Parasitenk.* 14: 426-431.

Rapsch, I. (1955). Microsporidien als Parasiten von *Mochlonyx culicifromis* de Geer. *Mitteil. Munchner ent. Ges.* 44/45: 443-450.

Richards, C. S., and Sheffield, H. G. (1970). Unique host relations and ultrastructure of a new microsporidian of the genus *Coccospora* infecting *Biomphalaria glabrata*. *Proc.* 4th *Int. Colloq. Insect Pathol.*, 1970 pp. 439-452.

Smith, H. M., and Williams, O. (1970). The salient provisions of the International Code of Zoological Nomenclature: a summary for nontaxonomists. *BioScience* 20: 553-557.

Steinhaus, E. A. (1968). Centers for pathobiology. *J. Invert. Pathol.* 11: i-iv.

Stoll, N. R., Dollfus, R. Ph., Forest, J., Riley, N. D., Sabrosky,
    C. W., Wright, C. W., and Melville, R. V. (1964). *International
    Code of Zoological Nomenclature*. International Trust for
    Zoological Nomenclature, London.
Weiser, J. (1964). Type collections of Protozoa and taxonomy.
    Proc. First Inter. Conf. Protozool., pp. 64-65.
Weiser, J. (1968). *Plistophora scolyti* sp. n. (Protozoa, Micro-
    sporidia), a new parasite of *Scolytus scolytus* F. (Col.,
    Scolytidae). *Folia Parasit.* 15: 11-14.
Wilson, G. G. (1971). *Nosema juli* n. sp. a microsporidian parasite
    in the millipede *Diploiculus londinensis caeruleocinctus*
    (Wood) (Diplopoda:Julidae). *Can. J. Zool.* 49: 1279-1282.

GLOSSARY

The definitions presented below are quoted from Chapter 16 of the *International Code of Zoological Nomenclature* (ICZN) (Stoll *et al.*, 1964). Bear in mind that this terminology was developed for single specimens (ICZN, Article 72a) and not whole subpopulations as in Protozoology. However, the transition from "type-specimen" to "type-preparation" is not a difficult one to make (Corliss, 1972).

1. Type-series — "The type-series of a species consists of all the specimens on which its author bases the species ..." (ICZN, Article 72b)

2. Holotype — "If a nominal species is based on a single specimen , that specimen is the 'holotype'." (ICZN, Article 73a)

3. Syntype — "If a nominal species has no holotype ..., all the specimens of the type-series are 'syntypes', of equal value in nomenclature." (ICZN, Article 73c)

4. Paratype — "After the holotype has been labelled, each remaining specimen (if any) of the type-series should be conspicuously labelled 'paratype', in order clearly to identify the components of the original type-series." (ICZN, Recommendation 73D)

5. Lectotype — "If a nominal species has no holotype, any zoologist may designate one of the syntypes as the 'lectotype'." (ICZN, Article 74a).

6. Paralectotype — "A zoologist who designates a lectotype should clearly label any remaining syntypes with the designation 'paralecotype'." (ICZN , Recommendation 74E)

7. Neotype — "........, a zoologist may designate another specimen to serve as the 'neotype' of a species if, through loss or destruction no holotype, lectotype, or syntype exists." (ICZN, Article 75)

In the case of neotypes, there are stringent conditions laid down by the Code (Article 75a-f). Anyone considering the designation of a neotype should check these conditions carefully before proceeding.

Glossary for the Microsporidia[*]

JIŘÍ VÁVRA AND VICTOR SPRAGUE

CZECHOSLOVAK ACADEMY OF SCIENCES
INSTITUTE OF PARASITOLOGY
DEPARTMENT OF PROTOZOOLOGY
PRAHA 2, VINICNA 7, CZECHOSLOVAKIA

and

UNIVERSITY OF MARYLAND
CENTER FOR ENVIRONMENTAL AND ESTUARINE STUDIES
CHESAPEAKE BIOLOGICAL LABORATORY
SOLOMONS, MARYLAND 20688

[*]Contribution No. 670, Center for Environmental and Estuarine
Studies, University of Maryland. Supported, in part, by
National Science Foundation Grant No. GB-26519 to Victor Sprague.

   The only existing glossary for the microsporidia is a list
of 30 terms given by Kudo (1924a) in his famous monograph. That
glossary, whatever its original merits, has become hopelessly
inadequate during the half century that has elapsed since 1924.
This has been in no small measure due to the introduction of
many new terms, especially after 1960 when electron microscopy,
combined with ultrathin sectioning, has opened up a higher level
of insight into the morphology of the microsporidia. At the same
time, a few of the older terms that were originally applied in
the mistaken belief that microsporidia are essentially similar
to some other groups of parasitic protozoa, particularly the
myxosporidia, have become obsolete. In recent years the rapid
accumulation of new data, resulting not only in the introduction
of many new terms but also in frequent reexamination of old ones,
has been accompanied by a marked instability in the meanings
associated with terms. Different authors have used many terms
with widely different meanings with the result that it is now
difficult for an author to select appropriate terms for commun-
icating his ideas and just as difficult for the reader to
understand the sense in which the author used those terms. Clearly,
there is now an urgent need for a modern and complete glossary
that will give a generally understood meaning to the technical
terms currently in use and thereby facilitate communication
about the microsporidia.
   We have tried to include in the following list most of the
technical terms currently used in the microsporidian literature,
along with thoughtfully prepared definitions and, when appropriate,
some explanatory remarks. In doing this, we have encountered some
difficult problems and have suggested some solutions, although we
are aware that the solutions offered are not without flaws.
   One general problem is inherent in the fact that a few of the
important terms which long ago became established in our vocabulary were originally applied to other protozoan groups (mainly
SPOROZOEA) and can not always be applied with an exactly equivalent
meaning to these groups and the microsporidia. We believe the
only practical solution to this problem is to continue using those
terms that have become established in our vocabulary and which
still seem to be particularly useful, while modifying the definitions according to our needs. The difficulty of this problem
is alleviated by the fact that Levine (1971) recently published
a new glossary for the SPOROZOEA (plus some related groups that
he placed together in subphylum APICOMPLEXA). Levine's list
contains 72 terms, 10 of which (*merogony, meront, parasitophorous
vacuole, schizogony, schizont, sporoblast, sporogony, sporont,
sporulation, zygote*) appear in our list below. Most of these 10
seem indispensible to microsporidian terminology but about half
of them have been troublesome because they have been more or less
unstable with respect to the manner of their usage. The classical
examples are *Schizogony* and *Sporogony*. Levine's definition of

Schizogony will help to clarify our ideans of these 2 terms and some of the others as well: "Formation of daughter cells by *multiple fission*. If the daughter cells are *merozoites*, the schizogony may be called *merogony*. If they are sporozoites, the schizogony may be called *sporogony*. If they are gametes, the schizogony may be called gametogony. (The term *schizogony* is often limited to *merogony*)." (Italics ours.) Since *schizogony* literally means fission, either binary or multiple, and since microsporidiologists commonly use it with this meaning, it seems clear that, for our purpose, *binary fission* should be added to Levine's definition of *schizogony*. Probably microsporidiologists have usually limited *schizogony* to *merogony* but we advocate that they follow the sporozoologists in using the broad and literal meaning, fission during any stage in the life cycle. After adopting this meaning for *schizogony* it becomes easier to clarify a few other important terms whose definitions depend upon this one. (See *schizont, schizogony, sporont, sporogony, meront, merogony.*)

A second general problem arises from the fact that organelles look different at the light and electron microscope (e.m.) levels and have been given correspondingly different names. Sometimes the name is appropriate at the one level and not at the other. *Polar cap* vs. *anchoring disc* is a good example. The umbrella-like structure terminating the basal portion of the polar filament looks like a cap at the anterior end of the exospore when viewed with the light microscope. However, the e.m. demonstrates that this structure is located inside the exospore and suggests that its function is to anchor the filament in the spore during *eversion*. Thus, at this level the name *anchoring disc* seems more appropriate. Another example is the *anterior "vacuole"* which looks like a vacuole in the light microscope but is actually the *polaroplast*, not a vacuole at all, when properly resolved with e.m. We suggest that in cases of synonyms for structures demonstrated at different resolution level, we should follow the general rule of letting them coexist. However, we do not recommend the use of terms, like *anterior "vacuole"*, which are merely appropriate to the appearance but are now known to be inappropriate to the fact, when there is a good alternative. Perhaps, in this case, *polaroplast* is suitable at both levels because it corresponds to the known fact at both levels. Terms that we do not recommend for general use or which are obsolete or inappropriate are marked with an asterisk.

A third general problem relates to the use of different languages in the microsporidian literature. Although most of the terms are in English, our science is an international one and a very large part of the microsporidian literature is written in other languages, especially French, German, Czech, and Russian. Therefore, it would be convenient and proper for authors who do not write in English to use technical terms taken from their own language. To make this

feasible, however, and avoid difficulties in communication, our
glossary would have to be expanded to include equivalent terms
in each of these major languages. It seems premature to try to
prepare such a multilingual glossary at the present time but
maybe we should hope that a future revisor will prepare one.
Meantime, we recommend the use of either the terms in the English
glossary (derived mostly from Latin or Greek and generally
understandable) or their literal translations in the other
languages rather than the creation of new terms.

It is inevitable that we have overlooked many terms in the
literature which should appear in this glossary. We hope the
next one will be more nearly complete.

anchoring disc. A complex of membranes appearing as an umbrella-
like disc at the base of the *polar filament* and presumed to
serve for anchoring the everted filament to the *spore* while
the *sporoplasm* is being discharged. Coined by Vavra (1971).
In its original concept the anchoring disc is an integral
although specialized part of the polar filament. Thus the
polar sac (vide infra) and *polar aperture* are parts of the
anchoring disc. Recommended for use at the e.m. level, while
the *polar cap* is more appropriate for its manifestation at the
light microscope level. Other synonyms: **disque basal*
(Maurand and Loubes, 1973); **base of the filament* (Jensen and
Wellings, 1972); **corps polaire* (g.v.); **formation basale*
(Maurand, 1973); *polar sac* (Canning and Sinden, 1973).

anterior end. The end of the spore from which the polar filament
becomes everted (Kudo, 1924a).

*anterior "vacuole". A clear area at the anterior end of the spore
as frequently seen with the light microscope, interpreted by
Sprague and Vernick (1969) P. 268) as a "negative image" of
the Golgi apparatus. Equivalent to the *polaroplast* of e.m.
Synonyms: **organe polaire* (Debiaisieux, 1928); **eccentric
vacuole* (Burnett and King, 1962).

*assise externe. See *exospore*.

*assise interne. See *endospore*.

*autogamete. Large cell with large nucleus appearing as terminal
stage of the *merogony* and believed to undergo later an
autogamy (Weiser and Coluzzi, 1964). Synonym: **presporont*.

autogamy. Fusion of two daughter nuclei to form a *synkaryon*.

*base of the filament. See *anchoring disc*.

*capsule. See *polar capsule. Also used by Burnett and King
   (1962) and de Puytorac and Tourret (1963) as synonym of
   exospore.

*capsule enveloppante. See pansporoblastic membrane.

cauda.   Tail-like appendage.

*cavum. An non-existent "fluid filled cavity" in which the polaro-
   plast was supposed to be suspended (Sprague et al., 1968). Later
   study showed that the structure corresponds to the peripheral
   laminated portion of the polaroplast (Sprague and Vernick,
   1969).

*centre cinetique. See centriolar plaque.

*centriolar plaque. A thick, often invaginated, electron-dense
   area on the nuclear membrane which serves as an attachment
   point for the spindle apparatus. Coined by Robinow and Marak
   (1966) for a similar organelle in the yeast cell. Adopted by
   Perkins (1968) for Haplosporida and by Sprague and Vernick
   (1971) for microsporidia. Synonyms: *centrosome (Vavra,
   1965); *centre cinetique (adopted by Vivier and Schrevel,
   1973, from Hollande, 1972); *formation pseudo centriolaire
   (Maurand et al., 1971); *spindle terminus, *plaque (Sprague
   and Vernick, 1968a); *nuclear plaque (Vavra and Undeen, 1970);
   spindle plaque (Moens and Rapport, 1971).

cineses associees. Division of a diplocaryon into two daughter
   diplocarya (Debaisieux, 1931, P. 150).

cisterna, perivacuolar. See perivacuolar cisterna.

collective group. "An assemblage of identifiable species in which
   the generic positions are uncertain; treated as a genus-group
   for taxonomic convenience" (International Code of Zoological
   Nomenclature).

complex xenoparasitaire. See xenoma.

*corps polaire. See polar cap. Used in French literature also at
   the e.m. level for anchoring disc (e.g., Vivier, 1965).

cyst. (Gr. kystis, bladder, bag, pouch). Any bladder-like envelope.

cyst, durable. See durable cyst.

cyst, sporogony. See sporogony cyst.

dicaryotic cell. See *diplocaryotic cell.*

diplocaryon or *diplokaryon*, pl. *diplocarya*. (Gr. *diploos*,
double + *karyon*, nut, nucleus). Two closely adjacent nuclei
in very intimate morphological contact, their membranes
adhering to each other over a large area (Vavra, 1968). First
used by Debaisieux (1919, P. 55 et seq.) for a certain cell
containing such nuclei: "nous appelions donc *diplocaryon
autogamique* cet indivibu binuclee qui sert de point de depart
a la multiplication sexuee". Later used by the same author
(1928, P. 419) as it is generally used today, "un noyau
double ou un *diplocaryon*". Sometimes inappropriately used to
designate *diplocaryotic cell* (Liu and Davies, 1972). Synonyms:
dicaryon (Weiser, 1947, P. 12); *diplococcus arrangement of
nuclei* (Ormieres and Sprague, 1973); *dopplekern* (Mattes,
1928, P. (559, 560); *noyau gemine"* (de Puytorac and Tourret,
1963). Obsolete: diplokaryon coined by Boveri (1905),
fide Wilson (1925), for a tetraploid nucleus.

diplocaryotic cell. Cell containing diplocaryon. (New term,
Vavra.) Synonym: *dicaryotic cell.*

diplospore. A permanent assembly of two spores, as in
Telomyxa glugeiformis, into a single structural unit. Coined
by Codreanu, 1961. Apparently a special kind of pansporoblast
containing two spores (Codreanu and Vavra, 1970). (More or
less permanently coupled spores occur in several microsporidian
species. However, we feel that the use of the term
diplospore for such associations which do not represent a special
kind of pansporoblast is not appropriate.)

disporous. Originally referred to the fact that the two products
of a final binary fission in *Perezia lankesteriae* tend to
remain joined together while they develop into spores (Leger
and Duboscq, 1909). The meaning became modified after
Weissenberg (1913) found that a sporoblast mother cell (sporont)
in *Glugea anomala* undergoes binary fission to produce 2
sporoblasts that develop separately into spores. Thus, "disporous"
came to mean "Each sporont develops into two spores" (Kudo,
1924a, P. 66), without reference to whether the sporoblasts
tend to remain together during their transformation into spores.

disque basal. See *anchoring disc.*

durable cyst. Cyst with a thick, resistant wall, as in *Chytridiopsis* and *Hessea*. "Kystes durables a paroi resistente"
(Leger and Duboscq, 1909).

eccentric granule. See *polar cap.*

eccentric vacuole. See *anterior "vacuole"*.

endogenous sporogony. Sporogony within the limiting membrane of the *sporogonial plasmodium*, necessarily involving *de novo* production of sporoblast limiting membrane, as in the genus *Pleistophora*. (New term, Sprague.)

endospore. The chitinous inner spore coat or envelope. The term was long ago used for Sporozoa (see Labbe, 1899) but was recently adopted by Vavra (1966, 1968) for the microsporidia. Synonyms: *assise interne* (Maurand, 1966).

entennoir. Funnel-like structure formed by the *lame polaire* at the distal end of the *manubrium* in spores of Metchnikovellidae (Hildebrand and Vivier, 1971.

exogenous sporogony. Sporogony not within the limiting membrane of a sporogonial plasmodium, this membrane becoming apportioned to the resulting sporoblasts to provide their limiting membranes. To be distinguished from a superficially similar type of *endogenous sporogony* seen in the genus *Tuzetia*. (New term, Sprague.)

exospore. The proteinaceous outer spore coat or envelope. Proposed by Vavra (1968). Synonym: *assise externe* (Maurand, 1966).

extrusion apparatus. Vehicle for sporoplasm injection into the host. It is composed of *polar sac* (in the sense of *anchoring disc*), *polar aperture, polaroplast, polar tube, posterior vacuole.* Coined by Weidner (1972).

fragile cyst. A cyst consisting of a thin, delicate membrane (Sprague *et al.*, 1972). A cyst such as the *"pansporoblast membrane subpersistent* as a *polysporophous vesicle"* (Gurley, 1854, P. 194).

gemmule. Minute cell of doubtful significance but thought to represent a very early life cycle stage. Found by Sprague and Vernick (1968a) in *Glugea weissenbergi*, but so far not reported in any other microsporidian.

germ. (L. germen, seed.) Infective particle. A broad term that includes sporoplasm. Synonym: *keime*.

gland. Enlarged distal portion of manubrium in Metchnikovellidae. Coined by Vivier (1965).

inclusion body. A large, electron-dense body occurring near the posterior pole in sporoblasts of some species (Sprague *et al.*,

1968). Possibly represents part of the filament material
within a Golgi vacuole (Jensen and Wellings, 1972).

*inner sheath. Electron-dense, sheath-like structure encircling
(in cross-section view) the central portion of the polar
filament. Coined by Akao (1969).

insertion cavity. An inconspicuous impression in the inner contour of the endospore in which the top part of the anchoring
disc is situated. Coined by Huger (1960).

Karyogamy. Fusion of two nuclei to form a synkaryon.

*keime. See germ.

lame polaire. Membranous, leaf-like lamella at the distal end of
the manubrium of Metchnikovellidae (Hildebrand and Vivier,
1971). Synonym: *Queue prolongant le manubrium (Vivier, 1965).

life cycle. The complete sequence (or sequences) of morphological
patterns within a species.

macrospore. A spore of the large class(es) when polymorphic spores
are formed by a species. Coined by Leger (1897). Synonym:
*megaspore (Overstreet and Weidner, 1974).

manubrium. (L. manubrium, handle.) Any handle-shaped structure.
In spores of the genus Mrazekia, a thick rod-like basal part
of the polar filament (Leger and Hesse, 1916, Lom and Vavra,
1963) around which are organized some secondary structures
(de Puytorac, 1961). In spores of the family Metchnikovellidae,
a short tubular organelle presumed to be the homologue of the
polar filament (Vivier, 1965) and, therefore, partly homologous
with the manubrium of Mrazekia.

merogony. (Gr. meros, part + gonos, reproduction.) Schizogony
during the vegetative phase of the life cycle.

meront. (Gr. meros, part + ont, a being.) Coined by Stempell
(1902, P. 236, 244) for a stage that undergoes binary fission
or budding (now generally understood to include also multiple
fission) to produce infective forms; a schizont in the vegetative phase of the life cycle.

merozoite. The product of merogony. Used by several authors, e.g.,
Weiser (1957).

microspore. A spore of the small class in polymorphic species.
Antonym: macrospore.

*micropyle. A presumed opening in the anterior part of the spore
   wall. However, the e.m. shows only a thinner portion in the
   endospore at the apex of the resting spore. Used also for a
   more dense area in the apical spore wall (Codreanu et al.,
   1965).

microsporidian. (adj.) Pertaining to microsporidia. (noun)
   microsporidian, widely used in the sense of microsporidium.

microsporidiologist. A specialist in microsporidiology.

microsporidiology. The science or branch of biology dealing with
   microsporidia.

microsporidium, pl. microsporidia. Vernacular name for a member
   (or members) of the Microsporida and related orders.

Microsporidium. A collective group name. Introduced by Balbiani
   (1884) and later used by several authors.

mictosporous. (Gr. mictos, mixed + sporous.) Pertaining to a kind
   of sporont that produces a variable number of spores or to a
   species with such a sporont. (Modified after Kudo, 1924a).

minispore. Spore, usually small and spherical, in which a number
   of the organelles (particularly the polaroplast, the polar
   filament, and the endospore) are markedly reduced. Type of
   spore that is characteristic of members of the Minisporida.
   Example: Spore of Chytridiopsis. (new word, Sprague.)

monokaryotic cell. Cell containing single nucleus (New term,
   Vavra). Antonym: diplokaryotic cell.

*monosporoblastic. "Developing into a single sporoblast as in
   Nosema" (Kudo, 1924a. Obsolete).

*monosporous. Pertaining to Nosema bombycis and other species in
   which, after a certain number of binary fissions, each element
   (sporoblast) develops in isolation to give a spore (original
   meaning when coined by Perez, 1905, P. 30). Often understood
   now to mean "Each sporont develops into a single spore" (Kudo
   1924a, P. 65), a confusing and untenable definition because it
   introduces ambiguity into the meaning of "sporont". The
   monosporous condition in the sense that one sporont gives
   rise to one sporoblast has not been demonstrated in microsporidia.

mucocalyx. *(muco* + Gr. *kalyx,* hust or covering.) The mucus
layer on the surface of the exospore in some species. Thus,
the exospore surface may bear spore appendages (filaments,
tubules, etc.) or *mucocalyx,* or both. (New word, Vavra.)

Mutterzellen der Sporoblasten. See *sporoblast mother cell.*

*organe polaire. Coined by Debaisieux (1928, P. 431) for
*anterior "vacuole".

pansporoblast. A *sporogonial plasmodium* whose limiting membrane
(= *pansporoblastic membrane)* is destined to become a sachet
(= *cyst* = *sporocyst* in this case or *sporophous vesicle)* to
enclose the *sporoblasts* (and, finally, spores). Useful, and
often used, also for later stages after *sporoblasts* or *spores*
have developed within the *pansporoblastic membrane* (Perez, 1905).
Sporogony, being endogenous within the *pansporoblastic mem-*
brane, is necessarily accompanied by *de novo* origin of the
sporoblast membranes. (A *pansporoblast* is to be distinguished
from a *sporogonial plasmodium* that undergoes *exogenous*
sporogony with its membrane dividing to become the sporoblast
limiting membranes.) Coined by Gurley (1893, P. 408), when
microsporidia were considered to be a family in the Myxosporida,
and defined in terms that do not fit the microsporidia well.
Nevertheless, used by Gurley for the sporogonial plasmodia of
Pleistophora and *Thelohania,* this use being completely consistent with the definition given here. Used by Debaisieux
(1928, P. 424) as a synonym of *sporocyst,* in the sense of
pansporoblastic membrane, an inappropriate and objectionable
usage followed by some later authors.

pansporoblast(ic) membrane. The limiting membrane of a *pansporo-*
blast, becoming a *sporophorous vesicle.* Coined by Gurley (1893,
P. 104.) [Used both by Labbe and by Tuzet *et al.,* (1971) as a
basis for dividing the microsporidia into two major groups.]

parasitophorous vacuole. Vacuolar space occurring around some
microsporidian parasites and becoming more prominent during
sporogony. The membrane delimiting the vacuole is of *host*
origin. Term currently used in sporozoan terminology (Levine,
1971) and adopted for microsporidia by Barker (in press) and
Canning and Nicholas(1974). Not to be confused with *sporophorous*
vesicle where the limiting membrane of the vacuolar space is of
parasite origin. Synonym: *periparasitic vacuole* (Weiser and
Zizka, 1974).

perivacuolar cisterna. A giant cisterna of the host cell endo
plasmic reticulum closely applied to the surface of the microsporidian (Szollosi, 1971).

planont. (Gr. *planos*, wandering + *ont*, being.) Coined by Stempell
   (1909, P. 298) for objects that he presumed to be amoeboid
   stage of *Nosema bombycis*, supposedly arising directly from the
   extruded germ, wandering around and reproducing extracellularly
   in the gut lumen, tissues and haemolymph. Although these
   observations of Stempell have not been generally confirmed,
   it is possible he saw in the blood some *secondary infective
   forms*.

plasmode sporogonial. See *sporogonial plasmodium.*

plasmodium. A multinucleate mass of protoplasm, syncytium. A kind
   of somatella.

polar aperture. Terminal portion of the polar filament at the site
   where it merges into the anchoring disc. Enclosed by a series
   of (usually 4) parallel septa (**renforcement basal* of Maurand,
   1966). Coined by Weidner (1970).

*polar body. Synonym of *polar cap.* Also used by Huger (1960) as
   synonym of *polaroplast.*

polar cap. A chromophilic body at the anterior end of the spore
   and contained within the *polar sac.* Proposed independently
   by Hiller (1959) and Vavra (1959, 1960). Found independently
   by Huger (1960) and Vavra (1959) to be PAS positive.
   Synonyms: *McManus positive polar cap* (Vavra); *PAS positive
   polar cap* (many authors); **polar granules* (Huger); **polar
   mass* (Kudo and Daniels, 1963); **corps polaire* (Debaisieux,
   1928); **disque basal* - see this term; **eccentric granule*
   (Burnett and King, 1962); *anchoring disc* (part) (q.v.);
   *base of the filament (q.v.); **polar body* (Dissanaike and
   Canning, 1957); **Polkorper* (Zwolfer, 1926).

polar cap-polaroplast complex. The term used by Lom and Corliss
   (1967) to express the fact that the *polar cap* and the *polaroplast* are closely related structurally.

*polar capsule. An obsolete term used in early days of microsporidian research when it was believed that the microsporidian
   spore is structurally similar to the multicellular spore of
   myxosporidia. See *posterior vacuole.*

polar filament. A tubular organelle, usually long and fine,
   anchored at one pole (the anterior) of the spore and coiled
   within; more appropriate, *polar tube.*

*polar filament base. See *base of the filament.*

polar filament complex. Complex of structures representing together the whole *polar filament: polar sac* (in the sense of the *anchoring disc)*, straight basal part of the filament and its coils. Coined by Canning and Sinden (1973).

polar filament-polaroplast complex. The term expressing that *polar filament* and *polaroplast* are intricately related in their development and structure. Coined by Jensen and Wellings (1972).

polar ring. *Polar cap* when punctured in the middle by evaginating filament. Coined by Vernick *et al.,* (1969).

polar sac. Term coined by Petri and Schiedt (1966) for a membrane at the base of the *polar tube* that encloses the *polar cap.* Frequently used as synonym for the *anchoring disc.*

polar tube. Term introduced by Weidner (1970) to replace *polar filament,* the latter term being less appropriate for an organelle now known to be tubular.

polar vesicles. Small vesicles probably of Golgi origin observed sometimes in the vicinity of the spindle *plaque.* Coined by Youssef and Hammond (1971).

polaroplast. A laminated complex of smooth membranes situated in the anterior end of the spore and demonstrable with the e.m. Interpreted by Sprague and Vernick (1969, 1974) as a major part of the Golgi complex. Often seen with the light microscope as an *anterior "vacuole",* the *organe polaire.* Coined by Huger (1960).

posterior body. Membranous, electron-dense structure (probably of Golgi origin), occurring in some microsporidia within the posterior vacuole. (Coined by Weiser and Zizka, 1974). Synonym: *inclusion body* (Sprague *et al.,* 1968); *membrane complex* (Sprague and Vernick, 1971).

posterior end. The end of the spore opposite the anterior end (Kudo, 1924a).

posterior vacuole. A large clear area that is often present in the posterior end of the spore and around which the polar filament is coiled. Synonyms: *posterior vesicle* (Ishihara, 1968); *capsule polaire* (Debaisieux, 1928).

presoporont. Cell with a *diplocaryon* from which the sporont is believed to arise by fusion of the two nuclei (Canning, 1960).

prosporoblast. An incipient *sporoblast;* one of the elements being produced during *sporogony,* still connected to the *sporogonial plasmodium* but in the process of becoming a *sporoblast.* Coined by Weiser and Zizka (1974).

schizogony. (Gr. *schizo,* split + gonos, *reproduction.)* Fission, binary or multiple, of a cell or plasmodium to form daughter cells. Levine (1971) points out that there are three kinds of schizogony (not necessarily all occurring in microsporidia); *merogony,* gametogony, and *sporogony.* Often used in micro-sporidian terminology for the part of the life cycle up to the formation of sporonts or, in a more limited sense, as a synonym of *merogony.*

schizont. A stage in the life cycle that divides by *schizogony* (Levine, 1971). Often used for stages preceding *sporont* or, in a more limited sense, as a synonym of *meront.*

schizontenschlauche. Ribbon-like arrangement of *schizonts* not yet fully separated by cytokinesis. Coined by Weissenberg (1913).

secondary infective form. Coined by Ishihara (1969) for a small binucleate form in *Nosema bombycis* that leaves a host cell, migrates, penetrates another cell and is, therefore, responsible for spreading the parasite from one cell to another within the host. Possibly the *planont,* in part, of Stempell.

secretion. Transitory structures of medium to high electron density and of very variable form (tubules, filaments, grains, aggregates or particles) at the surface of sporonts and sporoblasts and/or in the space between pansporoblast and the sporont or sporoblasts (Vavra, 1965). Synonyms: *granules de differentiation"; *granules intercalaires chromatiques"* (Debaisieux, 1919). Maurand and Loubes (1973) name this type of secretion *somatic secretion* (consisting of proteins rich in SH groups) and distinguish it from another type of secretion which occurs exclusively during the formation of sporoblasts and contains acid mucopolysaccharides.

spindle plaque. Synonym of *centriolar plaque.* For reasons dis-cussed by Moens and Rapport (1971) for similar structures in yeast, the *spindle plaque* is a less confusing term which should be preferred.

spore. (Gr. *spora,* spore, seed.) An infective stage, consisting
essentially of a generative cell *(germ)* enclosed in one or
more somewhat resistant envelopes and serving to initiate a
new infection, usually in a new host individual.

spore appendage. Any of various protuberant structures (filaments,
caudae, tubules, etc.) on the exospore. Synonym: **spore
projection* (Vavra, 1963).

*spore coat. An ambiguous term that usually refers to the
endospore (Liu *et al.,* 1971).

*spore membrane. An ambiguous term that usually refers to the
endospore, used in this sense by Kudo (1924a) and many other
authors.

spore morphogenesis. Transformation of the *sporoblast* into a
spore. Apparently introduced by Sprague and Vernick (1968b).
Synonym: *sporogenesis.*

*spore wall. The *endospore.*

sporoblast. A cell formed by the division of the sporont (Levine,
1971). A cell which develops directly into a *spore* (Kudo,
1924a).

sporoblast mother cell. Cell that undergoes sporogony to produce
sporoblasts (Weidner, 1970). Synonyms: *Mutterzellen der
Sporoblasten* (Weissenberg, 1913, P. 127); *sporont.*

sporocyst. In microsporidian terminology, an envelope or cyst
containing spores (Debaisieux, 1928); *sporophorous vesicle.*
The most familiar example is that formed by the *pansporoblastic
membrane* of *Pleistophora* and *Thelohania.*

sporogenesis. See *spore morphogenesis.*

sporogonial plasmodium. Any multinucleate body that divides
directly into sporoblasts (undergoes *sporogony).* It may have
a variety of shapes such as roughly spherical, ovoidal,
cylindrical, or moniliform. It may or may not be a
pansporoblast. Synonym: *plasmode sporogonial* of Tuzet
et al. (1971).

sporogony. The *schizogony* that produces sporoblasts. Often used
more broadly to mean *sporulation* (q.v.), a practice to be
discouraged.

sporogony cyst. Thick walled or thin walled cysts produced by the *sporogonial plasmodium* in Chytridiopsidae (Sprague *et al.*, 1972).

sporogony vacuole. The vacuolar space enclosing sporogional stages in some genera, as in the genus *Glugea,* being a particular example of a *parasitophorous vacuole* (Weissenberg, 1968).

sporont. An individual which gives rise to one or many sporoblasts (Kudo, 1924). A cell whose immediate division products are sporoblasts (Sprague *et al.*, 1971). A cell that divides directly into *sporoblasts;* identical with zygote when latter is present (Debaisieux, 1928, P. 419-420). Synonym: *sporoblast mother cell.* Minchin (1922, footnote P. 181) gave the following history of the word: suggested by Butschli to replace "sporadin", a word coined by Schneider to denote the adult spore-forming phase of a cephaline gregarine; since this form produces first gametes, "sporont" then came to mean a gamete-producing form. Meanings given by Minchin are not at all applicable to the microsporidia but the definition given by Debaisieux is both applicable and still widely used. Furthermore, the concept of *sporont* as *zygote* corresponds with Levine's recent (1971) definition of this term for the Coccidia.

sporont appendages. Filamentous or acicular appendages occurring at the surface of the *sporophorous vesicle* in some species (e.g., *Trichoduboscqia, Mitoplistophora).* Coined by Codreanu (1966).

sporont mother cell. In some species a distinct type of cell that divides into *sporonts.* Coined by Kudo (1924*b*) for a certain kind of cell in *Thelohania legeri* that was thought to divide into two sporonts. Probably usable also for a cell that develops into a plasmodium which then divides into sporonts (as in *Glugea).*

sporophorous vesicle. Any cyst, particularly the *pansporoblast membrane,* containing spores. It is octo-, poly-sporophorous, etc., according to the number of spores it contains. Coined by Gurley (1893, P. 410).

sporoplasm. The *germ* of the spore (Debaisieux, 1928, P. 428). The differentiation into **endo-* and **exosporoplasm,* introduced by Popa (1964) is not substantiated.

sporulation. The process of spore production. *Sporogony* plus *spore morphogenesis.* Meaning only roughly comparable to that given by Levine (1971) for Sporozoa, "The process of sporozoite production, i.e., sporogony".

sporulation stages. *Stages* in the process of *spore* production,
   beginning with *sporont* and ending with *spore.* Synonym:
   sporulating stages (Kudo, 1943).

stage. "A single step or degree in a process" (The Random House
   Dictionary).

subpersistent membrane. A *fragile cyst,* such as the *"pansporoblast
   membrane subpersistent* as a *polysporophorous vesicle"* (Gurley,
   1894, P. 194).

synkaryon. *Zygote* nucleus.

terminal sac. A vesicle appearing at the end of the everted polar
   filament in which the *sporoplasm* is located (Erickson *et al.,*
   1968.

tetra-, polysporous, etc. Pertaining to a sporont that produces
   the corresponding number of spores or to a species with such a
   sporont (modified after Kudo, 1924a). (Continuation of the
   series that starts with *disporous.)*

*trophozoite. Commonly used term for not exactly specified
   developmental stages but probably meronts. (Used, e.g.,
   Kudo, 1943, and Weidner, 1970).

*umbilicus. A not well-defined specialized region in the sporoblast
   where the cell is separated from another cell at the end of the
   last division. Anterior part of the spore is differentiated
   near the *umbilicus.* Coined by Sprague and Vernick (1969).

*vacuole cells. *Sporonts* ("die Mutterzellen der Sporoblasten") of
   Glugea anomala located in *sporogony vacuole.* Term created by
   Weissenberg (1913). Not applicable to most genera.

vacuole, parasitophorous. See *parasitophorous vacuole.*

vacuole, posterior. See *posterior vacuole.*

*vegetative form. Term used by Kudo (1924a) in all his summaries of
   species descriptions (but, strangely, not listed in his glossary)
   for all life cycle stages excepting the spore. An inappropriate
   term, which, unfortunately, tended to render obscure several
   distinct life cycle phases that it covered.

vegetative stages. Stages in that part of the life cycle when the
   organism is actively feeding and proliferating before entering
   into the *sporulation* sequence (Kudo, 1943). Commonly called
   "schizonts".

xenoma. The symbiotic complex formed by the hypertrophying host cell and the multiplying intracellular parasites (Weissenberg, 1949) as in *Glugea anomala* and *Mrazekia caudata: "complexe xenoparasitaire"* of Chatton (1920). The concept of *xenoma* has recently been broadened and applied also to other cells hypertrophied by microsporidia (Maurand, 1973).

zygote. Cell resulting from *autogamy* or from fusion of gametes. *Zygote,* when present, equals *sporont* (Debaisieux, 1928).

SUMMARY

This is the first glossary that has been prepared for the microsporidia since Kudo published a brief one in 1924. Kudo's glossary contained 30 terms and this one contains over 4 times that many. The additional terms include several older ones that Kudo did not list but most of them have been introduced during the past 50 years by students using either the light or the electron microscope. Special attention has been given to clarifying the meanings of a few terms that have long been established in the vocabulary for both microsporidia and sporozoa but which cannot be used with exactly the same meanings in both these groups.

REFERENCES

Akao, S.(1969). Studies on the ultrastructure of *Nosema cuniculi*, a microsporidian parasite of rodents. *Jap. J. Parasitol.,* 18, 8-20.

Balbiani, G. (1884). Les psorospermies des articles ou microsporidies. Pages 150-168, 184 *in* O. Doin, ed. "Lecons sur les sporozoaires," Paris.

Barker, R. J. **Ultrastructural observations on** *Encephalitozoon cuniculi* Levaditi, Nicolau & Schoen, 1923, from mouse peritoneal macrophages. *Folia Parasitol.* (Prague) 22, (in press).

Burnett, R. G., and King, R. C. (1962). Observations on a microsporidian parasite of *Drosophila willistoni* Sturtevant. *J. Insect Pathol.,* 4, 104-112.

Canning, E. U. (1960). Two new microsporidian parasites of the winter moth, *Operophtera brumata* (L.). *J. Parasitol.,* 46, 755-763.

Canning, E. U., and Sinden, R. E. (1973). Ultrastructural observations on the development of *Nosema algerae* Vavra and Undeen (Microsporida, Nosematidae) in the mosquito *Anopheles stephensi* Liston. *Protistologica* 9, 405-415.

Canning, E. U., and Nicholas, J. P. (1974). Light and electron microscope observations on *Unikaryon legeri* (Microsporida, Nosematidae), a parasite of the metacercaria of *Meigymnophallus minutus* in *Cardium edule. J. Invertebr. Pathol.,* 23, 92-100.

Chatton, E. (1920). Sur un complexe xeno-parasitaire morphologique et
    physiologique, *Nereisheimeria catenata* chez *Fritillaria pellucida*.
    C. R. Acad. Sci., Fr., 23, 92-100.
Codrenau, R. (1961). Sur la structure bicellulaire des spores de
    Telomyxa cf. *glugeiformis* Leger et Hesse, 1910, parasite des
    nymphes d'*Ephemera* (France, Roumanie) et les nouveaux sous-
    ordres des Microsporidies Monocytosporea nov. et Polycytosporea
    nov. *C. R. Acad. Sci., Fr.*, 253, 1613-1615.
Codrenu, R. (1966). On the occurrence of spore or sporont appendages
    in the Microsporidia and their taxonomic significance. Pages
    602-603 *in* A. Corradetti, ed. "Proceedings of the First Inter-
    national Congress of Parasitology," Roma, 21-26 Sept. 1964,
    Pergamon Press, New York.
Codreanu, R., Popa, Al., and Voiculescu, R. (1965). Donnes sur
    l'ultrastructure des spores de microsporidies. *Bull. Apicole*,
    8, 5-16.
Codreanu, R., and Vavra, J. (1970). The structure and ultrastructure
    of the microsporidian *Telomyxa glugeiformis* Leger and Hesse,
    1910, parasite of *Ephemera danica* (Mull.) nymphs. *J. Protozool.*,
    17, 374-384.
Debaisieux, P. (1919). Microsporidies parasites des larves de
    Simulium: *Thelohania varians*. *Cellule*, 30, 47-79, 3 pls.
Debaisieux, P. (1928). Etudes cytologiques sur quelques Microsporidies.
    Cellule 38, 389-450, 3 pls.
Debaisieux, P. (1931). Etude cytologique du *Mrazekia argoisii*.
    Cellule, 40, 147-168, 2 pls.
Debaisieux, P., and Gastaldi, L. (1919). Les microsporidies parasites
    des larves de *Simulium*. II. *Cellule*, 30, 187-213, 3 pls.
Dissanaike, A. S., and Canning, E. U. (1957). The mode of emergence
    of the sporoplasm in Microsporidia and its relation to the
    structure of the spore. *Parasitology*, 47, 92-99.
Erickson, B. W., Jr., Vernick, S. H., and Sprague, V. (1968). Electron
    microscope study of the everted polar filament of *Glugea
    weissenbergi* (Microsporida, Nosematidae). *J. Protozool.*, 15,
    758-761.
Gurley, R. R. (1893). On the classification of the Myxosporidia,
    a group of protozoan parasites infesting fishes. *Bull. U.S.
    Fish Comm. for 1891*, 407-420.
Gurley, R. R. (1894). The Myxosporidia, or psorosperms of fishes,
    and the epidemics produced by them. *Bull. U.S. Fish & Fish.
    Comm. for 1892*, 190-205.
Hildebrand, H., and Vivier, E. (1971). Observations ultrastructurales
    sur le sporoblaste de *Metchnikovella wohlfarthi* n. sp. (Micro-
    sporidies), parasite de la gregarine *Lecudina tuzetae*.
    Protistologica, 7, 131-139.
Hiller, S. R. (1959). The morphology and life cycle of *Plistophora
    scatopsi* sp. nov., a microsporidian parasitic in the mid-gut of
    Scatopse notata Mg. (Diptera). *Parasitology*, 49, 464-472.

Hollande, A. (1972). Le deroulement de la cryptomitose et les modelites de la segregation des chromatides dans quelques groupes de Protozoaires. *Annee Biol.*, 11, 427-466.

Huger, A. (1960). Electron microscope study on the cytology of a microsporidian spore by means of ultrathin sectioning. *J. Insect Pathol.*, 2, 84-105.

International Commission on Zoological Nomenclature (1961). "International Code of Zoological Nomenclature Adopted by the XV International Congress of Zoology." Trust Zool. Nomen., London. 176 pp.

Ishihara, R. (1968). Some observations on the fine structure of sporplasm discharged from spores of a microsporidian *Nosema bombycis. J. Invertebr. Pathol.*, 12, 245-258.

Ishihara, R. (1969). The life cycle of *Nosema bombycis* as revealed in tissue culture cells of *Bombyx mori. J. Invertebr. Pathol.*, 14, 316-320.

Jensen, H. M., and Wellings, S. R. (1972). Development of the polar filament-polaroplast complex in a microsporidian parasite. *J. Protozool.*, 19, 297-305.

Kudo, R. (1924a). A biologic and taxonomic study of the Microsporidia. *Ill. Biol. Monogr.*, 9, 1-268.

Kudo, R. (1924b). Studies on microsporidia parasitic in mosquitoes. III. On *Thelohania legeri* Hesse (=*Th. illinoisensis* Kudo, 1921). *Arch. Protistenkd.*, 49, 147-162, 1 pl.

Kudo, R. R. (1943). *Nosema termitis* n. sp., parasitic in *Reticulitermes flavipes. J. Morphol.*, 73, 265-276 + Pls. 1-2.

Kudo, R., and Daniels, E. W. (1963). An electron microscope study of the spore of a microsporidian, *Thelohania californica. J. Protozool.*, 10, 112-120.

Labbe, A. (1899). Sporozoa. *In* O. Butschli, ed. "Das Tierreich. 5," Friedlander, Berlin, 180 pp.

Leger, L. (1897). Sur une nouvelle Myxosporidie de la famille des Glugeidees. *C. R. Acad. Sci., Fr.*, 125, 260-2626.

Leger, L., and Duboscq, O. (1909a). Sur les *Chytridiopsis* et leur evolution. *Arch. Zool. Exp. Gen. Notes Rev.*, Ser. 5, 1, 9-13.

Leger, L., and Duboscq, O. (1909b). *Perezia lankesteriae* n. sp. g., microsporidie parasite de *Lankesteria ascidiae* Ray-Lank. *Arch. Zool. Exp. Gen. Notes Rev.*, Ser. 5, 1, 89-93.

Leger, L., and Hesse, E. (1916). *Mrazekia*, genre nouveau de microsporidies a spores tubuleuses. *C. R. Soc. Biol.* (Paris), 79, 345-348.

Levine, N. D. (1971). Uniform terminology for the protozoan subphylum Apicomplexa. *J. Protozool.*, 18, 352-355.

Liu, T. P., and Davies, D. M. (1972). Fine structure of developing spores of *Thelohania bracteata* (Strickland, 1913) (Microsporida, Nosematidae) emphasizing polar-filament formation. *J. Protozool.*, 19, 461-469.

Liu, T. P., Darley, J. J., and Davies, D. M. (1971). Preliminary
    observations on the fine structure of the pansporoblast of
    Thelohania bracteata (Strickland, 1913) (Microsporida, Nosema-
    tidae) as revealed by freeze-etching electron microscopy. *J.
    Prozool.*, 18, 592-596.
Lom, J., and Vavra, J. (1963). Contribution to the knowledge of
    microsporidian spores. Pages 487-489 *in* J. Ludvik, J. Lom,
    and J. Vavra (eds.) "Progress in protozoology," Proc. First
    Int. Congr. Protozool., 22-31 Aug. 1961, Prague, Academic
    Press, New York.
Lom, J., and Corliss, J. O. (1967). Ultrastructural observations
    on the development of the microsporidian protozoon *Plistophora
    hyphessobryconis* Schaperclaus. *J. Protozool.*, 14, 141-152.
Mattes, O. (1928). Uber den Entwicklungsgang der Microsporidie
    Thelohania ephestiae und die von ihr hervorgerufenen Krankheit-
    serscheinungen. *Z. Wiss. Zool.*, 132, 526-582, pls. 9-12.
Maurand, J. (1966). *Plistophora simulii* (Lutz et Splendore 1904),
    Microsporidie parasite des larves de *Simulium;* cycle, ultra-
    structure, ses rapports avec *Thelohania bracteata* (Strickland
    1913). *Bull, Soc. Zool., Fr.*, 91, 621-630.
Maurand, J. 1973). Recherches biologiques sur les Microsporidies
    des larves de Simulies. Ph.D. Thesis. Academie de Montpellier,
    Universite des Sciences et Techniques du Languedoc. 113 pp.,
    21 pls.
Maurand, J., and Loubes, Cl. (1973). Recherches cytochimiques sur
    quelques Microsporidies. *Bull. Soc. Zool., Fr.*, 98, 373-383.
Maurand, J., Fize, A., Fenwick, B., and Michel, R. (1971). Etude au
    microscope electronique de *Nosema infirmum* Kudo, 1921, micro-
    sporidie parasite d'un copepode cyclopoide; creation du genre
    nouveau *Tuzetia* a propos de cette espece. *Protistologica*, 7,
    221-225.
Minchin, E. A. (1922). "An introduction to the study of the pro-
    tozoa," Edward Arnold, London. 520 pp.
Moens, P. B., and Rapport, E. (1971). Spindles, spindle plaques,
    and meiosis in the yeast *Saccharomyces cerevisiae* (Hansen).
    J. Cell Biol., 50, 344-361.
Ormieres, R., and Sprague, V. (1973). A new family, new genus, and
    new species allied to the Microsporida. *J. Invertebr. Pathol.*,
    21, 224-240.
Overstreet, R. M., and Weidner, E. (1974). Differentiation of micro-
    sporidian spore-tails in *Inodosporus spraguei* gen. et sp. n.
    Z. Parasitenkd., 44, 169-186.
Perez, C. (1905). Microsporidies parasites des crabes d'Arcachon.
    Note preliminaire. *Soc. Sci. Arcachon, Trav. Lab.* 8, 15-36.
Perkins, F. O. (1968). Fine structure of the oyster pathogen
    Minchinia nelsoni (Haplosporida, Haplosporidiidae). *J. Invertebr.
    Pathol.*, 10, 287-307.
Petri, M., and Schiødt, T. (1966). On the ultrastructure of *Nosema
    cuniculi* in the cells of the Yoshida rat ascites sarcoma.
    Acta Pathol. Microbiol. Scand., 66, 427-446.

Popa, A. L. (1964). Donnees concernant la morphologie et la
pathogenie du parasite *Nosema apis* Z. *Bull. Apicole*, 7,
93-105.

Puytorac, P. de. (1961). L'ultrastructure du filament invagine de
la Microsporidie *Mrazekia lumbriculi* Jirovec 1936. *C. R.
Acad. Sci., Fr.*, 253, 2600-2602.

Puytorac, P. de, and Tourret, M. (1963). Etude de kystes d'origine
parasitaire (Microsporidies ou Gregarines) sur la paroi interne
du corps des vers Megascolecidae. *Ann. Parasitol. Hum. Comp.*,
38, 861-874.

Robinow, C. F., and Marak, J. (1966). A fiber apparatus in the
nucleus of the yeast cell. *J. Cell Biol.*, 29, 129-151.

Sprague, V., and Vernick, S. H. (1968a). Light and electron microscope study of a new species of *Glugea* (Microsporida, Nosematidae)
in the 4-spined stickleback *Apeltes quadracus*. *J. Protozool.*,
15, 547-571.

Sprague, V., and Vernick, S. H. (1968b). The Golgi complex of
Microsporida and its role in spore morphogenesis. *Amer.
Zool.*, 8, 824. [Abstr. 405].

Sprague, V., and Vernick, S. H. (1969). Light and electron micro-
scope observations on *Nosema nelsoni* Sprague, 1950 (Microsporida,
Nosematidae) with particular reference to its Golgi complex.
J. Protozool., 16, 264-271.

Sprague, V., and Vernick, S. H. (1971). The ultrastructure of
Encephalitozoon cuniculi (Microsporida, Nosematidae) and its
taxonomic significance. *J. Protozool.*, 18, 560-569.

Sprague, V., and Vernick, S. H. (1974). Fine structure of the cyst
and some sporulation stages of *Ichthyosporidium* (Microsporida).
J. Protozool., 21, 667-677.

Sprague, V., Ormieres, R., and Manier, J. F. (1972). Creation of a
new genus and a new family in the Microsporida. *J. Invertebr.
Pathol.*, 20, 228-231.

Sprague, V., Vernick, S. H., and Lloyd, B. J., Jr. (1968). The fine
structure of *Nosema* sp. Sprague, 1965 (Microsporida, Nosematidae)
with particular reference to stages in sporogony. *J. Invertebr.
Pathol.*, 12, 105-117.

Stempell, W. (1902). Ueber *Thelohania mulleri* (L. Pfr.). *Zool. Jahrb.
Anat.*, 16, 235-272, pl. 25.

Stempell, W. (1909). Ueber *Nosema bombycis* Nageli. *Arch. Protistenkd.*,
16, 281-358, 7 pl.

Szollosi, D. (1971). Development of *Pleistophora* sp. (Microsporidian)
in eggs of the polychaete *Armandia brevis*. *J. Invertebr. Pathol.*,
18, 1-15.

"The Random House Dictionary of the English Language," Unabridged.
(1966) Random House, Inc., New York.

Tuzet, O., Maurand, J., Fize, A., Michel, R., and Fenwick, B. (1971).
Proposition d'un nouveau cadre systematique pour les genres de
Microsporidies. *C. R. Acad. Sci., Fr.*, 272, 1268-1271.

Vavra, J. (1959). Beitrag zur Cytologie einiger Mikrosporidien.
Acta Soc. Zool. Bohem., 23, 347-350.

Vavra, J. (1960). *Nosema lepiduri* n. sp., a new microsporidian
    parasite in *Lepidurus apus* L. *J. Protozool.*, 7, 36-41.
Vavra, J. (1963). Spore projections in Microsporidia. *Acta
    Protozool.*, 1, 153-155.
Vavra, J. (1965). Etude au microscope electronique de la morphologie
    du developpement de quelques microsporidies. *C. R. Acad. Sci.
    Fr.*, 261, 3467-3470.
Vavra, J. (1966). Some recent advances in the study of microsporidian
    spores. Pages 443-444, 453-454 *in* A. Corradetti, ed.,
    "Proceedings of the First International Congress of Parasitology,"
    Roma, 21-26 Sept. 1964, Pergamon Press, New York.
Vavra, J. (1968). Ultrastructural features of *Caudospora simulii*
    Weiser (Protozoa, Microsporidia). *Folia Parasitol.* (Prague),
    15, 1-10.
Vavra, J. (1971). Ultrahistochemical detection of carbohydrates in
    microsporidian spores. *J. Protozool.*, 18(Suppl.), 47.
    [Abstr. 179].
Vavra, J., and Undeen, A. H. (1970). *Nosema algerae* n. sp.
    (Cnidospora, Microsporida) a pathogen in a laboratory colony
    of *Anopheles stephensi* Liston (Diptera, Culicidae). *J.
    Protozool.*, 17, 240-249.
Vernick, S. H., Sprague, V., and Lloyd, B. J., Jr. (1969). Further
    observations on the fine structure of the spores of *Glugea
    weissenbergi* (Microsporida, Nosematidae). *J. Protozool.*,
Vivier, E. (1965). Etude au microscope electronique, de la spore de
    Metchnikovella hovassei n. sp.; appartenance des Metchnikovellidae
    aux Microsporidies. *C. R. Acad. Sci., Fr.*, 260, 6982-6984.
Vivier, E., and Schrevel, J. (1973). Etude en microscopie photonique
    et electronique, de differents stades du cycle de *Metchnikovella
    hovassei* et observations sur la position systematique des
    Metchnikovellidae. *Protistologica*, 9, 95-118.
Weidner, E. (1970). Ultrastructural study of microsporidian develop-
    ment, I. *Nosema* sp. Sprague, 1965 in *Callinectes sapidus*
    Rathbun. *Z. Zellforsch.*, 105, 33-54.
Weidner, E. (1972). Ultrastructural study of microsporidian invasion
    into cells. *Z. Parasitenkd.*, 40, 227-242.
Weiser, J. (1947). *Caudospora simulii*, n.g., n. sp., Microsporidie
    parasite des larves de *Simulium*. *Ann. Parasitol. Hum. Comp.*,
    22, 11-15.
Weiser, J. (1957). Mikrosporidien des Schwammspinners und Goldafters.
    Z. Angew. Entomol., 40, 509-527.
Weiser, J. and Coluzzi, M. (1964). *Plistophora culisetae* n. sp., a
    new microsporidian (Protozoa, Cnidosporidia) in the mosquito
    Culiseta longiareolata (Maquart 1838). *Riv. Malariol.*,
    43, 51-55.
Weiser, Jr., and Zizka, Z. (1974). Stages in sporogony of *Pleisto-
    phora debaisieuxi* (Microsporidia). *J. Protozool.*, 21, 476.
Weissenberg, R. (1913). Beitrage zur Kenntnis des Zeugeungskreises
    der Microsporidien *Glugea anomala* Moniez und *hertwigi*
    Weissenberg. *Arch. Micros. Anat.* 82, 81-163, pls. 4-7.

Weissenberg, R. (1949). Cell growth and cell transformation by intracellular parasites. *Anat. Rec.*, 103, 517-518.

Weissenberg, R. (1968). Intracellular development of the microsporidian *Glugea anomala* Moniez in hypertrophying migratory cells of the fish *Gasterosteus aculeatus* L., an example of the formation of "xenona" tumors. *J. Protozool.*, 15, 44-57.

Wilson, E. B. (1925). "The cell in development and heredity," 3rd ed., Macmillian, New York.

Youssef, N. N., and Hammond, D. M. (1971). The fine structure of the developmental stages of the microsporidian *Nosema apis* Zander. *Tissue and Cell*, 3, 283-294.

Zwolfer, W. (1926). *Plistophora blochmanni*, eine neue Microsporidie aus *Gammarus pulex* L. *Arch. Protistenkd.*, 54, 261-340, 5 pls.

INDEX

MARSTON SCIENCE LIBRARY

Date Due

Due	Returned	Due	Returned
	FEB 1 1 2017		

Renew online @ http://www.uflib.ufl.edu

Select: Renew Books Online / View Account

Loan Policy Information @

http://www.uflib.ufl.edu/as/circ.html